DOING CHURCH

a practical guide,

by those who do it...

Other Resources by William D. Watley
- 10 Steps to Financial Freedom
- African Presence in the Bible
- African American Pulpit
- Are You the One?
- Breaking Financial Barriers
- Bring the Full Tithe
- Exalting the Names of Jesus
- From Mess to Miracles
- God Wants You To Grow
- Less Than Tipping (book)
- Less Than Tipping (guide)
- Poems of a Son, Prayers of a Father
- Preaching in Two Voices
- Preparing Joshua
- Roots of Resistance
- Sermons from the Black Pulpit
- Sermons on Special Days
- You Have To Face It To Fix It

CDs / DVDS

DVD Set
William Watley at The Potter's House

DVD Series - *"Vision for Recovery"*
Don't Underestimate Yourself
Ingredients for Recovery
More than Meets the Eye

Individual DVDs
From Being Taken to a Takeover
"Men Are Builders" Conference

CD Series "Vision For Recovery"
Facing People When We Have
  Been Damaged
When It Won't Go Away
Broke But Not Broken
Obedience Will Not Leave You
Empty Handed

Individual CDS
From Being Taken to a Takeover
The Foolishness of the Cross

CD Sets
10 Steps to Financial Freedom
William Watley at the Potter's
  House

DOING CHURCH

a practical guide,
by those who do it...

VOLUME I

Edited by

William D. Watley, Ph.D.

New Seasons Press
Newark, New Jersey

All scripture quotations are taken from the New Revised Standard Version (NRSV), New International Version (NIV), or the King James Version (KJV) of the Bible unless otherwise noted.

For copies contact:

Rev. Dr. William D. Watley, Senior Pastor
St. James A.M.E. Church
588 Dr. Martin Luther King, Jr. Blvd.
Newark, New Jersey 07102
(973) 622-1344, Ext. 111 (office)
(973) 622-6912 (fax)
www.williamwatley.org

New Seasons Press, 2010
Printed in the USA
ISBN 978-09972409-9-3

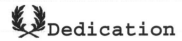
Dedication

Mrs. Carolyn Elizabeth Ferrell-Scavella

Thank you for your faithfulness and friendship across the years.
Thank you for your generous and caring spirit.
Thank you for your invaluable and priceless assistance in helping to birth this publication.

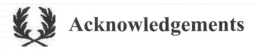 # Acknowledgements

I am grateful to my friend of long standing and editor of more publications than she cares to remember, Mrs. Carolyn Scavella. She has helped birth, and shape this publication in a variety of ways. Over the past twenty-six years you have served as sounding board, first reader and primary redactor for every publication I have written. I am extremely grateful for the blessing you continue to be to me personally, my family and to the Lord's cause. You are an outstanding example of classy Christian womanhood and loyalty. This, along with so many other reasons provides the rationale for my dedicating this work to you. My prayer is that the Lord will pour back into your life everything and more for all that you give to so many of us who are privileged to know you, to love you and respect you.

I am also grateful to Rev. Marcia Sapp Salter who did so much of the preliminary and non-glamorous grunt work that turned this dream into a deliverable. I am grateful for your love for the Lord, your enthusiasm, commitment and creativity as you execute your responsibilities, as well as your teachable spirit. I am also grateful for the keen eye and anointed gifts of the Executive Minister of St. James A.M.E. Church, Dr. Raquel St. Clair, who also did some of the proof reading for this work. My gratitude further extends to my daughters beloved, Mrs. Jennifer Watley-Maxell and Mrs. Shawna Watley, for their invaluable contributions to the editing process.

The people of St. James A.M.E. Church in Newark, New Jersey have grown, struggled and suffered with me in my efforts to *do church* among them…and sometimes on them. I am truly blessed to have had the privilege of serving as pastor to such a supportive flock of Christ.

Last, and certainly not least, I am grateful for my spouse and companion of over 40 years, Mrs. Muriel Annette Lewis Watley. You have never wavered in your support and understanding down through the years, as I have sought to make full proof of the ministry entrusted by God into my care. Thank you for looking after our family when I was not around, and for praying for me in season and out of season. Thank you for your particular contribution to this work in terms of your proof reading and helpful questions and suggestions.

To God be the glory! Great things God has done and continues to do in all of our lives as we attempt to *do church* in a way that honors our Lord Christ.

Contents

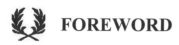 **FOREWORD**

Ministry in the 21st century has been a new and challenging experience. Fundamentalists and liberals alike have to retool themselves to meet contemporary challenges. The old scripts are being abolished and the new ones scrutinized as leaders grapple over what stays and what is to be excluded from the crock pot of post-modern leadership.

As much as we attempt to maintain our image of intellectual absolutisms, the reality is, uncertainty is one of the tools God uses to create a thirst for knowledge. It is there, at the humility of plaguing questions, that seeking, knocking and asking begins. To be sure we have new challenges, some of which even the Bible doesn't directly address, yet its truths help to fence in our debate within the scope of orthodoxy.

The idea of collective reasoning isn't new. You will remember that the early church used it to keep them from deviating too far from their brand and mission. The first experience they had with Jerusalem that brought about Pentecost must have been amazing! Imagine the enthusiasm in which the disciples left Jerusalem filled with fire and armed with the demonstration of the Holy Spirit. These men, who had been trained at the feet of Jesus Himself and filled with His Holy Spirit, must have been confident that they were ready for the challenge of their day.

However, it wasn't long before they found themselves bombarded with questions about inclusion, interpretations and protocol: Who would be required to be circumcised and who wouldn't? How did they prepare for a church whose diversity threatened the traditional ideas of sanctity and holiness? What role would women play in this new and exciting organic church

i

whose growth was paramount with its rampant division? How could they garner the strength of its people when so much compartmentalization threatened to divide the baby born on the cross?

Quickly these sagacious men learned that the fire of Pentecost alone wouldn't be enough to hold the church together. Neither the oratorical skills of Peter, nor the intellectualism of the newly converted Apostle Paul were equipped to circumvent the constant bombarding of distracting ideas. Yes, there were reports of great miracles and yes, there were great movements growing out of desert lands and city streets alike, but there was also dissension and egotism that corroded the underbelly of the movement.

Jerusalem Again
It was under the staggering weight of these and many other responsibilities that a cry was made to gather again in Jerusalem. This time it wasn't to wait on a great demonstration of the Spirit, nor was it to hear the burning sermons of those touted to be gifted with swelling words, and inspirational monologues. No, this time they came to Jerusalem with the best of the best. Like Olympic champions gathering to win the cup, these men came to pursue the prize of a deeper understanding for the future and to benefit from their collective debate. Like the Passover bread shared by the twelve, each one had a part of the whole. Jesus had well demonstrated to them that each of them held within himself a part of the mystery of the memorial body of Christ!

So they gathered again. From camel backs to worn sandals, every mode of transportation was employed to bring together pieces to a place of wholeness. The outcome would determine whether Holy Days would be observed, or whether meats offered to idols would now be consumed. They wanted to know how to proceed with the organizational infrastructure of the church in a way that didn't virally contaminate or corrupt the living organism of the church for which Christ died.

I shudder to think what might have happened had they not loved the church more than they romanced their perspectives. They sought common ground for the sake of the coming generation. Their return to Jerusalem would inevitably create debate. It would assuredly cause discourse. But at the end of the day, they hoped to anchor ideas from which they could extrapolate a new creed and lift the old rugged cross no longer weighted by the uncertainty that drove them there.

The sun was hot, the room crowded, and dust filled the air as they sat, like Native American chiefs around the evening fire, to openly debate each other for the sake of theological posterity. Sometimes the debate might have been like frolicking children, but more often than not, the debate would likely stir the fire of incivility. And only their shared love for Christ, his cross, and the church would keep it from erupting into an argument akin to a bar room brawl! The reward they sought from this crossfire of ideas was a clarion call to new and heightened direction. It was from this premise that the New Testament and its burgeoning church would survive its embryonic stages and emerge out of the embers of debate with the blueprint for leadership and living! They succeeded and the church moved forward, trimmed of the fat meat of archaic ideals and toned by reasoning on issues not addressed by any teaching to which they had previously been exposed. Today, we are the benefactors of that debate.

Fast forward to our days and times. This is a needy time in which we live. Many leaders in the church have lost their way. Some have imitated what they couldn't create. It is a day where the vision, purpose and goals of the church seem unclear. What is clear, however, is that someone has to act now. My friend and brother Dr. William Watley has been commissioned by the Master Himself to gather a collective pool of reasoning for our times and leave these thoughts in a book for the coming generation. He, himself, is no lightweight thinker. So many react when he blows the trumpet in Zion and reaches for the collaboration of the unified perspectives of highly respected clergy!

I met Dr. Watley personally several years ago and knew almost immediately that we would be friends. Perhaps because I was in part mesmerized, no actually I was stunned, by the profundity of his rationale and his often uncanny ability to be planted on principles sacred to the church while still able to transition to a message cut to the continuity of contemporary relevance. His ability to intellectualize without becoming entombed in the shrine of humanistic self-aggrandizement, opened up the way for a crossbreed of inspirational and yet intellectual comrades from various circles of thought to engage in this work, since he, himself, is not a limited man.

Who better than a man steeped in church leadership for over forty years and yet trained by the scholarly, without acquiescing his convictions for his credentials, to determine who would be the select group of thinkers that would be gathered together in this work called, **DOING CHURCH**?

I welcome every reader to eavesdrop on the ideas and concepts shared in every turned page, like hungry minds gathered at the windowpane of an upper room, filled with the aroma of a well-prepared smorgasbord. Listen with your heart while you read with your eyes the collective reasoning of this hand-selected team of thinkers, to grace every page in this book with a rich and substantive discussion. But greater still, is its ability to move the discussion to conclusion. For I am sure you realize, as I do, that discussion without conclusion is engaging but ultimately fails to be gratifying. What this book and its varied authors provide is a template far beyond the parading of ideas into the goal of an absolute conclusion. It is written to the intent that it might cure the ills of this critical moment.

Dr. Martin Luther King Jr. spoke of the fierce urgency of now. This is a new "now" with a new "fierce urgency." That is why my heart leaps in joy as I watch Dr. Watley's rapid and yet regal response in this critical work to the fierce urgency of our "now" moment! His thoughts are like a drum major with his baton held high. He sets the pace and rhythm to which we march. His book blows the whistle to which each reader will march into the mausoleum of truths, the museums of theological warriors, and the mosaic cross-pollenization of ideas from which the church will increase its impact without reducing the blood of Christ to the cherry red Kool-Aid of mediocrity! Without this father of the faith's commitment, our impact globally will weaken to water and never evolve to the rich wine of a process worthy of the church itself. We will, through his teachings, think globally and not be limited to an asphyxiatingly narrow manipulation of thought that keeps us channeling a universal God into a city councilman whose vision is for a small region. God's leaders need a message that transcends the community and goes on to transform a generation!

I am therefore proud to lift my pen to push forward Dr. Watley's march into leaving both a legacy and pointing to an absolutely irrevocable destiny to which the Holy writ says is the inheritance of the remaining leaders who would usher its followers into the place where hearts and minds touch and agree. For it is there where asking anything, is possible from that union. I only ask that you, with an open mind, prepare to shift into high gear as you have been invited to join the voyage to the bottom of absolute truth and thereby know with all certainty that we preach the doctrine of the apostles with the flare of our contemporary generations no less artfully than our spiritual ancestors did. But our focus must be tailored, and custom designed to an abiding understanding of our times.

Bishop T. D. Jakes,
Senior Pastor, The Potter's House Dallas, Inc.

Preface

When the Day of Pentecost had come, they were all together in one place. And suddenly from heaven there came a sound like the rush of a violent wind, and it filled the entire house where they were sitting. Divided tongues, as of fire, appeared among them, and a tongue rested on each of them. All of them were filled with the Holy Spirit and began to speak in other languages, as the Spirit gave them ability.

Now there were devout Jews from nation under heaven living in Jerusalem. And at this sound the crowd gathered and was bewildered, because each one heard them speaking in the native language of each. Amazed and astonished, they asked, "Are not all these who are speaking Galileans? And how is it that we hear, each of us, in our own native language? Parthians, Medes, Elamites, and residents of Mesopotamia, Judea and Cappadocia, Pontus and Asia, Phrygia and Pamphylia, Egypt and the parts of Libya belonging to Cyrene, and visitors from Rome, both Jews and proselytes, Cretans and Arabs---in our own native languages, we hear them speaking about God's deeds of power. All were amazed and perplexed, saying to one another, "What does this mean?" But others sneered and said, "They are filled with new wine."

But Peter, standing with the eleven, raised his voice and addressed them, "Men of Judea and all who live in Jerusalem, let this be known to you, and listen to what I say. Indeed we are not drunk, as you suppose, for it is only nine o'clock in the morning. No, this is what was spoken through the prophet Joel...

Now when they heard this, they were cut to the heart and said to Peter and to the other apostles. "Brothers, what should we do?" Peter said to them, "Repent, and be baptized every one of you in the name of Jesus Christ so that your sins may be forgiven; and you will receive the gift of the Holy Spirit. For the promise is for you, for your children, and for all who are far away, everyone whom the Lord our God calls to him." And he testified with many other arguments and exhorted them, saying, "Save yourselves from this corrupt generation." So those who welcomed his message were baptized, and that day about three thousand persons were added. They devoted themselves to the apostles' teaching and fellowship, to the breaking of bread and the prayers[1].

So reads the account of the Day of Pentecost according to the New Revised Standard Version of the scriptures. The Day of Pentecost has traditionally been called the birthday of the church. Of course the events of Acts 2 is not the first time that the community of faith or baptized believers in Christ is referenced in the scriptures. As early as Matthew 16: 17-18 in response to Simon Peter's confession of faith that the Lord Jesus Christ is the Son of the living God, the Master replies, "Blessed are you, Simon son of Jonah! For flesh and blood has not revealed this to you, but my Father in heaven. And I tell you, you are Peter, and on this rock I will build my church, and the gates of Hades will not prevail against it." However, even though the Lord had referenced the church and expressed an international vision for the work of the church before the momentous events of Acts 2, the Day of Pentecost is still considered the birthday of the church in a number of traditions because of the outpouring, infilling and empowering presence of the Holy Spirit. On that day the Holy Spirit saturated the 120 worshippers who were gathered in the upper room. The coming of the Holy Spirit to the whole church, and not simply to a few scattered individuals who were in the mix, meant that the church became the corporate evangelical voice and gospel body of Christ in the world.

Since the first three thousand souls were joined with the 120 worshippers on that day, the record of growth and the sphere of influence of the church over the past 2000 years are beyond measure. The number of Christians runs into the billions while the number of congregations and communities of believers can easily reach the hundreds of millions. The organized church denominational structures and para-church fellowships is mind boggling, and the educational, medical, economic, and outreach institutions that minister to the poor, the victimized and the voiceless is staggering. When one looks at the stellar record of the church over the past 2000 years one can truly proclaim, "Look at what the Lord has wrought through the efforts of those

---

[1] Acts 2:1-16; 37-42

viii

who represent and proclaim him as Lord and Savior to the world." The church has indeed come a long way since the Day of Pentecost.

Any casual reading of history, as well as ordinary observation of the current times, also recognizes that the church has had anything but a stellar record over the past two millennia. When one looks at some of the dastardly and shameful things we as followers of the Lord have done in his name; and, as we have represented his cause, we can often be accused of crucifying the Savior again and again and again. Too often we have twisted and perverted the Gospel to suit our own ends. We have all too often portrayed ourselves as more petty than powerful; as the envious rather than the excellent, and as the compromised rather than the committed. There have been times when the church has been the church that strengthened the arms of oppressors rather than the voices of the oppressed.

In our own times we have seen the image of the church and the body of Christ damaged and fractured time and again because of misunderstanding, bickering, turf wars, doctrinal fights and scandals. We as the followers of Christ have managed to fight over everything from the traditional church-dividing issues of baptism, Eucharist and ministry to newer issues such as music and liturgy, sexuality and alternate lifestyles, prosperity and a plethora of justice issues. When one looks at the litany of abuses done at the hands of the church in past and present times, one is also tempted to raise one's hands in horror and proclaim, "Church of the living Christ, your sins are legion!"

Why does the church have such a contradictory and checkered history as well as a turbulent present? Reasons include human sin, pettiness, greed, error and doctrinal disagreement. The spiritual warfare that evil wages against the church to prevent the spread of the kingdom of God, in a domain that evil has mistakenly claimed for itself, is also a theological factor. When one looks at the impediments to the church becoming the bride and body of Christ, without spot or blemish; when we consider the church's greatest blessing and bane we humans who administer, serve and represent it, the reality is that even after glorious achievements and a two thousand year history of existence, many times we still don't know how to do church very well.

We know how to sing about church. We know how to pray for the church. We know how to preach about the church. We know how to express our faith and belief in the church. We know how to defend and fight for the church. We know how to write about the church in both poetry and prose. We know how to study, research and analyze the church. We know how to quote the Bible regarding the church. We know how to organize and structure churches. We know how to do everything but live out the implications of the gospel as the church. Even after all this time and experience in being the church, we still don't know how to *do church*, live the church and even be the church very well.

From the oldest among us to the youngest, from the most seasoned to the least experienced, from the most sincere to the most selfish, from the most giving to the most exploitive, from the most degreed to the least formally educated, whether we are clergy or lay, male or female, rich or poor, no matter what our ethnicity, we as members of the body of Christ called church, still have trouble doing church. We still make a number of plain old ordinary human and even stupid mistakes administratively, in spiritual formation and development, in formulating, expressing, and implementing vision, and in our normal dealings with each other as human beings.

To put the matter succinctly and plainly, we as church people, whether leaders or followers; whether we are in the pulpit, the pew, the classroom, or the administrative office as support staff or denominational officials, we do some really foolish things. Too often in our attempts to stand up and represent the Lord, we stumble over our own feet and end up on the ground looking up, scratching our heads and licking our wounds, as we ponder how we got ourselves into some situations. We question, how did something that started out so well and felt so good and so right, end up in such a mess?

Hopefully, this book will help address some of the common, ordinary issues and challenges we as the people of God face in our efforts to do church. We have drawn together some of the best minds and practitioners of our time who have established themselves as imperfectly proficient in doing church. While none of our contributors is perfect, each has impeccable credentials, credibility, and a proven track record in the areas in which they have written. I am sure that you as a reader will appreciate both their personal and transparent writing style and their authoritative and academic contributions.

Although each of these writers is African American by ethnicity and although they write from the perspective of the cultural milieu of the African American religious ethos, the quality of their ministry, the poignancy of their insights, the serious and studious nature of their articles, and the integrity of their walk and witness, bring a message and has valuable insights for the kingdom of God as a whole and for the church universal. I shall forever be grateful to each of the contributors whose offerings have made this publication the living reality that it is, and the blessing to the kingdom it promises to be.

William D. Watley
Spring, 2010

DOING CHURCH:
the personal journey

Building Ministry As a Single Black Woman

Cynthia L. Hale

Time Magazine calls African American women the most *"unpartnered"* group in America. Recent statistics show that 70% of Black women are single and I am one of them. I am single, never married and in all honesty, no one has ever seriously asked to marry me. At the time of this writing, I am 57 years of age, celebrating 30 years in ministry and 24 years as the Senior Pastor of the Ray of Hope Christian Church.

I never intended to build ministry or anything else as a single Black woman. I always dreamed of being married with children. I wanted 5 boys, a starting line up for a basketball team. I just knew that I would be married one day, that is, before I acknowledged my call to ministry. I can remember as if it was yesterday, having a conversation with God about my life and purpose. It was during that encounter that God confirmed what my pastor and others had been telling me. They told me that I had the gifts and graces for ministry. I was called! As a woman, this call was hard for me to wrap my mind around. I had never seen a woman in ministry, never heard one preach. At that time I struggled with believing that a woman should preach.

What did all of this mean? How was I supposed to do this? God assured me that He would lead and guide me in the way I should go. God also promised to meet all of my needs. I knew that God would be faithful and take care of everything, but there was one thing that concerned me; there was this thing that haunted me. I said to God, "You aren't going to give me a husband, are you?" God said nothing in response to my question. There was complete silence! I had this feeling that God's silence meant that I would be doing ministry alone.

Nevertheless, I proceeded to try to find someone to marry. I was a normal young adult who enjoyed dating to get to know someone. I dated wonderful men for the most part. I dated one in college and another while in seminary that I thought were great prospects except that they were both ministers. Having accepted my call to ministry, I knew that marrying either one of them could potentially pose a problem. I wasn't called to be a pastor's wife, though being a pastor's wife is an honorable calling. I knew that I was called to be a Senior Pastor of a church just like the brothers I dated were aspiring to be.

While some would argue that I could have married and later developed a partnership in ministry with my husband, there was no such thing as co-pastors back then. I felt at that time that I needed to choose ministry over marriage. What later became clear to me was that in making that choice, I was claiming my call and establishing in my own mind and heart clarity about my call. It is important in ministry, especially as a woman, to know who you are and your unique purpose and assignment in the Kingdom of God. It is when we are walking fully in our purpose, even in partnership with others that we are the most effective and can do the most significant ministry. I knew I had the calling and gifting to be a pastor, and I wasn't willing to compromise the call and settle for less. I needed to be obedient to the call of God on my life even at the sacrifice of what I wanted most – marriage. I knew deep in my heart that I was to build a ministry alone. Though God has given me wonderful partners in ministry as colleagues, friends, staff, leaders and members, there has been no husband, no soul mate with whom to share the ministry.

Nevertheless, ministry has been incredible. As I look back over my life, I could not have imagined achieving what God has privileged me to achieve, developing the ministry God has used me to develop as a wife and a mother in addition to my role as Senior Pastor.

I entered pastoral ministry as a developer of a new Disciples of Christ church. The "Ray" started with 4 persons meeting for Bible study in my apartment. Developing this church from scratch, as my grandmother would say, was a full time job. There was no time for anything else. I worked 24/7 getting involved in the Metro-Atlanta community, making contacts with young professionals (my target audience) through power lunches, working out at the Athletic Club, networking through community organizations, speaking at various functions and reaching out to anyone and everyone, wherever I found myself. In addition to this, I had the normal pastoral and administrative responsibilities of a new church start or any church for that matter.

Being single was truly an asset then and continues to be today in a number of ways. First of all, being single meant that I could devote my time and energy to my work. The word "devote" means steadfast and single-minded fidelity to a certain course of action. When you are a wife and a mother, your primary responsibility is to your husband and children. Though things are changing and there are a lot more men who are involved in the raising of children and sharing of household chores, for the most part, it is still largely the wife's responsibility. Being the Senior

Pastor of a church, building a dynamic and successful ministry as a wife and mother is a daunting task. Someone may argue that married men do it all the time. Yes they do, but they have wives, who even when they work outside the home are still responsible for the household. I said it before, I will say it again, I am sure I could not have accomplished all God has allowed me to accomplish if I had been married with children.

Paul was on to something in his letter to the church in Corinth when he commended marriage, but put the single life on par with it by encouraging men and women to remain single if they could and not marry, especially in light of the imminent return of Christ. He says in I Corinthians 7:32ff, (NIV)

I would like you to be free from concern. An unmarried man (woman) is concerned about the Lord's affairs—how he/she can please the Lord. But a married man (woman) is concerned about the affairs of this world—how He/she can please his/her wife/husband—and his/her interests are divided.

When building ministry as singles, we have freedom from family responsibilities (unless we have children) to devote ourselves to full time ministry. We have the freedom to focus. Anyone who has ever built ministry knows that in order to be successful and effective, one needs to focus.

One of the things that keep people, ministers in particular, from being as sharp as we can be in any endeavor is the fact that we find it hard to focus. We are easily distracted. We take on too many tasks that are unrelated to our primary purpose. We get involved with too many activities that have nothing at all to do with what we are assigned to do. Many of these activities are good, and worthwhile, but they are usually not what we need to be doing at that moment.

When you are not focused, you are like Jesus' description of Martha in Luke 10:38-42. You know the story. Jesus and his disciples were on their way to Jerusalem when they stopped at a village called Bethany at the home of Mary and Martha. Martha, being the consummate homemaker and hostess busied herself making an elaborate dinner for Jesus while her sister sat at his feet and listened to his teaching. Martha, after a while became annoyed by the fact that while she was running around preparing the meal, her sister could just chill in front of Jesus and enjoy his company. She complained to Jesus and inquired about how he could let her do this.

Martha, Martha, the Lord answered, you are worried and upset about many things, but only one thing is needed. Mary has chosen what is better and that will not be taken away from her.

Now this story says a lot about our lives as women. The text says that Martha was "distracted." The Greek word for "distracted" means "pulled apart in many directions," which is the very opposite of being focused. To be focused is "to center one's attention, one's activities on one thing." To be distracted is to divert one's attention to different objects or different directions at the same time.

Even for those of us who are good at multitasking; we can only focus on one maybe two things at a time and be effective. But the reality is most of us have too many irons in the fire; we are pulled in many directions at one time. We are burdened with too many commitments that we have made because we didn't know how or just couldn't say no, got caught off guard, or we are trying to fill the empty space of not having a significant other or a family.

Therefore, we become in the words of Jesus, "worried and upset about many things." Thus, we are not focused. It is impossible to be focused and distracted at the same time. The two are polar opposites; they are mutually exclusive.

If we are truly going to be effective in building ministry we must focus. Real power is focused power. Haven't you noticed how powerful a stream of water becomes as it flows through a hose that has a nozzle on it? Forcing water through the small hole of a nozzle causes it to become focused and powerful. It has been said about focus – the sharper it is, the sharper you are.

As single persons with what some people assume is a lot of time on our hands, we have to be careful not to get caught up with other concerns and responsibilities that could easily become distractions. There are a myriad of ministry responsibilities that clamor for our attention. There are exciting opportunities that are always being presented to us. There are lots of people who have their own ideas about what we should be doing with our time.

Some of us, particularly as women, are people pleasers and will do anything to keep others happy. This is dangerous in life, and even more so in ministry. There are too many demands from people with legitimate and sometimes not so legitimate needs that are always coming to us. As I just said, people have this tendency to think that when you are single, you have plenty of time on your hands to respond to whatever needs and requests they may have. Members used to say to me all the time, "*You can do this, Pastor. You don't have anything else to do but go home, read or watch television.*" It's as if singles don't deserve or need to have time to do nothing or to have time to relax and refresh themselves. Some of us share this same view of the single life. We depend on those who are single in our ministry to do much more than we expect of persons who are married.

Unfortunately, as single women we operate as superwomen (it takes one to know one) trying to be all things to all people, a Jill of all trades, a woman for all seasons. We act as if we can handle it all. Some of us also have a Messiah complex, we think we can save, heal and deliver everyone or at least fix what is wrong with him or her.

No doubt, the greatest disappointment in ministry has been the realization that after all the sermons, prayers, time spent listening and counseling people, folks still fall short, refuse to change and fail to live a holy and healthy life. I had to learn early on that I couldn't save everyone. I am not Jesus. There is no S on my chest. I don't know why it's so hard for us to get this. The scriptures make clear that we have this treasure in earthen vessels, but the all-surpassing power belongs to God. (II Corinthians 4:7)

We are vessels of clay; someone called us "cracked pots." You are only one person. You only have so many gifts, so much time and energy. There is no way you can be everything people want you to be and do all they would have you do.

The other thing we struggle with as single women in ministry is a need to be needed. Ministry is lonely; it is even lonelier when you have no significant other in your life, when you have no one to go home to, no one with whom to share stresses and struggles as well as the joys and the celebrations of ministry. Given the loneliness of ministry, the void that many of us experience in life, because there is no spouse or significant other, we often throw ourselves into ministry activities and meeting the needs of others to fill the void. We need to be needed and we take great delight in responding to the needs of others, but we have to be careful with this. Too many of us become workaholics and unhealthy as we seek to meet the needs of others, often to the neglect of our own.

There have been times in ministry when I have been so physically exhausted and emotionally drained that I wanted to walk away from it all. Clergy burnout is real and has no gender bias. Whether we want to admit it or not, we are human and not indestructible. We will self-destruct, if we are not careful and don't take better care of ourselves.

If we are going to be effective as well as healthy as single women in ministry, we must focus our efforts by practicing certain principles. First of all, we have to set priorities. One has to determine the essential things you need to be doing relative to what you are trying to accomplish, concentrate your efforts there and delegate the rest. We need to focus our time and energy by spending 70% of our time on areas of strength, doing those things we are uniquely gifted to do, 25% on new things, so that we are always on the cutting edge of ministry, continually growing and reaching new levels, and 5% in our areas of weakness. Too many of us spend too much time and energy trying to do what we are not gifted to do. Not only is this a waste of time and energy, it is also frustrating.

I have discovered that if I am not gifted to do a certain thing, even when people insist that I need to do it, it is healthier for me and better for the overall good of the ministry for me to delegate it to someone else. I am not the only gifted person in the ministry. There are both staff persons and laypersons that are gifted in areas we are not. We always need to surround ourselves with people who are strong in our weak places. At this stage in ministry (I wish I had begun this sooner) I try to only do what I am uniquely gifted to do and what no one else in the church can do.

When I started the Ray, it was clear to me, that I could not handle the ministry all by myself nor was I supposed to do it all by myself. We had no money for staff, so I took the scriptures seriously when it talks about the church as the body of Christ with many members, each gifted for the common good (I Corinthians 12). I immediately began the practice of selecting gifted men and women to partner with me in ministry and developed them into great leaders, some of whom eventually became staff. The laypersons helped run the church by staffing the ministries, employing the abilities they use in the world everyday to build the kingdom of God. Even today, the paid staff continues what I started, by facilitating the work of laypersons who partner with us in ministry. As Senior Pastor, I focus on what I am specifically called and gifted to do: preaching, teaching, visioning and leadership development. When you build the leadership, the leaders partner with you in equipping the membership, so that each one discovers his or her gift, finds their place of ministry and helps to build the church as each one does his or her part. (Ephesians 4:11-16)

Secondly, if you are going to be effective and healthy in ministry, you must learn to set boundaries. Boundaries stop us from over committing, freeing us to focus on what we value most and what is the most important. Boundaries help others understand what they can reasonably expect of you and what they can't. (What you are willing to give and what you aren't!) One of the biggest benefits of setting boundaries is learning how to say "no." Saying no is difficult for most of us, because we then have to admit that we are not indispensable, and that folks can get along well without us. The program can go on without us. People can manage without us. Some of us feel guilty saying no to people because we fear they will be disappointed or become angry with us.

This is the problem with those of us who are people pleasers. We live to make people happy and we live for their approval. Through the years, I have had to learn the hard way that you cannot please everyone. Jesus couldn't do it, so you know you can't, either. Jesus didn't spend his time doing what everyone else wanted him to do. His mother and brothers were unhappy with his choice of career. They thought he was nuts. The Pharisees didn't like what he believed; they were always criticizing his teachings. The disciples tried to stop him from going on his suicide mission to Jerusalem, but he went anyway. Now all these people were well intentioned like the people in our lives. They just wanted him to do what they thought was best. But, Jesus said "no" to the pressure to be what everyone else wanted him to do because he was focused. He kept the main thing the main thing. Jesus realized that the only One he had to please was his Father. He could say at the end of his life as recorded in John 17:4, "Father, I have brought you glory on earth by completing the work you gave me to do."

Third, if you are going to be effective and healthy in ministry as a single Black woman, you must get a life. I mentioned earlier that I got to a place in ministry where I wanted to walk away from it all. I was tired; I was emotionally drained and I was constantly giving out but not taking the time to refresh and to just live apart from the church. All my time was spent in ministry or working at the church. I rarely took a day off; I didn't go home until late at night, there was no one to go home to. Even on the weekends, I would find ministry opportunities to engage in. Finally, I got tired and fed up with ministry, but before I followed through on my threat to walk away, someone said to me "get a life" and I heard them.

I started taking my day off, committing only to 2 nights a week at the church and never on a Friday. I said to myself, though you don't have a family and you are not in a serious relationship, you still need to take time for you, to be with you. I started asking friends to go to dinner, to the movies, a play or a concert. Sometimes I went by myself. After church, I loved going to one of my favorite restaurants for dinner and then across the street to the mall to shop. I had to let that go, it was too expensive. I began to travel by myself, going anywhere and everywhere I thought I wanted to go all over the world. I prayed and asked God to send me some good girlfriends, sisters with whom I share things in common who would love me unconditionally and sharpen me as I helped to sharpen them. He sent me Elaine Flake, Claudette Copeland, Jo Ann Browning, Jessica Ingram and Renita Weems, initially. All of these women are married, which allowed me to live the married life through them and their experiences. When I turned 50, the Lord gave me a group of single women to walk with me as well. I also have developed through the years, wonderful male friends and colleagues in ministry who are like brothers. *I got a life and I'm living it like its golden.*

Being a single Black woman in ministry has also proven to be an asset because many of the persons that have been attracted to our church through the years are single. Though many churches do not realize it, at least a third or more of younger congregations are single persons with and without children.

Being single has helped me to identify intimately with them and their stresses and struggles. The church has traditionally focused on married people and families in its preaching, teaching and programming. But I have made it a practice while preaching to talk freely about being single, using illustrations that speak to where singles live, move and have their being. Often I have been told how refreshing it is to have a pastor who acknowledges the presence of singles in the congregation. When you are single,

11

you know what it is to feel left out of the sermon; because the sermon talks exclusively about husbands and wives or lifts up the married life as the only legitimate one. Being single is not a curse, as many of us have been led to believe with comments from too many (including the pulpit) that suggest that we are less than whole. A colleague and friend of mine once suggested in a sermon that a wise woman has to be a married woman because she is connected to a wise man and that a woman finds her sense of worth when she is finally connected to man whose rib she is.

With this kind of preaching and suggestions about one's worth being tied to having a spouse, it is important that as single black women in ministry, we preach an inclusive gospel that helps singles see themselves as whole and complete because of their connection to and position in Christ. We must also help persons to discover and celebrate their dignity and worth as single persons both in the church and in the world.

Of course, this will require us to settle our own questions about our singleness and see ourselves as whole and complete. We must be clear in our own minds and hearts about what we think and how we feel about our own singleness. We have to believe that our singleness is not a curse for mistakes made or promises to God not kept. Some have suggested that if one is not celibate, it could be we have not been chosen because we did not keep ourselves pure until marriage. My mother used to say, "No man is going to want you, if you give yourself away" or "Why buy the cow when you can get the milk free." God is a loving and forgiving God and your singleness is not punishment for sin or indiscretions.

Nor is singleness a consequence of our being too picky or of having high standards for what we want in a mate. One has to have standards. You cannot settle for less than God's best for you nor for what you really desire. God does delight in giving us the desires of our hearts, while at the same time knowing what is best for us and wanting the best for us. The Bible talks about being unequally yoked and while we certainly want to be open, there are certain qualities one must have in a mate when he/she is in ministry.

There is no question in most of minds that our mates need to be saved, though many of us can remember a time in our lives when we experimented with dating people who were not. We thought we could get them saved enough to marry them only to have them show out on us before we could get them to the altar, making it clear that we could not settle. Some of us have settled and now that we are single and free again, we dare not go back unless it is worth it. One would think that it is important that we have a mate who is a mature committed Christian, who is prepared to partner with you in ministry, at some level. While it is not required that he be an officer of the church, it is desirable that the person be fully supportive and not a hindrance to ministry.

For some of us singleness appears to be a mystery; because, we are not sure why we are single. Though we talk about the fact that many are single because of a lack of eligible men, the truth of the matter is, there are sisters who are finding their soul mate every day. Why we are not among the ones who are partnered, no one knows for sure. I struggled with this for years, feeling rejected, undesirable and unwanted. Then I came to the conclusion that for many singleness is a choice. If we wanted to be married we could be. Some of us have made a conscious choice to be single, at some point in our lives (like the choice I made while in college and seminary) to pursue ministry, our professional careers, and to follow our dreams. This does not mean that we will never be married. Singleness for some is a season! It is a wonderful time to discover and get in touch with you, pursue your passions and the ways that you can make a significant contribution to life and ministry.

Having clarity about your own singleness allows you to minister effectively to others who are single in the congregation and to model healthy living as a single person, particularly a woman. We are called to practice what we preach.

While I have talked about singleness in ministry as an asset, there are some churches that do not see singleness in a pastor as an asset. Most of us have heard of churches that refuse to call single men and women to be their pastor. We all know that there was some concern that a single person would have a more difficult time operating with integrity in regards to their sexuality and might have a tendency to run through the congregation in an attempt to date persons and meet their needs.

As I was completing seminary, I applied to a small Disciple's of Christ church whose pastor had been there for over 30 years and had died. They were interested enough to invite me to preach and to be interviewed. The interview was interesting in that they asked a lot of questions about my personal life, who was I dating and the nature of the relationships. They wanted to know if I had a boyfriend and whether or not we planned to get married. They were trying to see if I was sexually active. I wasn't sure that this line of questioning was appropriate. I wondered if they asked these same questions of men.

They interviewed me, but they didn't hire me. They were honest with me. They didn't want a woman, even though they loved my preaching and the fact that I was seminary trained. They didn't want a single Black woman. This was devastating to me because they chose a married Black man who at the time was a barber and going to seminary part time. I decided that I would not allow the experience to hinder me. Though it angered me, I dealt with the anger appropriately. This was not the first experience of rejection as a woman in ministry and it would not be the last. I decided early in my life that no matter what I experienced in ministry, I would not be an angry Black woman.

Developing a church shielded me from having this kind of experience again. The people who came to our church, in the beginning, were for the most part new Christians and first time members of a church. This gave me an opportunity to develop an understanding of what it means to be single in ministry and to model how one can be single and live life to the fullest with integrity. This has required through the years that I operate with emotional health and honesty, sharing appropriately with the congregation my challenges and struggles as a single person as well as setting appropriate boundaries personally and professionally.

Sharing appropriately my challenges in life and ministry as a single person has meant being only as transparent as necessary to minister to the needs of the congregation. In the context of preaching, that includes a well-placed relevant illustration about however I happen to be feeling about my singleness at the moment, and how God and the Word help me to resolve or find comfort during these times. One of these times, I preached a sermon on loneliness and how one works through his/her loneliness.

Ministry can be a lonely place. Loneliness can be a challenge for all persons, whether single or married. Living alone with no one there to share with in an intimate and personal way can be difficult. Loneliness is actually a result of our humanness, of the fall of humans, of our separation from God. When Adam and Eve sinned in the Garden, they ruined their perfect union with God and one another, causing estrangement that resulted in feelings of loneliness.

What I have come to realize is that loneliness is an attitude; it is a state of mind. One can be lonely in a crowd. Loneliness is a decision. We can choose to be lonely. When we are lonely, it may mean we have not yet learned how to enjoy our own company. We have not yet realized the gift of aloneness. Everyone needs time to be alone. Aloneness is an investment. A time to recharge our emotional and spiritual batteries, a time to think and pray, a time to gain insight or a solution to a pressing problem, rest after a battle, grace to deal with life, time to hear from God.

Someone said that we must learn how to turn our loneliness into solitude and our solitude into prayer. There were times in Jesus' life when he looked for opportunities to be alone. As a matter of fact, he withdrew from the crowds and went off to a solitary place where he prayed. (Mark 1:35, 6:31-32)

I now love living alone. The time I enjoy most is Sunday afternoon or evening after I have preached and entertained as many people as I desired to interact with after church, gone to dinner, and have finally arrived home. It is a joy to walk into my home, shut the door on the world, and let go of all the cares and concerns of the day. I have a second floor in my home with a deck that allows me to sit and rock, look up at the sky and be mindless. I look for times when I can hide away and not have to be anything other than what I want to be. Even if I had a family, I would still desire and need those times to myself.

I have not always felt this way. There was a time when loneliness consumed me and caused me to be discouraged and perhaps, even a little depressed. I had to make some healthy decisions to deal with my loneliness as well as well as my need for intimacy. The experience I had in seminary shaped my life in this regard, I never wanted the members of the congregation to see me as a loose woman, someone of whom they would be ashamed or have questions about my integrity.

When I started the church, I was sexually active with the men that I was in relationship with, though I was not guilt free. I have always had the conviction as a Christian that God reserved sex for consummation of the marriage covenant and the way that married couples expressed their love for one another, physically. Though I had always preached that, I had not always lived it. Now it was time for me to practice what I preached. Little did I realize what a difference this would make in the lives of the single women in my congregation who wanted to be healthy and make right choices for their lives as Christians, but needed to see it modeled in a healthy and wholesome way.

The other thing that I needed to do was to be clear about my relationships within the church and how I would date. One of my practices in the past was not to date men in my denomination, as a single black woman, who held some important positions within the church. For example, I was the first female and the youngest President of the National Convocation – the Black fellowship group of our denomination – I didn't want anyone to be able to say that they had slept with the sister President. They may have said it, but it wasn't true.

I adopted this same policy in my congregation. I made a decision not to date any of the men in the congregation. I believe one has to exercise some professional distance from the members of one's church. Professional distance suggests that one responds pastorally to the needs of the congregation without becoming too intimately involved in their lives. While it has always been important for me to have friendly relations with members of the church, I have had to learn to set appropriate boundaries with men and women, too.

In dating relationships, you are becoming emotionally and sometimes, physically involved with an individual. It is difficult to maintain a level of professionalism and objectivity in dating relationships. One never knows how long the relationship will last and how the other person will handle the break-up. Unfortunately, I had to learn this the hard way. Though I said I would not date a member of the congregation, I became friends with one and we started going out just for fun. Eventually, it turned serious, at least on his part When he realized that I did not feel the same about him, he became hurt and angry. He walked around the church sulking. He was a leader and so he attended meetings I was conducting displaying his angry feelings. It was a mess. I handled him as lovingly and as professionally as I could and eventually he was able to work through his feelings and move on. He even found someone else in the church, and I performed his wedding. But, I learned my lesson and never did that again. As a matter of fact, I have made a point of telling men who come to the church to pursue me that I don't date members of my church.

When men belong to other churches, I am very discreet in dating them. While I have nothing to hide, I think it best not to parade men before the congregation or even acknowledge a dating relationship with one until after one is engaged. In many ways, I am the mother of the church and as I tell my single women with children all the time, you don't need to parade men before your children or constantly mess with their emotions as one man after

17

another gets emotionally involved with them and anticipates a permanent relationship with them.

My interaction with the men in my church whether single or married has always been pastoral and professional. I am aware that I am an attractive woman with a winsome personality. People, male and female, are drawn to me. They want to be in relationship with me. That is true of most of us as women in ministry. However, as women, we have to be aware of the way we operate with men. I enjoy being a woman, dressing and operating in feminine ways. I am careful though about not dressing or operating in a seductive or sensual way. I do not use my femininity to get what I want from men. I do not flirt with the men in my church, even when I find them attractive. When I have found men in my congregation attractive, even though I have a policy not to date a member, I pray about it and talk to friends and colleagues, whose opinions I trust, to see if it is something I really want to pursue. Pursuing my interest in a member of the church would mean that if he shared my interest, we would need to make a decision about how to proceed in dating. Either he would have to leave the church or I would have to dismiss my policy.

Men in my church have for the most part been very respectful, but I have had a few married brothers to make comments or gestures that were totally inappropriate to me. One such comment was made when I asked a brother how he was doing. His response was "without!" I turned and walked away. He later came up to me and asked my forgiveness, admitting he was out of line. He said it would never happen again. Another brother gave me a full body hug, pulling me close to his body in the middle of worship. I pulled away and gave him a look that let him know that was not acceptable. He also later apologized. I was offended by these gestures, and would have dealt with the behavior if the brothers had not come to me first. I have had to learn through the years not to totally demoralize a person who acted in an inappropriate way towards me. I have been known to do that with a razor sharp tongue that cut to the quick. I may have made my point in the past, but in many instances, I demoralized a man, possibly lost not just a member but also a family and severed a relationship that did not need to be severed. I have had to determine the most loving but firm approach for all persons involved, always remembering that I am an attractive single black woman but I am also the person's pastor who has been given responsibility for that person's soul.

Sometimes, I will admit, it has felt much like walking a tightrope as I have sought to build ministry as a single Black woman responsible for the lives of others as well as her own. The primary thing that has guided me in my thoughts, my decisions and my actions has been a desire to be in the perfect will of God as I serve both God and God's people. At the risk of ending this like a sermon, my mantra has been,

A charge to keep I have
A God to glorify
An ever dying soul to save
To fit it for the sky.
To serve this present age
My calling to fulfill
O may it all my powers engage
To do my Master's will.

19

On Being Male and Single in the Ministry

Jerry Sanders

I have always felt that my life was being directed on a path that was not my choosing. Preaching is my calling but not my choice. I tried to escape ministry long before I embraced preaching. Even as a child I felt called to preach but I had no desire, and yet I have always felt that the life I lived was leading me to the pulpit. I cannot say that I have always been a good man but I do believe the Lord has ordered my steps. I do believe that that where I am is where the Divine would have me to be. Even when I'm not sure if I'm doing the right thing, I'm sure I'm in the right place. I have no doubt I was called to preach and ordained to pastor. The pulpit is where God placed me.

When I accepted my calling and gave in to God's will I made a pact with the Divine and promise to myself that what ever door God opened for me I would walk through. I have never knocked on a door, or tried to break down a door. I have never selected a door nor was overly curious about a door that was closed. In my ministry I have only walked through the doors God has opened up for me. One thing I have strived to do in the 32 years I have been in ministry is accept God's open door and even though I have gone through some doors I did not appreciate, I have always had the peace that comes from believing I was in God's will. Many times I was not where I wanted to be, but I found comfort knowing I was where God placed me. Even when I was not in a safe place, I felt safe being in God's will. One thing that has been my anchor for 32 years is my belief that where I am, is where I am supposed to be. This assurance and this peace are not based on success or acceptance. It's not connected to how others perceive me or praise me. By no means can I make the claim that I have not fallen nor that I have not failed. I know about moral failure and broken promises. There have been times when I did not live up to the calling and when I didn't reach my own goals. I have never been as faithful as I should or done as much as I could, and yet I have had peace knowing that where I am is where I am suppose to be.

I believe that when I made the decision to accept my calling, that delivered me from the need to struggle with other choices. Because I made the supreme decision, I don't have to wrestle with making decisions. Saying "yes" to God set me free from having to deal with other questions. Accepting God's will for ministry enabled me to trust God with my life. Knowing that where I am is where I'm suppose to be helps me to be at peace with myself. Since I have been called by God and since I have given myself to God, I've come to believe it's alright to be me. I want to be all I can be, but I have no need to be other than me. I strive to give my best, but I have to give my best being me. I want to be a better me, but it's me that I want to be.

Somewhere on my journey I learned that it's all right to be different and it's all right to be me. Whatever success I have had, it's not because I have been better, it's because I have been me. I have never intended to be different but being me made me different. I'm not the best at anything but I can only do my best being me.

I do not believe that being single in ministry has been a great help, or a major hindrance. I do not believe I have had greater obstacles or better opportunities. For some, a single pastor is an oddity and something that isn't well received but how I see myself has been more important than how others see me. You can't be a single pastor and your singleness not be discussed. You cannot pastor a church as a single and not have plenty of candidates running in an undeclared election to be *First Lady*. You can't be a single pastor, and for some your singleness not be an issue, but how you see yourself is more important than how you are seen by others. Self-perception is more important than public image. Being true to yourself is more important than trying to convince others about who you are. Making peace with yourself enables you to provide ministry for others. When you are sure of your calling, you can be comfortable in your skin.

I cannot say, like Jeremiah, that I heard the Lord say "not to marry" (Jeremiah 16:1-2), yet I have no doubts that being single is where I need to be in my ministry. I have never made a conscience decision to not marry but neither have I felt being single is a hindrance. I know for some it is an issue but for me, it's the right thing to be. For some it's not the proper image but for me, it's the best way.

Somewhere along my journey I learned it's all right to be different and as I have been at peace with myself, I have been able to bless others in ministry. Being comfortable in my own skin has helped others to be at peace in my presence. I know there are some who have issue with a single pastor, but there have been many who have let me be their pastor with no qualms about my singleness. Somewhere along the way I learned that it's all right to be different.

Now, as a single pastor I have come to realize there is a price to pay for being different. You don't have to do wrong to be suspect; you can be under scrutiny just for being different. You don't have to commit a wrong act, just be a unique being. Those who ride the bandwagon have trouble with those who march to a different beat. When others try and blend in, they have issue with us who stick out. People who only go with the flow have an attitude with us who swim against the current. Those who need the approval of the masses are not happy around those who have no concern for the Gallup Poll. As a single pastor, I have learned that there is a price to pay for being different. There are those who want to question your reasons for being single and there are others who want to help deliver you from your perceived loneliness. There are issues one will face as a single pastor, but how you see yourself is what will determine how you cope with the problem. Somewhere on my journey I learned it's all right to be different.

Paul the Apostle says that, "He who marries does well, but he who stays single does better" (1 Corinthian 7:38). There's no sin in being married and there's no shame in being single. Being single is a challenge but it's not a curse. A single pastor has issues but they are not problems that can keep a sincere pastor from being successful if he/she seeks to be faithful. The word makes clear that marriage is not the only game in town. Not only does God need husbands, God needs bachelors. God can use the married and the single. He used the marriage of Hosea and he used the singleness of Jeremiah. He told Hosea to marry a prostitute and He told Jeremiah not to marry a daughter of Zion. He wouldn't let Hosea divorce a tramp and He wouldn't allow Jeremiah to marry a saint.

I know and believe that some of us have been called to singleness. It is a part of God's plan and it is the Divine will that some of us be single. Some of our pain is because we have been kicking against the pricks. We have tried to make happen for some, what God never intended. We've made a mess of our reality trying to fulfill a fantasy.

23

Somewhere along life's journey I learned it's all right to be different. Being single is a challenge but not a shame. You have not been denied you have been entrusted. You are not missing something; God gave you what others can't handle. It's a challenge but not a shame. When I read the word, I see that everybody used by God didn't have a marriage license. He was with Hagar, a single mother. He used Rahab, a single prostitute to save His people. He used Elijah, a single preacher to bless a widow woman in a time of drought. He sent John the Baptist into the wilderness with the Holy Spirit but no wife. He made Paul an Apostle to the gentiles but He didn't make him a husband. He made Jesus a Savior but the only bride He has is the church. Being single is a challenge but not a shame. It's a privilege and not a punishment. Somewhere along life's journey, I learned it's all right to be different. You have to be comfortable in your own skin.

It's hard to relate to others when you have trouble dealing with yourself. It's nigh impossible to be at peace with those around you when you are at war with yourself. You can't get along with others when you can't get along with you. Jesus says, "Love your neighbor as you love yourself". Jesus says how you feel about yourself dictates how you feel about others. How you see your neighbor is greatly affected by how you see what's in the mirror. To pastor as a single you have to be at peace with yourself. It's not good to be stuck on yourself; but it's important to be comfortable with yourself. You can be whole by yourself. You can be complete while being alone. You can have peace in your solitude.

I learned as a single pastor I am free to be free; and as long as I am content with myself, I am able to be a help to others. God can use me in my uniqueness. My being single does not make me a better pastor, but being single does not keep me from being the best pastor I can be.

Being single as a pastor has its challenges, but being single is not a shame. Now I have encountered those who rather to label you, than to learn of you. They would rather prejudge you than get to know you. They would rather talk about you than talk to you. There are those who have trouble with you when you are different. Because we like sameness, we are uneasy around uniqueness. Wear a different color but make sure it's the same style. Have a different tune so long as you're singing the same lyrics.

I rejoice in knowing that the God I serve loves us the same, but makes us different. He'll walk with anybody and yet we don't have to travel the same road. God loved Adam so much that He gave him a wife, and yet He loved Paul and gave him a throne. God permits us to be different.

For some reason I have never let being single cause me to feel as if I was less than others. I know there have been doors closed in my face by those who feel they can't trust a single pastor, and I also know my being single has not kept God from opening the doors that were for me to enter. Being a single pastor is a challenge but not a shame.

During my lifetime I have seen much in the church that is not good and is not right. I know for myself that the sin of hypocrisy is a concern in every church. We as believers are guilty as charged, but I also believe the real problem are not hypocrisy but happiness. It's not too many sinners; it's too many sad believers. Many in the church and even in the pulpit are sad and miserable. We do heavenly talk while we feel like we're catching hell. We say "Amen" to the gospel even as we choke on the world's garbage. We wear a happy mask to hide a sad face. We're more hurt than we are bad. We're more down on ourselves than we are running with the devil. We either want to blend in or hide out. Go with the flow or escape from the world. I know a lot of saved folks who are sad. There are single saints who are not happy with themselves. They are confused with God and mad at the world. Some people suffer from a terminal case of the blues. Their joy is short lived and their sadness is terminal. They are saved but not satisfied, and redeemed but not real. They have a smile on their faces, but no joy in their hearts. They've been miserable all their days and in the pits for a long time. They are in pain because they have no one, and a pain in the neck to every one they we have. Being single as a pastor is not a shame but it's a challenge. Because the church tends to overlook singles, the church is not at ease with single pastors.

I do not believe that being single has been a hindrance but it has been a challenge. I think being single has helped me to grow in spiritual gifts. You need the gift of discernment when more than ten sisters tell you that God spoke to each of them about being your wife. You need to know how to not be paranoid thinking every sister is looking for a romantic relationship. You have to get beyond your ego and realize that some folks are after the position you hold and not really infatuated with you. As a single pastor you need to have a healthy view of self and a clear understanding of your calling because how you see yourself will have impact on your success.

There are many of us in the pulpit that are not happy with self. Not being clear on our calling causes some of us to try and live up to an image. Having doubts about self forces us to hide self. Not being sure about who we are makes us sensitive to what others think. Any success I have had in ministry is due to God's goodness and my being at peace with myself.

Somewhere on my journey I learned to be content with me. It's hard to relate to others when you're having trouble with yourself. As a single pastor I learned the value of liking myself. Too many endure a loveless marriage and an abusive relationship out of dread of being alone. We would rather be in misery with somebody than agonize by ourselves. We prefer to have somebody to fight with than have to wrestle with ourselves. We will endure somebody who will put us down, so we don't have to do it ourselves.

We don't know that it's all right to be who we are and what we are in Christ. Some cannot see that it's all right to be by oneself and to be happy with oneself. Somewhere on my journey I began to realize that to survive the world you have to know how to make it with yourself. Not only do you have to make it on your own, you have to make it with yourself. Self-love is a part of survival, loving self is connected to salvation, and loving God and loving your neighbor are tied up in loving yourself. If you do not love self, you cannot love the God in whose image you are made. Those who do not love self will not love those who look like them or those who are different from them. Loving God, loving your neighbor and loving self all go together.

As a brother of color and as a single pastor, I've learned the value of loving me. My race does not make me inferior and my singleness does not make me wrong. I'm not lacking because I'm different, and I'm not strange because I am alone. I can be complete in Christ without somebody by my side. Somewhere on my journey, I learned it's all right to be different.

Since I have learned it's all right to be different, I no longer see myself as being *that* different. The issues I face in my ministry and in my life are the same ones my friends struggle with who are married. The temptations that come to me are the same that face my brothers who have a wife. The problems that arise in the church I pastor, happen in the churches that have a first lady. Being single does not give me an upper hand and it does not give me an added burden. I believe being at peace with self has helped me to be at peace in ministry.

By no means do I see myself as the voice for singleness. God has not called me to be the Apostle to the Singles. I feel I have what I need to teach and pastor married couples and single folks. God gives me what I need to minister to others whatever their personal situation. My being single is not a curse and it's not a crusade. It's a part of me, but it's not all there is to me. I have my issues as a single but I don't see it as a burden.

I rejoice knowing that I have a God and I have a people who have allowed me to be grateful for who I am, and what I am. I learned to thank God for what I can do and for what I can offer. I thank God for the life I've lived and the road I've traveled. Who I am in Christ Jesus is what I'm thankful for. I'm not a carbon copy; I have the choice to be an original. It's not just

27

what I have, it's how I am. It's more than what God did for me; it's what the Lord did through me. I rejoice in how God has used me in my singleness.

In 32 years of ministry I've learned it's all right to be different. Being single as a pastor is a challenge, but not a crime. It has been learning how to be content with myself that has helped me to minister unto others. I have learned that who I am in Christ is all I need be in life. If I am what God made me, that's all I need to be. I should not settle for less than what God intended, but neither should I try to be what I'm not or what I cannot be. I need to be what God made me. I need no label from others and no title from society. I need no one outside of me to shape me or mold me. I shouldn't be less and I can't be more. I shouldn't lack what God has promised and I shouldn't seek what God says for me is off limits. I should accept all God gives me and I shouldn't whine about what God will not allow. I realize it's all right to be different.

I see no need to make disciples and I have no need to be what others want me to be. I don't have to defend me, and I'm not under obligations to explain me. I don't have to look for a mate and I have the right to choose my own friends. *Me* is all I have to be.

I need to be saved, but I still need to be me. I need a Christ, but I need to be *me* in Christ. I see singleness as a privilege and not something to pity. It's not something I endure; it's something I enjoy. I don't cry about it, I think it's all right to celebrate it. I'm not living in limbo and I don't believe I missed out on something. Being a single pastor is a challenge but not a crime. For me it's more of a calling than it is a cross.

Sometimes I believe I was singled out to be single. Perhaps I was chosen to stand alone. Instead of being a pigeon, confined to a flock, I have the chance to be an eagle that can soar alone. For me it's not a disease, I believe it's the will of the Divine. It's not something to overcome; it's something to trust God with. I'm not ashamed or afraid. In the society of the world, and even in the church of the redeemed, we deal with marriage, and overlook singles. When we talk about family, we mean husband and wife with kids, not a man or woman who struggles alone. For most, family values means married life. We think marriage is the ultimate goal and being single is an awful shame. Marriage is celebrated and singleness is belittled. Some think the only way to live holy is to be married. Single women fear becoming old maids and single men are afraid of being mislabeled. As a single pastor I've learned it's all right to be different.

Because my singleness is not a curse, I'm not looking for a cure. I've seen too many single folks live their lives in fear of singleness. They see every man as a potential husband and every woman as a potential mate. Their mindset is, "If I can't marry you, I don't want to be bothered with you," "If we can't share a marriage license, we can't have any kind of relationship." Because some see singleness as a curse, they are always looking for a cure.

They sleep around and mess around trying to deal with the curse. They spend their lives and mess up their living trying to find a cure for the curse. They can't enjoy work and can't enjoy life because they are burdened down with the curse. They are jealous of married friends and ashamed of single buddies. There are some who see singleness as a shame. There are those who think that if you are a single pastor something is wrong. You can't preach and you can't serve being single. They feel you're not a role model and you're not a good witness if you are single. No matter how much good you do, some act like you've done wrong just by being single. Your living a full life will not keep folks from thinking you're missing something because you're single. There are those who think being single is a curse. They see it as a sin and a shame, but I believe it's all right to be different. God has not denied me, and I like to believe God trusts me. God lets me do as a single, what I cannot do with a spouse. The Lord gets from me as an individual what cannot be produced by a couple. I've come to realize it's all right to be different.

29

When I look into the word, being single is not a problem and not a shame. If you are in God's will, being single is just as good as being married. In the Bible, God does as much with individuals as He does with couples. The same God who made a woman for Adam never made a wife for His only begotten Son. In fact, Adam was doing fine when he was single, but got into trouble when he had a wife. God didn't give Jesus a mate; instead God gave Jesus a mission, and he lived up to it, single. Well, I do believe that Jesus is a better role model than Adam.

In the bible it's all right to be single. The word does not say that being by yourself means you're all alone. For the believer being married or being single is a calling. Neither one is your decision; it should be God's will. Neither one is better than the other, but it's based on the will of God. You don't need a better half if you're following God's will for your life. There's no need for someone to make you complete if the life you're living is in line with God's will for your life. No one should be married or single outside of God's will.

Everybody shouldn't be married, and everybody shouldn't be single. Some of us can't live with others, and some of us shouldn't be living alone, but none of us should be living outside of the will of God. We want to live in God's will. You can wake up by yourself and not feel lonely if you wake up in God's will. You can have somebody in your bed, but if it's not God's will you're just miserable with company. I want to live life in God's will.

Somewhere along life's journey I learned it's all right to be different. Being single is a challenge but not a curse. It's not free from burdens, but it's more blessing than shame. You are no better and you are no worse. I decided that instead of trying to get out of being single, I would try and get something from my singleness. Instead of trying to change my status I will trust God in my life. It's a challenge but not a curse.

What I have learned in 32 years as a single preacher is, it's all right to be different. God loves you in your uniqueness. God loves you the way you are. It's all right to be different. Go on and be who you are, just be it in Christ Jesus. Go on and be who God made you to be. Thank God for the you that you are. I thank God for what he has done in my life and for what He does with my life.

I know being a single pastor makes me different, but I thank God. I know I'm odd, but I thank God. I know I don't blend in, but I thank God. I know to some I am weird and strange but I thank God. I am grateful that God has trusted me to be different. I am no better, and I am no worse, I'm just free to be me. To quote Sly and the Family Stone, I say to the Almighty. *"I just want to thank you for letting me be myself—again."*

ع

"If God is Pleased:"
Surviving and Overcoming Public Attacks
Frank A. Thomas

In 1978, I sat as a young seminarian listening to a lecture given by Vincent Harding. It was the meeting of the National Black Seminarians Organization and Harding asked a question about the readiness of young seminarians, many of us not yet in our thirties, for a role of public leadership. He tried to conceptually lay a foundation of the responsibilities of public leadership, but in truth, though I was tremendously overwhelmed by the lecture, I was not sure that I knew what he meant. He talked about the weight and responsibility of the role of public leadership and the maturity that leadership required. Thinking back on it now, I heard what he said, but I did not have the experience to know what he meant. But, after thirty years of public leadership, I sure know what he means now. Based on my experience in the role of public leadership, I would like in this essay to address one aspect of the responsibility of public leadership that Harding tried to explain many years ago: the inevitability, the survivability, and the overcoming of public attacks.

In the role of public leadership, a leader will be the subject of many and varied public attacks. How one handles those attacks is, as one of my major mentors said, "the key to the kingdom." I want to state up front and directly how I have survived public attacks and have been victorious over attacks through the years: first, leaders survive and overcome public attacks because of a philosophy of leadership that allows the leader to place public attacks in a larger context, and as a result take them less personally. Secondly, leaders survive and overcome public attacks based upon the depth of their spiritual lives and their relationship and commitment to God.

In breaking down the subject of public attacks, I would first like to state the stark reality of public attacks. Next, I would like to discuss my thinking about leadership because how one approaches the question of public attacks has to do with one's broader thinking and understanding of leadership. Then, after stating one of my personal experiences with public attacks, I would like to approach the spiritual side of personal attacks and clearly place public leadership and the attacks that come with it in the context of faith, trust, and belief in God. I believe leaders have the ability to not only survive public attacks, but to be victorious over them, grow and mature from them, and ultimately thank God for them. I begin with the reality of public attacks.

The Stark Reality of Public Attacks
As a young seminarian, I was naïve to the reality of public attacks. I had no idea they could be so vicious and so painful. To help young leaders be less naïve, I would like to state openly and clearly the inevitable reality of public attacks. Public attacks are part of the price one pays for a role of public leadership. At some

level, if one does not receive any public attacks, one must question the effectiveness of one's leadership. Or as one of my close friends would encourage me with during one of the public attacks I suffered: "You would not draw so much enemy fire, if you were not right over the target." To help dismiss any naiveté, I would like to state the reality of public attacks in a series of "You will be attacked" statements.

First, you will be attacked because you cannot fulfill all the demands for relationship of the people you lead, especially when many of those demands are unrealistic, unexamined, vague, and for the most part entirely emotional. I often say that people are playing their home movies on my clergy collar. In other words, people do not see me – they see the reflection of the minister they grew up with, or the minister at their last church, or many see my predecessor, or any other combinations of perceptions that have nothing to do with me. Many do not see me at all. You will be attacked because you cannot meet all of the unrealistic demands for relationship that come with being a leader.

Second, you will be attacked because criticism is a form of pursuit of relationship. Many people are pursuing relationship with the leader and when they cannot get the relationship they want, they act out in order to receive attention. I have noticed that if I am not paying enough attention to some people, group, or ministry in the church, they will create a crisis so that I will have to come to the meeting, spend time with them, or in other words just pay attention to them. A public attack in the form of criticism is often a perverted form of pursuing relationship with the leader.

Next, you will be attacked because many people will not agree when you make a decision. The root of the word decision is "cision," to cut. When you make an in-cision, you cut into something, as when a surgeon makes an incision to operate. When you make a de-cision, you cut away something. There were two or more options, and when you make a de-cision, you cut away other options. Most people in most organizations want to have it all. For example, taxpayers want to have it all –

34

convenient services and low taxes. When the leader has to make the difficult choice between lowering services and raising taxes and chooses one, then the leader will be attacked. Not only do taxpayers want to have it all, so do teachers, children, parents, congregants, and everyone else. When the leader makes a decision, those that experience the decision as a loss will attack the leader. When a leader is decisive, he or she will be attacked.

Fourthly, you will be attacked because jealously is part of the human condition. As a leader, I underestimated the insecurities of people. My wife had to open my eyes to see that one of the most insidious and hidden sins in the church is jealousy. People are insecure about who they are and the progress and momentum of their lives. Many times, if they perceive you doing well, based upon their own insecurity expressed as jealousy, they will attack you. Many of us have learned to be very careful about sharing our blessings based upon the jealous attacks we have received. In the role of public leadership, I say never underestimate jealousy as a part of human nature.

Additionaly, you will be attacked because most people are automatically resistant to change. The moment you change something, people will attack you for it. Change is hard work and rather than do the hard work of change, people will consider the change agent an irritant and seek to force the change agent to change things back to the way they were. I have noticed that it takes the human family a significant amount of time to change, and many leaders have been attacked and even killed trying to secure change. Public attacks are part of any process that makes significant change in any organization, and change in organizations and people take significant time.

Next, you will be attacked because leadership in this time is more difficult than ever. In this present environment, people have so much anxiety and it comes out in so many ways. We see the screaming and unbridled emotion at microphones in public forums, the increased levels of violence such as the recent attention give to the levels of youth violence in Chicago, and the rants of scattered and unsubstantiated opinionating that perpetrates as serious discussion on some talk radio. America is more divided than ever. Given the fractionalism, divisiveness, and the levels of violence of the present moment, I sometimes wonder if our nation is governable, if leadership is possible. There are some places and times where groups of people are so divided and fractionalized that they refuse to be lead, and rather than face their un-governability, they attack the leader.

Finally, you will be attacked because in spiritual terms, "we wrestle not against flesh and blood but against principalities and powers and spiritual wickedness in high places."[1] In other words, there are spiritual forces that are against the positive work of God. Some are suspicious of me when I say that I believe that institutions and the physical plants of institutions have hidden ghosts and spirits. The spirits of the founders and the spirits of people who have come before are encased in the very walls of institutions. Some of these spirits are helpful, but some are not. Some are against change and seek unhealthy traditions to cover family secrets. Any attempt to move the organization to overcome the pathos that has gone before will force those spirits to quake and quiver. Those spirits will find some human(s) to act as agents to protect their interests. This is why the Bible says that we wrestle not against flesh and blood, but against spiritual wickedness in high places. Leadership for good is a positive spiritual force and there are negative spiritual forces that work against positive change. Never be naïve to the negative spiritual forces that you stir up when you are bringing positive change.

With a basic understanding of the certainty that we will be attacked in leadership, I want to now move to discuss my theoretical concept of leadership that broadens my perspective on the question of public attacks and allows me the freedom to take them less personally.

---

[1]Ephesians 6:12 (NIV). All Scriptural references will be from *The Holy Bible, New International Version*, (Grand Rapids: Zondervan Publishing House, 1973,1978, 1984.).

Leadership as a Healing Modality

Edwin H. Friedman has heavily influenced most of my thinking on leadership.[2] It was from Friedman that I began to understand the connection between leadership and the maturity of the leader. Friedman taught that leadership had more to do with a leader's presence and being than a focus on techniques and habits; with the emotional and spiritual maturity of the leader than the education and data available to the leader; with a leader's ability to be decisive more than the environment in which one was placed to lead. Most leadership theory focused on how to persuade, convince, and move followers, but Friedman focused on the leader and the maturity of the leader. At its core, Friedman's leadership theory was to help leaders increase their maturity; and upon an increase of their maturity, leadership was more effective and decisive. Based upon an increase in maturity, from Friedman's perspective, leadership was a "therapeutic modality." I change the word "therapeutic" to "healing." Based upon an increase in maturity, I believe leadership is a healing modality.

Regarding public attacks, Friedman taught that 90% of all criticism of the leader was a "red herring." It was not the real issue. He warned against getting caught up in the content of those issues. He argued that it was never the content, but the relationship and the emotional processes that were operating in the relationship. For example, several anxious members of the congregation go to the leaders and complain that they believe that the pastor is not working hard enough. They cite several examples of the pastor out of town or on vacation and they complain that the needs of the flock are not being met. The leaders of the church come to the pastor and say that they have a concern that the pastor is not working enough hours. Friedman argued that most of the time it was not about the hours at all, but

---

[2] Edwin H. Friedman, *Generation to Generation: Family Process in Church and Synagogue*, (New York: Guilford Press, 1985) and *A Failure of Nerve: Leadership in the Age of the Quick Fix*, eds. Margaret M. Treadwell, and Edward W. Beal (New York: Seabury Books, 2007).

there was a disturbance in the relationship between the pastor and this group that could only express itself in some content issue like the number of hours that the pastor works.

An anxious church leadership will get caught up in the content of the issue, like obsessively wanting to do a "time study" of the pastor's hours, or taking a poll to see if the members are happy with the number of hours that the pastor is working. They will want the leader to write their hours down and turn it into them for analysis and further discussion. Now there is nothing wrong with an objective discussion of the pastor's workload. The issue is that it is not objective; it is the result of the anxiety of several people in the congregation that have a disturbance in their relationship with the pastor. And when there is a disturbance in the relationship, it is not resolved by facts and reports on the number of hours.

Friedman taught that if you did not take matters personally and feed into them, get anxious oneself, and respond with the same level of anxiety, but treated the attacks factually and objectively while understanding that the relationship is the real issue, he believed that most of them would melt away. He taught that the leader had to feed back into the anxiety of the congregation for the congregation's anxiety to impact the leader. He called the ability to stay outside the anxiety of the congregation a "non-anxious" presence. It was very important to be non-anxious and connected.

Let me give you an example that helped me to understand this issue of being connected. Consider two porcupines with a coat of sharp spines or quills, which defend them from predators. If two porcupines are too close together, they will stick each other, but if they are too far apart, then they are not able to generate enough heat in the cold to stay warm. (For purposes of this illustration, staying warm is a metaphor for working together to accomplish some goal of task.) The key to two porcupines working together is to be far enough away not to stick each other, but close enough to get enough heat. Such is the relationship between people – if we are too close, we will stick each other, and if we are too far apart, then we will not get enough heat to stay warm. The relationship between a pastor and church leadership or a pastor and members, or a pastor and staff revolves, or any leader and people revolve around the critical question of how do we get close enough to stay warm, but not close enough to stick each other. Public attacks happen because you are either too close in the relationship or not close enough.

In the case of not being close enough, Friedman would say that if you do not stay in contact with your leadership on a regular basis or something like monthly, then you are asking for an attack. He would say call them for no reason, take them to lunch, send them a card, give them a compliment, etc. – if you do not maintain the contact, then you are not close enough and you will be attacked. Remember, criticism is a form of pursuit in the relationship. People attack you to have some sort of relationship because they do not know how to work toward the healthy relationship that they want. He would say voluntarily close the gaps in relationship on your own terms. He often said that many leaders shied away from this because they considered it a kind of "glad-handing." We have several unflattering terms for this, such as "brown-nosing," but he consistently emphasized that if you did not stay in contact, you were asking for trouble down the line. He reframed my thinking from a negative view of glad-handing to staying connected.

On the other hand, Friedman would say that if you were too close, or too connected, you will be attacked because a leader loses their own sense of self, a sense of their own values and priorities. Most people like to glob together into group think. And when people are globbed together, they act like a herd of animals. In a herd of animals, anxiety travels very quickly. If one animal becomes anxious and starts to run, then the whole herd will take off running without ever having established the initial threat or reason. Such it is with the anxiety in groups of people. Anxiety will start somewhere in the group; someone will feel threatened and will cause the entire group to be anxious. People will start to panic (run) and if the leader does not have a sense of his/her own self, priorities, and values, the leader will pick up the anxiety from the group. People do not know where to dump the anxiety, so they dump it on the leader, and if the leader does not have a sense of self, then the leader will carry the anxiety for the whole group. This is one of the prime sources of the stress and the attending health issues that many clergy face. They are not able to maintain a healthy distance, and a result, carry the anxiety of the group. For Friedman, carrying the anxiety of the group is a form of attack. If the leader is too connected, then the leader cannot get outside the anxiety of the group and maintain a non-anxious presence.

One of the keys to leadership then, is to be close enough to be connected, but not too close, and be distant enough to be objective, but not too distant. Friedman taught that leaders must have enough objective distance to be decisive, but also close enough to stay connected. My example of this is a mother who has to say no to her son's request that mom pays his rent. She calls to inform him of her decision that she will not pay his rent any longer, and he gets angry and accuses her of not loving him. Usually, they talk every Tuesday, but after this Tuesday's decision and the incident of his behavior, they do not talk for weeks. I believe that she must have the objective distance to make the best decision in regards to his rent, in this case saying no, but also, as far as it is possible with her, to not let distance develop in the relationship as a result of her decision. She is to call him every Tuesday as she does normally. She must continue to cultivate the relationship and though he might change the relationship based upon the decision, she must continue to be her normal self. It does not always work that the relationship can return to it's before decision state. But if a person will not take responsibility for their own rent, and manipulatively connect a mother's love with their immature stance that a mother should pay a grown man's rent, then it was simply a matter of time before the relationship would experience stress anyway. The mother is to do her own work of maturity and continue to strive to maintain her part in continuing the relationship.

One of the keys of successful leadership is to be objective enough to make a decision and personal enough to stay in touch with those that might attack and disagree with the decision. This level of maturity helps the leader to deal with public attacks or what Friedman called "sabotage." People will outright sabotage the agenda, vision, and the leader. This is one of the inevitable dynamics of leadership. People will say to you that they want you to lead them; what they will not often say is that some of the group will do everything in their power to prevent you from leading. Again, I am not speaking of everyone, but there is always a vocal minority that will sabatage the program and attack the leader. I am not certain as to why, but the negative vocal minority has more influence than their numbers allow because, at least in my experience, so many of the supporters are silent supporters. Friedman taught that sabotage could be overcome if the leader did not react to it, but stayed on track with the vision, direction, leadership, message, etc. Sabotage was only effective if the leader was anxious in his/her response to it.

Admittedly, I have found the work in the leadership role of pastoring difficult, demanding, and challenging. If all of what I have said above is true, why haven't I quit leadership after thirty years? The reason I have not quit is because leadership is a healing modality. Recently, I went to lunch with a Rabbi friend, and he passionately and poignantly articulated his belief that congregational leadership was damaging to one's body and soul. I immediately chimed in with agreement, and we listed some of the pitfalls that made congregational leadership dangerous to one's spiritual, physical, and emotional health. We identified that it is possible to lead worship, and so regularly meet the needs of others in worship, that one rarely gets the opportunity to worship oneself. We identified that when one teaches prayer and Bible as consistent and regular parts of one's work all day, many times the last things one feels like doing at home are prayer and Bible devotions.

We identified compassion fatigue, the irrepressible exhaustion that comes from being compassionately and regularly available to the needs of people. We acknowledged the deep and agonizing pain that goes with the inevitable conflicts and public attacks that arise, the emotionally draining mountaintop highs and the dismal valley lows that come often within the same hour or day in the normal flow of congregational life. Because it was so painful, we could only barely mention the gargantuan stress on family life from the long hours and the unrealistic expectations. And then we talked again about the attacks and the sabotage. In general, we concluded that one could be so busy working for God that one could lose his or her relationship with God.

We concluded that the only way to redeem the damaging nature of the clergy position is to operate from the mature perspective that one's service to God through the congregation is an opportunity to discover and develop what one deeply believes about God, life, and the world. We decided that the development of our maturity was a significant step in increasing the level of our satisfaction, fulfillment, and contentment in the pastoral role. We concluded that traveling the road of maturity involved spending less time complaining about the difficulty of the position, and more time taking responsibility for our healthy and unhealthy responses.

Friedman, in his classic work, *Generation to Generation: Family Process in Church and Synagogue*, suggests that congregational leadership can be a "therapeutic modality." I have substituted the word "therapeutic" with the word "healing." I believe that congregational leadership can be a healing modality. I have come to understand him to mean that if a leader can treat his or her transitions and crises as opportunities for growth, rather than hostile experiences that victimize and require escape, then the leader will increase his or her level of spiritual and personal maturity. And when the leader has increased his or her personal maturity, then leadership is a "healing modality." I am thankful that I have come closer to the place to view my experiences in congregational life as opportunities for growth. I want to now look at the spiritual side of public attacks. I want to look at faith as a resource in surviving and overcoming public attacks.

Faith as a Resource in Surviving and Overcoming
Public Attacks

I want to discuss faith and belief in God as a resource in surviving and overcoming public attacks, but first I want to detail one of my experiences with public attacks.

On a typically fall Monday afternoon, I received an emergency phone call that a group of church members had filed a lawsuit against me as the pastor and the church leadership. It had been threatened, several times, but not in my wildest dreams did I think it would become a reality. I immediately went into shock, and was even more dismayed when I found the lawsuit and myself on the cover of the newspaper the next morning. There is a ministerial email group in the city, where one person takes the responsibility to email any religious news in the paper to every preacher on the list. By the next morning, I knew that every preacher in the city would have the news, and it would not stop there because emails would be sent all over the country. The next morning, my phone, as the kids say, started "blowing up."
Folks from everywhere began to call the church, my house, my cell phone, and my wife. I was not embarrassed then, because basically I was in shock. The public attack intensified based upon the fact of the instant speed of communication and I barely held myself together as I received encouragement from the church members, family, friends, and preachers. And truthfully, prayer was hard. My prayers were emergency prayers, but it was the sustained prayer of others that kept me sane.

Several days later the embarrassment hit. I was embarrassed and in the depths of shame. I was supposed to be a skilled pastor. This kind of stuff happens to people when they start out in ministry, not to someone who has years of experience, and successful experience at that. I remember my first preaching opportunity, one week after the lawsuit. I turned the corner coming to the church and they had advertised widely and had my name on the side of the building. When I saw my name, I broke into tears because I was embarrassed and ashamed. I was in the pastor's study and I thought that no one would come that night. I thought no one would come to hear me preach. When I stepped out and the place was full, I was appreciative that they would come. I was dealing with all of the rumors, grapevines, etc. You begin to hallucinate and you think that everyone knows – even when people do not know or do not care or do not believe what they hear, the enemy convinces you that everyone knows and everyone believes it. Aside from the strategies of how to deal with this kind of massive and open conflict in the church, the most difficult part was the feelings of embarrassment and shame.

There is so much more that I could tell, but let me make a long story short. Ultimately, we were victorious and the lawsuit was sent back to be resolved as a matter in the local congregation. The church exclusively had the right to address any issues and the court had no "subject jurisdiction." The church addressed the issues with those members and we moved on to do the ministry God had given our hands and hearts to do. But after time and honest reflection over the whole experience of such a public attack, I came to this conclusion: I needed what happened to me. I needed to be sued. I needed to have my face plastered on the front on the newspapers. I needed to be an item on the television at 5pm, 6 pm, and 10 pm on three stations. I needed the pain – the hurt – the disappointment – the doubt – I needed it to learn that the most important thing in life is if the Lord is pleased. Up to that point, I had been a deep people-pleaser and I really tried hard to please people. I discovered in my soul, in the indescribable pain and loneliness of those hours that one thing mattered in life: if the Lord is pleased. I needed it because God delivered me from the opinion of people. I learned that if the Lord is pleased with us, God would lead us to a land flowing with milk and honey.

In the Bible, there is a text that saved my life as I was going through the public attack. It was a text in Numbers 14 verse 8: "If the Lord is pleased with us, he will lead us into that land, a land flowing with milk and honey, and will give it to us." (NIV)

The Hebrew people have come out of slavery in Egypt and are out in the wilderness. Moses and Aaron had sent twelve spies out to the scout the Promised Land. When the spies returned, they gave their report to Moses and Aaron and all the people. The collective group of the spies could not agree on one report so they submitted a majority and minority report. The majority report said that the people in the land were like giants and they were like grasshoppers, therefore "We cannot go up and possess the land." The minority report given by Joshua and Caleb said, "The Lord our God is able and we should go up and possess the land." The people believed the majority report and anxiety swept the camp. The people raised their voices in 14:1, wept aloud all night, and grumbled against Moses and Aaron: "We should have died in Egypt rather than out here in this barren land. Why did the Lord bring us to this land to let us fall by the sword?" In verse 4, they even suggested, "We should choose a new leader and go back to Egypt." Based upon their anxiety, the people were at the edge of almost being ungovernable.

In verse 5, Moses and Aaron fall face down in front of the whole people. Joshua and Caleb tore their clothes. Moses and Aaron pleaded with the people not to rebel against God. In verse 8, Joshua and Caleb say: **"If the Lord is pleased with us, we will possess the land."** They pleaded with the people not to rebel against God and not to be afraid of the people in that land. Joshua and Caleb encouraged the people to have faith in God because, if the Lord was pleased with them, then the people would possess the land. Joshua and Caleb were suggesting that the ultimate factor of victory was not money, intelligence, experience, management skills, etc. – *the critical factor was is if the Lord was pleased with them as a people.*

In verse 10, the people respond to Joshua, Caleb, and Moses' plea with verbal attacks. They wanted to stone them. Moses is preaching and trying to lead them in the spiritual way, and they were screaming, "Stone them!" And as they were screaming, God got involved. I tell leaders based upon my own experience, I do not care what happens; if God is pleased with you, they are not going to get you. They will howl, threaten, yell, and scream,

45

but if God is pleased with you, then God will show up. In the middle of the people's rage, God arises. The glory of the Lord shows up at the Tent of Meeting. God interrupts the violent plans of the people and calls for a meeting with Moses

In verse 11, God speaks to Moses and God is angry. God says, "How long will these people treat me with contempt? How long will they refuse to believe in me, in spite of all the miraculous signs I have performed on their behalf? God says: "I am going to destroy them and start all over with you. I will make you a great nation." In verse 13, Moses then pleads with God the way that he, Joshua, and Caleb pleaded with the people. Here he is pleading for them and they just wanted to stone him. Here he is begging God for their lives, when they have whined, complained, and despised him and his leadership. He says to God:

> the Egyptians will hear about it. They will get the report that you destroyed them. They know that you brought them out. They know that you go before them in a cloud by day and a pillar of fire by night. If you kill them, they will say that you were not able to do what you said and so you slaughtered them in the desert. What's more God, you are slow to anger, abounding in love and forgiving sin and rebellion. Yet you do not leave the guilty unpunished and you punish to the third and fourth generation. In accordance with your great love, forgive the sin of these people.

And because God is pleased with Moses, in verse 20 God relents. God forgives them – but even though God forgives, it does not release them from judgment – not one of them will make it to the Promised Land and they must wander in the wilderness until a generation dies off. Joshua and Caleb are the only ones that will walk into the Promised Land.

I am impressed with pastor Moses. He loves God and the people – he pleads for both even when the people have wanted to kill him. How does Moses plead for them though they have just wanted to stone him? You cannot help anybody if you are not delivered from the opinion of people. If you are still trying to please them – after all that you think you did for them. If you brought them out of rented facilities and built a virtual cathedral, and they are still talking about stoning you. You literally have your own blood on the walls of the sanctuary from what it has taken to move the ministry forward, and they do not even want you to put your son or daughter on staff without a fight. If you are into people pleasing, you will get mad. If you are into people pleasing, when they rise up to stone you, it will hurt so deep that it will cause you to hurt them. God will come up with a plan to destroy them, and you will not plead their case before God. You will take it personally and the people will not have a shepherd. And in your pain, God will say, "I am going to destroy them," and you will have a list of the ones you want to keep and the rest can go to hell. And you will reach out in unspiritual ways to crush the opposition. That is unspiritual management of conflict and the Lord will not be pleased. And how will God give us the victory if the Lord is not pleased with us?

What I am suggesting is that God will deliver if God is pleased with how the leader conducts himself or herself in the midst of public attacks. It is not what they do, but it is how one responds that makes all the difference in the world. One of my friends teaches the concept of 100% responsibility. I understand him to mean that I am not responsible for how people respond to me and what people do to me, but I am responsible for how one responds and what I do to people. Friedman taught that the leader's response either heightens the anxiety or lowers it. I have found the responsibility for my own behavior and actions gives me power in the most desperate situations. If I act in accordance with the mandates of Scripture, and God is pleased with my actions, then God will deliver. Moses did not attack them. Moses, at least in this text, did not complain about them. Moses went to God in prayer and pleaded with God on behalf of the people and pleaded with the people on behalf of God. Moses did not get anxious and maintained enough objective distance not to take their attacks personally but yet was close enough to them and cared enough about them to plead their case before God.

In closing, I want to articulate several of the tangible spiritual lessons I learned that helped me not only to survive the public attack, but to overcome them, grow from them, and ultimately thank God for them.

I remembered Jesus. God got a hold of me as I meditated on Hebrews 12: 2: "Let us fix our eyes on Jesus, the author and the finisher of our faith, who for the joy set before him endured the cross and despised the shame." The fact that he endured the cross got my attention. The word endured implies that he had a choice. He could have quit, given up, and gone back to heaven, but the text says that he endured it. He had a choice and made a decision to continue on with it. He had a choice and made a decision to go all the way to the end. When you make a choice, you have power in the situation. Based upon the power of his commitment to God, he tolerated, endured the cross. Secondly, the text says that he despised the shame. The cross is embarrassing. It is a place for criminals; the cross was shameful; he was a public spectacle; he was despised and rejected. The cross is embarrassing, but I noticed that he despised the shame. In the deepest and darkest moment of the public attack, God gave me this word that was a lifeline to a drowning preacher. God said about Jesus in this text-that he was not embarrassed by the embarrassment. Without question, it is embarrassing to go through public attacks, but we have to choose to be embarrassed. It is embarrassing, but we can choose not to be embarrassed. Being embarrassed is my choice and my decision. Jesus chose not to be embarrassed and I decided to not be embarrassed and ashamed. I despised the shame. Jesus was not embarrassed by the embarrassment and neither was I. God was pleased with Jesus and I thought God would be pleased with me.

No matter how personal it may appear to be, you cannot take it personally – public attacks are not personal. It is impossible to keep public attacks from happening in leadership positions. I heard one writer encourage readers to "not eat the emotional garbage of other people." He said that we would not dare or even think about going next door and eating the physical garbage of our neighbors, unless we were in the direst of circumstances. He asked, "Why then do we eat the emotional garbage of other people?" Why do we eat, take in, or entertain the emotional garbage of other people? Taking it personally is to eat the emotional garbage of other people. Do not take personal attacks personally, even if the attack is personal on the part of the perpetrator(s). I said to a young lady who had been molested by a family member that it was not personal. In other words, it was not about her or what she had on or how she looked. This violent act was about the family, and how the family organized itself and allowed a lack of protection for girls in the family. I said to her that it had to do with this man that perpetrated this act and the family more than it had to do with her. I asked her to not take the most personal act, sexual molestation, personally. Nothing was wrong with her. Something was wrong with the family. Conflict in the church is the exact same. Often, conflict is a family issue and is a result of the way the family has organized itself to provide or not provide a place of safety for effective leadership. God is pleased with the one who does not take the attacks personally, but pleads with God for the people and pleads with the people for God.

There are no victims, there are only volunteers – it helped me immensely when a friend said to me that "there were no victims in life, there were only volunteers." There are the exceptions to this rule, violent crime and especially children who are victims of sexual abuse. But when I looked closely at my situation, it helped me to realize that I was not a victim, I volunteered for leadership and could handle whatever came as a result of my attempt to lead. I made a choice to lead. I was not a victim, because I volunteered for the assignment. I am not a victim of my circumstances, I volunteered for my leadership assignment. I am not a victim of personal attacks; as a part of my service to God, I chose to be a leader. God is pleased when we take personal responsibility and do not blame. I am not a victim. I volunteered for this difficult assignment.

Vindication takes time – people can tear down in five minutes what it takes years to a lifetime to build. It is easy for people to throw mud on you, disparage your reputation and in the words of

49

the old Negro spiritual, "scandalize my name." I learned that sometimes it takes years to clean off the mud that people can throw on you in ten seconds. I had to learn to wait and depend on God. God will vindicate, but it takes time and you just have to wait. Some of these attacks are so deep and complex that you cannot vindicate yourself. God is pleased when we can wait and trust God to vindicate. In the words of an old preacher, "You cannot hurry God; you just have to wait." My vindication took several years, but I was vindicated.

Do not fight battles with unspiritual weapons – the Bible says in I Corinthians 10:3-4 that we do not fight with weapons that are carnal. We do not wage war as the world does. We fight. Now, I am not in any way implying that we should be passive and not fight public attacks. I am not suggesting that we simply cave in and let matters run their course. I am suggesting that we fight, but we fight with spiritual weapons and not with carnal ones. Utilizing unspiritual weapons leaves God out of the mix. I always reminded myself that my weapon was truth, unarmed truth. The poet said: "A lie cannot live forever and truth crushed to the earth will rise again." Truth will win. God will be pleased with my battle plan, if I base it on truth. And if God is pleased, then I cannot be defeated.

And finally, it took me a long time and a tremendous amount of maturity to come to be honest about the fact that **I needed it.** I needed it to happen. I was in counseling and the therapist asked me: "What lessons have you been avoiding all of your life that it took this kind of major calamity to reveal?" It took me several weeks to come up with a response, but this is what I came up with: It took all of this for me to learn that you cannot please people. It took all this for me to learn if God is pleased, then I do not have to worry about pleasing people. I am not proud to tell you all this; I am not posturing myself as some hero. I am just a person that grew up in a family that has issues and problems they could not handle and I learned some things that were not true and I lived them for a long time. But God helped me and delivered me. God delivered me from the opinion of people. I have some deliverance to go, but I thank God that though I am not where I want to be, I am not where I used to be. I thank God for the experience of public attack. I would not wish it on anyone. I would not want my worst enemy to go through all that I went through, but I thank God for it because I am stronger and better. Leadership for me has been a healing modality.

Being Comfortable In Your Own Skin
John K. Jenkins, Sr.

"I like livin' this kinda' life. I'm livin' a blessed life!"
So goes the chorus of a song sung by gospel recording legends, The Clark Sisters. With it's catchy tune, it continues: *"I'm blessed when I come and when I go. Everyday I'm livin', livin' in the overflow."*

These words permeate my being and represent my current state of contentment and self-assurance. However, they were not always words I could sing. Learning to be comfortable in my own skin has been a process for me. But it has been worthwhile and has brought me to a place where I thrive - life in The Zone.

Born and raised just outside of Washington, DC, I am the oldest of four children. As would be expected, my siblings looked up to me. I set the example and was the leader whether I wanted that responsibility or not.

As a young boy, I had a passion for church. I loved going and I was especially interested in listening to ministers preach. I was captivated by the stories they would tell and the way they would tell them. Those who listened would become enthralled in what the Bible had to say. I was among them.

"Did you hear that preacher tell the story about David and Goliath?" "Yeah, David wasn't afraid of an 'ole giant." My friends and I would spend hours standing on the street corners of our little town discussing the things we'd heard. We'd sing songs and dream dreams about our futures in ways that only young boys could do.

"Every great dream begins with a dreamer. Always remember, you have within you the strength, the patience, and the passion to reach for the stars to change the world." I didn't know those words of Harriet Tubman back then. But I had a dream. And my dream was to some day become a preacher. I often saw myself standing before others and explaining the Bible like I had seen so many do before.

Eventually the dream became something more. It turned into a burden. "They are listening but no longer hearing," I whispered to myself one day. I realized that going to church had become something different for me. My friends were no longer interested. But I was. I was extremely interested. I could comprehend the messages on a deeper level. And I wanted to. But I didn't want my friends to miss out.

I began to take the messages I had heard others preach and speak those same truths to my friends in my own words. But I would do it in a way that captured their attention. They listened to me. And they learned what they would have otherwise missed out on. This fueled me. It ignited something in me that caused me to do it again and again and again. I was passionate about it. I felt a sense of purpose whenever I did it. I later grew to understand that it was God's way of calling me. And I was answering.

Like oil and water, responding to the call was both burdensome and freeing. Anxiety about helping others in such a profound way carried a heavy weight. But it was offset by excitement and a sense of personal fulfillment.

By the time I was 15 years of age, I was licensed to preach and heavily involved in both ministry and church work. In addition to preaching, I also served as an usher. Although I was not much of a singer, I sang in the choir. I helped clean the church after services and dinners. And I was available to assist in any way I could. I loved church and everything about it. I loved being there. I loved the people there. And I loved to preach.

With the amount of time spent in church, it was inevitable that I would watch other preachers. "Can I get a *witneeeeees, weeeeeellll?*" spoken in a singsong melody was the call of many a "whooping" preacher. I was captivated by this style of preaching. The stories that were told and the challenges that were issued often pricked my heart and caused me to think.

I was fascinated. "I want to do that!" was the cry of my heart. "I want to preach so other people can understand the Bible and apply it to their lives. Can I *really* be a preacher? Can I help others understand the Bible and make an impact in their lives?" "Who would I become, as a preacher?" I wondered...

Being Comfortable
I've always wanted one thing from ministry and from life. I want to positively impact the lives of others. As a young preacher I felt pressure from family, friends, and church members to be like everybody else. And as great as the pressure was to please others, the internal pressure was even greater. I observed many preachers who were making a difference and I wanted to be like them. I wanted to sing like them, walk like them, and talk like them. So I began a journey to model myself after them.

Emulating others can be a good thing. It has been said that imitation is the greatest form of flattery. We identify role models and strive to be like them. We do what they do, read what they read, wear what they wear, and eat what they eat. It can be good to learn this way. Observing others who are successful and incorporating some of their practices into your own life can be an effective way to grow and develop. I encourage it but only to a point. It's possible to model yourself after someone to your detriment. This happens when you never take the time to develop your own style and find your own voice.

I remember an incident early in my ministry. A preacher was coming to our church and his reputation had preceded him. He was a very dynamic speaker. His style, presentation, and message were timely and very effective. I decided I wanted to be just like him. He would be my role model and I studied his style as if I were his protégé.

Once I vividly remember him doing something that was not the norm at our church. He preached with the accompaniment of a musician. This was fascinating to me. I had never seen or heard it done before. At just the right time, the musician would follow the spoken word with a musical chord that seemed to shout, "Amen, preach on!"

Needless to say, I was completely captivated. "I'm going to preach *just like that*," I thought. So my quest began. I started by having a conversation with a childhood friend who played the keyboard. I asked him if he would join me at my preaching engagements and play behind me. He, too, had witnessed the greatness of this preacher so he understood exactly what he was to do. He agreed and I was ready. Or so I thought.

I remember it like it was yesterday. I stepped to the pulpit, read the foundational passage of scripture that was my text, and stated the title of my message. Within the first minute of my message, I knew I was in trouble. My friend began to pound a series of chords on the organ after each sentence that I spoke. He did not strike an occasional chord here and there. No, he played after each and every sentence! This went on for the remaining twenty-five minutes of my allotted time. For me, it felt like an eternity.

The stunned look on the faces of the audience was the first indicator that perhaps I had made a mistake. The deafening silence was another. Certainly, the fact that they never invited me back again was the final indication that I had made a lasting impression. It just wasn't the one for which I had hoped.

In reality, I was seeking to do something other than what God would have me do. I was trying to "be like Mike". It was fine for him to share his gift with the accompaniment of a musician. It worked for him. And it served the congregation well. But not when I did it. The problem was more than my inexperience with the technique. The truth was that this was not my style of presentation. It was not the way I was created to preach. There were other things about this preacher God could've had me emulate. Having a musician to play as I spoke was not one of them.

The experience was uncomfortable and I was ineffective. But it taught me a valuable lesson: Always be yourself. The Bible states that each of us is fearfully and wonderfully made. The Lord would have us to be the person He created us to be, not someone else. Watching others as a means of developing your own personal style can be effective if you can take what you see and hear and package it in a way that fits your own gifts and call. I was forced to go back to the drawing board and wrestle with who I was as a person and who I was going to be as a preacher.

The 17th chapter of the book of First Samuel tells the familiar story of David and Goliath. David is the ultimate underdog who goes on to conquer the giant, Goliath, using only a sling and a few stones. Hidden within the story is a passage of scripture that has become a compass for me whenever I reach ministry crossroads in my life.

There comes a point in the story when David is preparing to face Goliath. Verses 38-39 reads as follows: "So Saul clothed David with his armor, and he put a bronze helmet on his head; he also clothed him with a coat of mail. David fastened his sword to his armor and tried to walk, for he had not tested them. And David said to Saul, 'I cannot walk with these, for I have not tested them.' So David took them off."

Saul wanted David to wear his armor. So he put his helmet, his coat of mail, and his sword on David. When David began to walk, he could not. He was unable to function as he was accustomed to doing. He had not tested Saul's armor and it had not been made for him.

The analogy is clear. You cannot toil in ministry wearing the armor of another even if it is glamorous. You can't even walk in it. The most dynamic and effective communicators are those who have learned to identify their gifts and function comfortably in them. This holds true for ministers as well.

The key is this: God has created armor for each of us. It is uniquely designed with each of us in mind. That armor fits your frame and your life in a way that nothing else can. It accentuates every aspect of your personality, your temperament, and ultimately your assignment in life. Try as you may to put on the armor of another. It may fit. But you will never be able to accomplish the full extent of all God has for you as long as you wear it.

The passage goes on to reveal that David set aside Saul's armor and picked up the weapons he was accustomed to using: his staff, his sling, and five smooth stones. And he proceeded on his journey. When he did this he was able to slay the giant. David experienced great victory, even against all odds.

In ministry leadership, we must do the same. We must set aside those things that can be classified as "Saul's armor" in our lives. The need to dress a certain way or drive a certain car, live in a certain community or have a church that looks a certain way, talk in a certain manner, or present according to a particular method – these things weigh us down and render us ineffective. Instead we must embrace what has been given to us, whether we view it as glamorous or not. And we must use it willingly. Then and only then can we, like David, be conquerors.

The New Testament also provides some insight. In the book of Luke, we read a story that on its surface appears to be about greatness. The 22nd chapter, verses 24-30 says:

^{24} *Now there was also a dispute among them, as to which of them should be considered the greatest.* ^{25} *And He said to them, "The kings of the Gentiles exercise lordship over them, and those who exercise authority over them are called 'benefactors.'* ^{26} *But not so among you; on the contrary, he who is greatest among you, let him be as the younger, and he who governs as he who serves.* ^{27} *For who is greater, he who sits at the table, or he who serves? Is it not he who sits at the table? Yet I am among you as the One who serves.*

"But you are those who have continued with Me in My trials. ^{29} *And I bestow upon you a kingdom, just as My Father bestowed one upon Me,* ^{30} *that you may eat and drink at My table in My kingdom, and sit on thrones judging the twelve tribes of Israel."*

In this passage of scripture the disciples get into a debate. They are bickering among themselves in an effort to determine which of the twelve was the greatest. However the controversy isn't over greatness at all. A deeper, and more significant conflict is taking place. What's really at stake is the Kingdom. The disciples are arguing over who will take over the ministry after Jesus dies.

Two very key points are presented that shed light on the significance of discovering your unique giftedness and operating in it. Understanding them will lead you to a place of contentment.

Point #1:
Your particular giftedness has already been bestowed upon you. In verse 29 of this passage, Jesus declares to the disciples that

each one of them had a kingdom bestowed upon them. Just as the Father had bestowed His Kingdom upon Jesus, Christ has bestowed upon each of us our gifts, our assignment for life, our very own destiny to fulfill. It is in you. Everybody has a mandate on their lives, that special something that nobody else can do. One of the keys to being comfortable in your own skin is realizing that God has bestowed, deposited, and granted to you your assignment for life. It is already determined and delivered.

The Bible is filled with examples of those who fulfilled their purpose. David, Elijah, Elisha, Peter, and Jesus are a few. While the world is filled with pastors and leaders in the ministry, there is only one you. And only you can fulfill that which God has bestowed upon you to do.

Point #2:
Your destiny is specific. Also in verse 29 Jesus tells the disciples that he has given them "a kingdom." By kingdom, Jesus means a walk, a purpose, a call. He has deposited in you gifts and abilities that are unique to you. I like to think of it as The Zone. God has put each of us in our very own Zones. When we get into them, nobody else can do what we do in the manner that we do it in.

Problems arise when we see others in their zones doing what they're supposed to be doing and we try to replicate them. We attempt to operate in their zone instead of in our own. This is prevalent in the church. There are people who fail to serve in the church but are quick to tell the pastor what he's doing wrong. Some should be working with the youth but they are trying to direct the choir. Still others are trying to teach classes when they are better equipped to evangelize. These are but a few examples. I'm sure you have a list of your own.

Jesus told the disciples they didn't have to fight amongst themselves to know who was great. Each person is uniquely gifted to do what no one else can do. When they compared their gifts with each other, it led to friction and tension. Anytime we compare ourselves with others, it will lead to problems. The revelation from Jesus to them was this: Each one of them was uniquely gifted and should celebrate their gifts and not be jealous of one another. That message applies to us today. Each of us is great when we function within our own Zone.

I've watched as peers have so fashioned their preaching after others that to close your eyes and listen would render you unable to distinguish who was actually speaking. Many go down this road to a point of no return. As a result they never develop their own style, their own personality. This makes them ineffective in ministry.

God uses all kinds of people to accomplish His will. He doesn't rely on one type of person. I have seen lives transformed by many different people using various preaching and teaching styles.

Your gifts must be discovered and developed. This is where God requires each of us to be wise stewards, and handle our talents responsibly, so that we might multiply and benefit His Kingdom. (See "The Parable of the Talents" in Matthew 25:14-30.) No matter where we are in ministry, we must continue to develop ourselves, to sharpen our skills, and to discover new and different ways God may want to use us in His service.

It has taken me several years to make this a regular part of my practice. I'm often asked, "Pastor, how do I know where my area of giftedness lies? How can I discover it?" The keys to discovering your Zone are quite simple.

First, your Zone will bring glory to God. You must learn to focus on those things that do just that. Take the time and ask yourself the question – "Is this glorifying Him?" As a pastor it's very easy to become encumbered by things that are nonessential. We do "good things" that are not necessarily "God things." Don't let this happen. And when it does, recognize it, adjust, and move on.

Second, your Zone is the place where you feel a burden. For me, it is shepherding others in the things of God. It is a part of my being. It is who I am. My life would be incomplete if I embarked upon a different calling.

Third, by serving you will discover your Zone. It is birthed there. It will never be discovered outside of service. In the passage of scripture from Luke, Jesus says that God had given Him a Kingdom and that he had come to serve. If Jesus served, then we should serve as well. This is our ultimate example.

Avoiding Discomfort
Ministry is hard. Works such as Anne Jackson's *Mad Church Disease: Overcoming the Burnout Epidemic* and "Why Pastors Leave the Ministry," by the Fuller Institute, George Barna, and Pastoral Care, Inc. point to one truth: pastors do burn out.

We are not immune to realities such as conflict, marital and family issues, health concerns, and financial frustrations. Seventy percent of pastors say that throughout the years spent in ministry they have a lower self-image than when they began. And seventy percent say they do not have someone who they consider to be a close friend. In addition to the personal statistics, 4,000 new churches begin each year and 7,000 close.[1]

With numbers such as these, it is no surprise that many pastors are leaving the ministry all together and seeking a "change in career". Those who remain feel the pressure. "Following the crowd" seems appealing.

While I have never seriously contemplated leaving the ministry, I have faced many challenges over thirty-six years. I've even burned out in the past. However, I never let it defeat me.

I have made several life style adjustments that have allowed me to maintain a level of contentment. I have become well

---

[1] Statistics compiled by The Fuller Institute, George Barna, and Pastoral Care, Inc.

acquainted with healthy eating and exercise. I embrace seasons of separation from church work and ministerial obligation. A home office enables me to be productive in an atmosphere that is more relaxed.

I have learned the importance of not allowing myself to become burdened by the ministry. More importantly, I have embraced the concept of rest. This has not been something I've always done. I've learned the hard way that God commands rest and that He does so for a reason. It has been said, "the more tranquil a man becomes, the greater is his success, his influence, his power for good. Calmness of mind is one of the beautiful jewels of wisdom."

During my early years in ministry I worked 12-18 hour days, 7 days a week. And with all that is required, this is not a difficult thing to do. The list of responsibilities is extensive. It includes Bible study and sermon preparation, attending staff meetings, board meetings, ministry meetings, and community-related meetings. There are conflicts to resolve, issues to address, and questions to answer. There are phone calls and email messages to make and return, events to attend, visitations to make, and people to see. And none of these involve time spent in personal devotion or with my family.

On any given day, I would engage in many, if not all, of these activities. This was not the exception. It was the rule. I had to be freed from feeling like I had to do something all the time. It is said that ninety-four percent of clergy families feel the pressures of the pastor's ministry. I am certain that my family did.

Rest is not passive. It is an act of the will. According to Psalm 116:7, we must return our souls to a place of rest. In stark contract to my early days, I have learned that everyone needs to engage in activities that take their minds away from responsibilities and obligations. There needs to be something you do that is just for yourself. Take up a hobby. Learn a craft or develop a skill. For me, it is aviation.

Flying gives me a chance to defy gravity and soar high above the things that keep me occupied. The exhilaration felt at take-off and the peace that meets me in the sky are unlike anything that can be felt on the ground. It is during these times that my soul is quieted and at rest. I exhale.

True Comfort
Living in the comfort zone comes with risks. You must have the courage to allow God to develop you, even if it costs. God develops me on a regular basis. He uses everyday circumstances, people and relationships, and the challenges of life to conform me to His image. They teach me to be flexible as I manage on various levels. He calls me to be compassionate as I'm allowed into the intimate details of the lives of others. He requires me to be accountable as others look at me and examine the way I live my life. Through these experiences I am forced to see myself for who I really am and to embrace my need for Jesus.

You must also be willing to be a trendsetter, to mark a course through uncharted territory; to be different. There are countless times in my life where I took a risk at being different. And in each instance, I learned about myself and about the power of God.

In 1992, First Baptist Church of Glenarden [Maryland] entered into an undertaking that was far from the norm. We were rapidly outgrowing our worship facility and in need of more space. We took an old warehouse and converted it into a 105,000 square foot church. During that time, this was rare. Since then, many churches have followed suit. Warehouses have been converted and given new uses.

It wasn't long before we outgrew this facility and began plans for new construction. Again, we diverged from the norm and did something different. Against all odds, we served as our own general contractor in the building of a 4,000 seat, 205,000 square foot worship center. In the fall of 2007, we cut the ribbon at our new location.

Experiencing Comfort While in The Zone

Comfort, is defined as a state of physical ease and freedom from pain or constraint. It brings to mind a sense of ease, contentment, and tranquility. How does one arrive at a place of comfort in their giftedness so that they can be effective? It is done through proper priorities, perspective, and principles.

Priorities: As a young pastor with a young family I often failed to do the right thing. My priorities were out of order. This occurred at the expense of my family. It was not intentional but it happened nonetheless.

Like a game of tug-of-war, there is a pull that ministry has. It is constant and it is real. The inability to recognize it and brace yourself against its strength will cause you to be dragged across the line. At that time in my life, I didn't realize I was in a game of tug-of-war. I thought I was "doing the work of ministry." And I was. But I was also missing milestone moments in the lives of my wife and children, moments I'll never have the chance to experience.

Things are quite different today. I have learned to put my wife and family first and we are all the better for it. I am able to attend ball games, go on family outings, and take vacations. I enjoy the intangible pleasures of family life and experience the growth of my children and grandchild, first-hand. *Proper priorities are necessary for life in The Zone.*

Perspective: Having a right perspective is a gift. It enables you to see the three sides of a coin - heads, tails, and the edge. As a pastor I am confronted with problems to solve, conflicts to resolve, and questions to answer on a daily basis. They have taught me the value of being a fact-finder. I have learned to be deliberate in decision-making, giving equal consideration to all sides, at all times, no matter what the cost. With Christ as my example, I do my best to search for truth and I strive to do so without making judgments. He is the ultimate judge.

Like the grandest of courtrooms, pastoral leadership places the issues of others' lives before me. I must be very careful to create an environment that fosters trust and the discovery of truth. When I have been deliberate, thoughtful, and prayerful in all that I do, I am able to rest well at night. *Proper perspective is key to life in The Zone.*

Principles: You are either leading men and women to God, or you are driving them away. I recognize the impact that my role as a pastor can have on the lives of others. I strive to be a bridge and not a wall. Luke 12:48 tells us that if we are given much, then much will be required of us. For this reason, I do my best to live with integrity. I strive to be honest before God and transparent as a leader. I have mentors who hold me accountable and faithful friends who keep me grounded. And I do my best to operate with proper motives.

Great preachers or those who are different from myself do not intimidate me. Instead, I am helped and blessed by them. I learn from them and then I bring them before the First Baptist family so that they can learn as well. I like exposing the members of my congregation to different ministries. Like a grand tapestry, it allows us to experience the fullness God has placed within the Body of Christ. *Proper principles are paramount to living in The Zone.*

Final Thoughts...

The Christian life is one that evolves around the God of the universe. The life that is focused, purposeful, and meaningful does not function apart from Him. Are the things that you're doing bringing glory to God? Is your heart set on being of service to others? Are you *livin' a blessed life?* As a minister of the one true God, I believe that you should be. And as a fallible man with faults and flaws of my own, I serve as an example that you can be

Becoming the Pastor

Ralph West

In the Fall Semester of 1980 I was a senior at Bishop College in Dallas, TX, majoring in Philosophy and Religion. At the time I was studying sociology under the tutelage of Dr. Joseph Howard, a Ph.D. from Baylor University. Dr. Howard recognized something of value in me. He invited me to come and preach at Fruitdale Baptist Church where he pastored. This would be the first time I preached in a multicultural congregation. The membership of Fruitdale had dwindled down to fewer than two hundred parishioners on Sunday morning worship. The atmosphere was different from any church at which I was accustomed to preaching. The people were warm, winsome and "quiet." After the sermon, Bro. Joe, as the members of Fruitdale Baptist Church affectionately referred to him, asked me to consider sharing the preaching responsibilities at Fruitdale. Then he invited me to preach a spring revival to give the members of Fruitdale the opportunity of considering me to become the senior pastor of the declining congregation.

In May 1981, Dr. Howard retired from Fruitdale and Bishop College and asked the leadership of the church to consider accepting me as their next pastor. I was excited to be considered for the pastorate of the church. In a June meeting the church elected me as pastor of Fruitdale Baptist Church.

Fruitdale was located in a densely populated South Oak Cliff community. The church was seen as a "white church" with a newly elected "black pastor" for the first time in its fifty-year history. The church had a 900-seat auditorium with a new nursery (that served as storage) and an unused educational facility. The first item on my pastoral agenda was to put bodies in the empty seats of this declining church.

Things seemed to be going great. At least that's what I thought. New people were coming to the church. We incorporated a program called "telemission." Securing a key map and manually going through a telephone book, a few college classmates and I began to call people in the neighborhood to come and worship with us. Keep in mind this is long before email, Facebook, and cell phones. But the efforts were paying hefty dividends. People were responding to our unsophisticated method of evangelism.

Fruitdale had elected me as pastor and preparations were being made for me to be installed in that position. I didn't realize, until too late, that not everyone in the church was thrilled about the new pastor. There were some who had another preacher they wanted to be their pastor. In July 1981 the church's deacons and several influential members took charge of the church and asked me to leave as the pastor of Fruitdale Baptist Church. I had been *elected* pastor but I hadn't *become* the pastor.

For many years I never rehearsed this experience, neither would I talk about it because it was too embarrassing and demeaning.

But I learned several lessons for any young preacher desiring to serve as pastor of a local congregation. In this context, I learned that just because the church elects you as pastor or the title is given to you doesn't mean that you have become the pastor.

Becoming the Pastor is a Process.
One question often asked is, "When do you become the pastor?" I can't assign a time to the question. Sometimes becoming the pastor happens immediately; other times it takes years and still other times you never become the pastor of a particular congregation. D. Elton Trueblood has written a useful book, *The Common Ventures of Life*[1]. In this book, Trueblood discusses the common venture people journey. For instance, he talks about the birth of a child, marriage, death and funerals and people journeying through the difficult times of life. I have learned that pastoral care is often neglected but at no time does the preacher move from the preacher to the pastor of the church than when he involves himself in the common ventures of his/her people.

I am not suggesting that because you are present and priestly in these moments you will be viewed as the pastor. I am only suggesting that they substantiate you as the pastor. I have been involved in ministry for 35 years. I began my preaching ministry during the era when the gifted preacher or communicator was almost guaranteed a steeple to pastor. The paradigm has shifted. Today it takes more than a good sermon or a preaching gift to become the pastor of people in need of shepherd.

Make sure when a church elects you to the office of pastor that the church confirms that election in an official document. And before you accept the position of pastor ask the pulpit committee or the church representatives to spell out carefully what your expected role as pastor will be in the context of that church. Keep in mind, you have nothing to lose, so be honest about your expectations of the leadership of the church and the church itself. Ask the church to put in writing what their understanding of the

---

[1] *Trueblood, Elton. The Common Ventures of Life.* New York: Harper & Row, 1949

pastor is. You will discover that most churches are unaware of the biblical and theological rationale of the pastoral role.

Most churches today are more interested in your credit score than they are your conversion. They are more concerned about your criminal history than they are your devotional habits. And they are more interested in whether you have a gambling problem than they are about your understanding of proclaiming the gospel. Don't allow your ambition to pastor any congregation to compromise the calling and consignment given to you by the Lord Himself.

Here would be a good place for you to be clear on the role and the responsibility of the pastor. One place where this is clearly defined is in the conversation between Jesus and Peter regarding the primary role of the pastor- Feed my lambs and feed my sheep.

After a brief hiatus from the pastorate I returned to Houston to recover from my brief embarrassing and hurtful pastoral encounter. I felt like Jeremiah rejected, defeated, disappointed walking through the streets of Houston (Jer. 20:7-13). But I was certain that like the prophet Jeremiah, God had called me to serve Him and to preach His Word.

Learning in the Village
Sitting in my home church (Lyons Unity Missionary Baptist Church) Deacon Whittaker approached me about preaching at his lodge brother's church. Have sermon will travel. I went. I drove up to Zion Hill Missionary Baptist Church, a small neatly kept church in Brookshire, Texas just twenty miles outside the Houston city limits. Although the Brookshire was close it seemed a world apart from the city of my youth. I met Deacon L. H. Bostick, the chairman of deacons. He was a short strong warm gentleman. It was evident L. H. was a churchman. He escorted me to the pastor's study, escorted me to the pulpit and introduced me to the congregation as the preacher for the morning.

I preached to approximately 150 people. They were very receptive and after the message Bro. Bostick asked me if I would consider becoming the pastor of Zion Hill. I had learned my lesson, a verbal invitation would not suffice; it would have to be spelled out in writing...a formal letter of invitation, written by Bro. Bostick, was sent to my apartment. I accepted the position as pastor of Zion Hill only after meeting with the entire church.

I served that congregation for 18 months. This was a good place for me. I learned some valuable lessons in this rural church. One lesson I learned is that every church, regardless of size, has a history. The wise pastor will learn as much as possible about the history and the people of the congregation. For instance, Zion Hill for most of its history was a first and third Sunday church. On the second and the forth Sundays the church attendance was low, the first and third Sundays were always significantly higher. I mention this because every church has its own idiosyncrasies. At first I tried to scheduled special events on these off Sundays. I learned quickly that this was a bad idea.

Out of Here
There are times the small town church appears resistant to change made by the new pastor. I learned that these churches have a suspicion about the new pastor: if he is young, gifted and talented, he is not going to hang around for long. These churches are slow to make shifts, not because they are resistant to change as much as they are aware of the new pastor's likely short tenure. Questions surrounding the longevity of the pastor cause the small town church to become hesitant to making emotional or pastoral investments in ministers who may not be there for long. If you find yourself in one of these churches don't get frustrated. Remember, many of these people are protecting their history.

The small town church is significantly different in several ways from the urban or suburban church. In the rural church almost always everybody knows everybody. The people in these churches intermarry, creating large extended family churches. Often to get things done you have to win the matriarch or the patriarch of the church to your side on major issues. In my case L.H. Bostick was the influence of Zion Hill. Fortunately, Bro. Bostick saw me as one of his children. Whenever I needed something done, I went to Bro. Bostick, explained to him what I wanted to do, what I envisioned for the church and let him take the lead. No one was going to oppose him.

At the same time I never exploited the relationship I had with Bro. Bostick. In 1983, as a college graduate and seminarian, I served that church as pastor with a salary of $150 a week. I was married and my wife was pregnant with our first child. I went to Bro. Bostick and told him I needed insurance and a raise. He took my concerns to the congregation on a Sunday and without one dissenting vote my raise and insurance were accepted.

Money is a servant, not a master. Jesus says, "No man can serve two masters" (Matt. 7:24). Nothing can destroy the pastor like an unhealthy understanding of money. The scripture has some sobering teaching about money. When it comes to money don't be afraid to negotiate for what you need. Rarely will you ever get what you deserve. Normally you get what you negotiate. Use money; don't let money use you or rule you.

Probably the most significant lesson I learned at Zion Hill was the power of relationships. My temperament as a young pastor was sharp and short. During dinner at Bro. Bostick's home one Sunday, his wife, Sis. Ruby Bostick, a wise woman, said to me, "Bro. Pastor, you can catch more flies with honey than you can with vinegar." I had heard those words spoken about other people but never to me, I'm *Mister Personality*.

Becoming a pastor involves relationships. Father Henri J. M. Nouwen in his book, *The Living Reminder*[2] speaks of pastoring with presence. There are times when your pastoral presence can make all the difference in a member's world. The pastor walking

---

[2] Nouwen, Henri J.M. *The Living Reminder*. San Francisco: Harper & Row, 1977.

into the hospital room of a member waking up from surgery can bring comfort. The pastor standing next to the casket of a grieving family can lift their bereavement. The pastor walking through the children's church and letting the babies grab you around your legs or your touching them on their heads develops the first stages of new unbreakable relationships.

Move To Town

After eighteen months in the rural I was called to pastor in the city of Houston. Greater Mt. Zion Missionary Baptist Church called and elected me to serve as their fifth pastor. The church once bustled with the laughter of children and the energy of youth. When I arrived at the church its once glorious past had long disappeared.

The congregation was made up of families that were raised in the church, intermarried within the church, divorced and remarried in the church. Well, you get the idea; the church was full of congregational messes. However, though Greater Mt. Zion was dysfunctional, they were rather normal as church goes.

Often you will hear the term "honeymoon" used regarding the new pastor and his initial tenure at the church. Take it from me I had no honeymoon. My first day on the job was a nightmare. The church had agreed to pay me a salary of $450.00 a week. When I received my first paycheck it was reduced by $50.00 with no explanation other than the treasurer saying, "The deacons told me to do it." That one act would be the beginning of three and half years of tension.

The next Sunday at the end of service I dismissed the visitors and met with the congregation. I informed them of the deacons' actions and then I dismissed the majority of the deacons. The church applauded my actions. The truth be told, I did what the enemies of these people were not courageous enough to do themselves. The same people who cried "Hosanna" were the same ones who cried out "Crucify him crucify him!"

One big influential family of the church frowned upon anything I attempted to do. On Sunday, when I was preaching, some of the deacons would come to church and read the newspaper. Others would conveniently go to sleep. Others would frown and smirk at me every Sunday when I preached. One Sunday morning in March of 1987 immediately following the worship service I went to my office, and I heard somebody scream "I can't believe they're doing this to my pastor!" The concerned church members had circulated allegations against me as grounds for why I should be dismissed as the pastor. Their reasons: "He wears a beard, he wears jeans under his robe, he fixed the leaking roof without the church's permission, he changed the carpet, and he wanted to cut down trees to put in more parking." I know you are saying, "West is using hyperbole." If that is your response, you haven't pastored a real "negro Baptist church" or any other kind of church.

This action would lead to my arriving at church on a Sunday morning to learn that the locks on the door had been changed. My wife was pregnant with our youngest child, and as we walked up to the church this particular morning we were met by an angry mob of church members. I felt like a lamb being led to the slaughter.

In a church meeting, the members voiced their primary reason for my dismissal, "Reverend West, we did not call you here to bring all of these other people to this church. This is our church." They were telling the truth. I asked a judge and he told me that, according to the legal document bearing the names of deceased trustees, the church in fact belonged to the people. I knew it was time to get out of a church where God and the Bible didn't have preeminence.

Lessons in a Hard Classroom
Here are a few lessons learned in the midst of a hostile church environment. First, in becoming a pastor you have to love people. This sounds easy but you have to love *all* the people. You have to love the ones that support you and those who openly oppose you. "Joe" didn't like me. This is not paranoia speaking;

he said it on a Sunday morning in worship. I tried to quiet him but he got louder. His last words to me were, "The Lord will handle this." I said, "So let it be." That week, while attending a Winter Board Meeting I received a telephone call that "Joe" had suffered a heart attack and died after struggling for his breath. These were the words from the lips of his wife (someone who knew me and taught my brother and sisters in High School). I returned home to be a good pastor and fulfill my pastoral responsibilities. The funeral was planned. I was not included on the program. I was not offended; I believe people have the right to choose whomever they desire to comfort their family.

The family asked a local pastor and friend of the family to deliver the eulogy. The funeral began; the minister hadn't arrived, and the program proceeded as printed. When it was time for the eulogy, the visiting minister still had not arrived and I asked that the choir to sing another song. By this time it was apparent the visiting reverend was not going to come. I rose, made a few comments about Joe's love for this church and commitment to the Sunday School. Then I made some references about his love for his family (all of this was true). The people were waiting on me to use the opportunity to turn negative and personal. They are still waiting. I had learned from my boyhood pastor to love people. Loving this family didn't win any support, but it allowed me to sleep well at night.

The natural tendency is to retaliate, but I could hear Mrs. Ruby Bostick, "Bro. Pastor, you can attract more flies with honey than with vinegar." I'm not implying that this was my temperament most of the time. My tendency is to fire back, but that day there were people in that family that were so moved by my kindness they would later become my best supporters.

You Can't Win Them All
I made several blunders as the pastor of Greater Mt. Zion. I thought in order to be the pastor you had to have your way all the time. That was my young adult misunderstanding of the role of the pastor. I had been fortunate to grow up in a healthy church environment. My uncle was the chairman of deacons and my

pastor was a well-polished preacher. I didn't learn until much later as a preacher that there was constant conflict during meetings with the pastor and the deacons. But this was always kept away from the congregation. When the meeting had ended, the deacons and pastor emerged as a "united front."

I thought this was the way all churches functioned. Not at Greater Mt. Zion! Every opportunity was taken to say something negative and combative towards the pastor. The deacons' board was split on every issue right down the middle. I didn't meet with these men with any regularity. That was a mistake. They met without me and they made decisions without me. I made decisions by myself and there was an ongoing tension. Would meeting with the deacons have made a difference? I don't know. But what I do know is that I would have learned how they thought, and more importantly, what made them think the way they did.

I was viewed as an outsider. I was nothing more than a hired preacher. I wasn't supposed to make any decisions. My role according to the board was to preach, visit the sick, raise the money (not spend any of it), take orders, shut my mouth and be glad I was the pastor. Unfortunately, this attitude towards pastors is not restricted to geographical regions. This is the attitude of many misinformed church leaders. Try in your pastorate to be prayerful about who you select to serve as a deacon, officer or leader in your administration. The Bible is very clear on the qualifications of the deacon. Unfortunately, too many persons are chosen because of their business acumen, or their status, education, longevity with the church and not their spiritual character. Jesus spent the night in prayer before he chose his disciples. Even then, one of his chosen was a devil.

I had thrown away a collection of books poorly stacked in the cabinets of the church. When the Sunday school teachers saw what I had done, they were livid. Their anger didn't move me an inch. I told them that if the material was that important to them then they would have stacked the material neatly and in order. This was a reaction from my earlier days of working in the

Houston Public Library. Hindsight is twenty-twenty. Someone purchased those books. There was a time when that Sunday School Department didn't have those books and I disregarded the sacrifice someone made for the children of that church to have religious material to read.

It Only Takes a Spark...

Inside of the sanctuary of the church hangs a picture of the Reverend Ed. Carrington. He was the iconic pastor of Greater Mt. Zion. I moved the picture (not the best idea) from the wall of the sanctuary to the foyer. I found a picture of Rev. Riggmaden and Rev. Cain and hung their pictures in the foyer also. When the church leadership voiced their disapproval, I said, "I only hung the pictures in the foyer so everyone could have a good look at our beloved pastors from the past." The pastor's picture is a sacred icon. I was viewed as an iconoclast. Something as innocent as moving a picture can become the spark to ignite a conflagration.

I wanted to spruce up the old church sanctuary. The floor was covered with indoor/outdoor carpet. The widows were colored glass: red, purple, green and yellow. The names of those who contributed the widows were affixed to the glass. You couldn't read the names because the paper had fallen off the window. For instance, Mrs. Barlow's name read "M s. Ba l w." I told the secretary to have brass nameplates made to replace the stencil. You would have thought I was trying to write graffiti on the wall. After I was long gone, someone had the brilliant idea to preserve the names of the donators by putting up brass plates. It may not come when you want it to, but when it arrives it's always on time.

We needed parking, as the church grew. The 450-seat auditorium was filled to overflowing. West 23rd Street was filled with cars. The neighbors complained that the people were parking in front of driveways. The removal of a couple of trees would allow us to have several more parking places. Several houses across the street from the church could have been bought and demolished to make room for the much needed parking. I introduced the idea.

Why did I do that? The Black newspaper featured an article describing a young pastor in the Heights wanting to evict senior residents to expand his personal agenda. Can you guess whom they were talking about?

Several years after I was removed as the pastor of Greater Mt. Zion, the trees were moved from the front of the church. And those houses that belonged to the elder members of the church were sold to developers. Today row houses have been built and are selling for $250,000 to $400,000. The church is land locked and the seats are empty. I find no delight in the present condition of this church. That's enough of Greater Mt. Zion. (Trust me, the half has not been told).

Follow the Star
In the middle of all of this pastoral drama, a healthy church in Beaumont, Texas was interested in me becoming their pastor. Star Light Baptist Church was the flagship church of the Golden Triangle area with a rich history and a promising future. I preached there in September 1987 and that same week I was elected as the next pastor. This church was different. Star Light was healthy and well organized. They had built a new edifice to the already existing church building. The 1100 seat auditorium had about 900 people present that day.

Unlike the previous churches, Star Light was ready with their questions. They interrogated me for hours about my savings, credit, legal history, etc. Then came the blockbuster question, "How much money will it take for you to be the pastor." Try not to answer this question to soon. You don't know how much it will take until you find out how much living expenses you will need to relocate, purchase a home, car, insurance. They proudly made me an offer of a $36,000 package. That was the first time the term had been used and I knew I was dealing with corporate minds. I laughed at the offer because I had done my research on the church. I said, "I know a church that invests with Paine Webber wouldn't insult me with an offer like this." They were more concerned with how I knew about their holdings than rejecting their initial offer. The retracted the offer and presented me with a $66,000 package, not including housing and insurance.

Confession is good for the soul but bad for the reputation. Honestly, I was through with the pastorate. I had made up in my mind I would take this church for one reason. I would negotiate the biggest financial package they would give, save my money and in a few years leave and go back to school, take a terminal degree and teach. The pastorate didn't like me and I didn't care very much for the pastorate. Going to Beaumont would be *a get out of jail free card* from Greater Mt. Zion. But the Lord would have another plan for my future. I came under a deep conviction. The Lord restrained me from exploiting Him and His church. I refused the offer even though those wonderful people were willing to give me forty-five days to pray and think about reconsidering the offer to accept Star Light.

Know When to Hold 'Em
At the same time, I had a group of young people who pleaded with me not to leave Houston but to start a church. No way! I was not made for a church start. To begin with nothing! I had one very optimistic man in my crew, Ralph O. Frazier, who said to me, "Pas, why don't you start a church?" We had a meeting in my small wood-framed two bedroom house in the 'hood. All of thirty-two people came to the meeting, which was about seventy people shy of what Frazier thought would come. I reached the decision to start Brookhollow Baptist Church after prayer and reading *The Road Less Traveled*.[3]

I am in my twenty-second year as the pastor of The Church Without Walls and I have learned and I am still learning what it means to become a pastor. In becoming a pastor I am learning to listen to the right voice. How do you know when you are listening to the right voice? How do you distinguish between the voice of God and the voice of your personal ambition?

---

[3] Peck, M. Scott. *The road Less Traveled: An New Psychology of Love, Traditional Values and Spiritual Growth.* New York: Simon & Schuster, 1978

In *Wishful Thinking*[4], Frederick Beuchner writes, "There are all different kinds of voices calling you, all different kinds of work. And the problem is finding out which is the voice of God, rather than of society, or the super-ego or self-interest. By and large, a good rule of finding out is this: The kind of work God usually calls you to is the kind of work, (a) that you need most to do, and (b) that the world most needs to have done. If you really get a kick out of your work, you've presumably met requirement. (a), but if your work is writing TV deodorant commercials, the chances are you've missed requirement (b). On the other hand, if your work is being a doctor in a leper colony, you have probably met requirement (b), but, if most of the time you're bored and depressed by it, chances are you've not only bypassed (a) but probably aren't helping your patients much either. "Neither the hair shirt nor the soft berth will do." I like the way Buechner concludes: "The place God calls you to is the place where your deep gladness and the world deep hunger meet."

The call of God is a distinguished call. In the same way God called Abraham to go west and Moses from the burning bush, the call to every pastor is distinct. He called Gardner Taylor from an inquest in Louisiana.

He called George Truett when he didn't want to be called.

He called G. Campbell Morgan even though the Methodist turned him down.

He called J. Alfred Smith from a bandstand; Smith put down his horn, walked out and rode a bus home.
God's call is a distinctive call.

---

[4] Buechner, Frederick. *Wishful Thinking: A Seeker's ABC*. New York: Harper Collins Publishers, 1973.

LONELINESS IN MNISTRY
Gethsemane, Golgotha, Galilee and God's Grace

Debra Haggins O'Bryant

Introduction

I begin this offering with a confession. I have reached a serious writer's block. My life at this point is a gift from God. My life today, with my husband, my adult children and grandchildren is beautiful. My God is real (intensely real), my faith is strong, my dependence on Him for everything is unwavering, and my love for my Father is seriously non-negotiable. Every day, I am privileged to have the kind of solitude, space and time that most people can only dream of having and that I have longed for in days and years past. No longer am I simply getting through life, praying that another day would begin long before the current day would end. Even with my life's ever present ups and downs, highs and lows, successes and failures, disappointments and discouragements, I finally feel good about *my* life. I am not alone and neither am I lonely. I am not wanting or needing anything but more and more of God in my life. My sincere prayer for my life and every life is that we would all get to the place of King David where he prayerfully reflected in this way and penned these beautiful and heartfelt words, *"One thing have I desired of the LORD, that will I seek after; that I may dwell in the house of the LORD all the days of my life, to behold the beauty of the LORD, and to enquire in his temple..*[1]*"*

I guess one would inquire, *well then preacher, why the block?* Why the hindrance and the hesitation if all is so well with you? To be honest, living through loneliness and being able to reach back, although not too far back, and give a two-minute testimony about having overcome and survived isolation is one thing. But going back and writing about it; sharing so deeply in such a public forum is another. Reflecting on loneliness means that you are forced to dig deeply; to participate in a kind of spiritual excavation, if you will, whereby you are asked to carefully disturb the new landscape of your now delicately settled-in life to remember the ugly details of the painful seasons you would not have survived had it not been for the Lord on your side. If I am to be true to this assignment, then I am duty-bound to remember long lonely nights, tear-soaked pillows, mascara-stained pillowcases, and rumpled sheets that bear witness to the evidence of tossing and turning well after the midnight hour; hoping for the joy to which I held fast because I staked my claim in the belief that it would come with the morning.

If I am to be true to this assignment, then I am determined to go back to a time when my only protection was the razor-sharp two-edged existence of self-imposed aloneness; a solitary isolative loneliness that was almost more than my heart could bear and my mind could handle. And as you read these words, you too have a responsibility. You are bound to take a spiritual journey with me into a virtual world of a kind of human anthropology of the spirit with the excavation site of your own mind, your own soul, your own spirit; hence your very life. For it is not the cold hard facts and uncovered relics of days gone by that set you free-relics that are buried like hidden yet forbidden treasure within your earthen vessel. Rather, it is the carefully preserved artifacts of God's revelatory truth that brings liberation of the soul and freedom of the spirit that the mind desperately needs to be transformed and renewed[2].

Upon accepting this assignment and delivering this offering to its publisher, I am forced to reflect upon those painful seasons in my life when I was lonely and alone, when a friend could not be found, and my betrayer was close at hand. For those of us who have traveled the road of loneliness or aloneness, we know that it is a difficult one. One cannot teach loneliness unless one has been lonely. One cannot preach about aloneness unless one has been alone. One cannot appreciate solitude unless one has been without the hearts longing for the silence of the world and the stillness of the voices within for just a few moments of intimacy with God. Even if only vicariously, our Father has this awesome and mysterious way of allowing me to somehow revisit or in some way experience the issues of life that I hope to come to aid others who are in need of healing in a particular area of life; indeed, I do go through. Yet, as we explore together the issue of loneliness in ministry, I will use one or two relevant experiences from my life in conjunction with the biblically chronicled life experiences of Ruth and Naomi and the ministerial loneliness experienced by the Apostle Paul to create a basis for our brief discussion. Within the context of a four-pronged nexus, inclusive of a view of the earthly life and ministry of our Lord and Savior Jesus Christ, I will attempt to elaborate on what I have discovered to be prevalent in our lives. I call it, **The Abandonment Cycle: Gethsemane, Golgotha, Galilee and God's Grace**.

It is my prayer that you will discover as you read this offering that I do not have any answers, only scars and personal life accounts. It is my prayer that you will discover that I have no cookie-cutter solutions. However, I am sure that you will easily discern that I have a few wounds that have yet to heal. I posit that God and God alone has the answers to any and all of man's needs. Yet, I am willing to allow God to use the totality of all that I am and the composite of my existence as an instrument to bring my fellow parishioners to that place of Grace, readiness for healing, and wholeness that is already on the inside of each of us. At this moment, I pray for the authority and the wisdom to draw out, and the power to heal through these words.

Bless Be The Tie That Binds

I have always been receptive to the beautiful biblical account of the lives of Naomi and Ruth. Naomi is a woman whose husband and two sons die. Naomi is now left alone in a strange land, among strange people who worship strange gods and live under even stranger customs. It appears as if Naomi has no hope of survival in Moab. When she hears that the famine is over in Bethlehem and the Lord is once again showing favor to His people, she strikes out alone to return to Bethlehem. Naomi has decided to abandon her life in Moab and begin the long solitary journey back to her homeland. She, by death's unyielding hand, has been forsaken and is determined to return to Bethlehem alone, live an isolative life and sketch out the rest of her days in a kind of obscure loneliness. Naomi is the seeking solitude within the familiar.

Ruth, on the other hand, is a young woman full of hopes and dreams who leaves or abandons the house of her own mother, in order that she might find a new life through the witness and the testimony of her mother-in-law, Naomi. Ruth is a young woman who needs not to be lonely anymore. Therefore, she pledges her friendship, love, devotion, commitment and loyalty to the one whom she has not abandoned, Naomi. Ruth does not forsake Naomi; she bonds to her. Naomi reluctantly receives the loyalty of Ruth after an impassioned plea of *entreatment*. And Ruth said, *"Entreat me not to leave thee, or to return from following after thee: for whither thou goest, I will go; and where thou lodgest, I will lodge: thy people shall be my people and thy God my God*[3]*"*.

Ruth takes care of and ministers to the needs of Naomi as if she were the mother of her birth. Ruth is a young widow from a foreign country who has abandoned the old life to face an uncertain destiny and possible isolation in a new land. How many pastor's spouses have set out with husbands and wives who have been called to strange lands filled with strange parishioners, who have set in place even stranger constitutions, bylaws and hidden laws not to mention the unwritten rules for pastors' spouses? It is a lonely life; abandoning the things and people you had finally come to terms with just to pull up stake and start a cycle of unfamiliarity all over again. Herein lies another face of loneliness and abandonment in ministry. It is the place where we find ourselves when we forsake our desires for the will of God in our lives. Abandoning oneself is not easy, but the call of Christ demands that we abandon all and forsake all.

In small towns most of the people know each other, go to the same churches all of their lives and rarely venture beyond more than a one hundred mile radius from home. To clearly make my point, some years ago I returned to my hometown after having moved away. Many of the people I knew had now relocated to other areas in search of a better way of life and most of all in pursuit of destiny. I had not lived in the place of my childhood in more than twenty years. Yet, I returned home to discover that the environment that had loved and nurtured me had not changed much; I had changed. My spirit, my mind, my body, my soul, my perspective on the world had all been renewed by the power of the Holy Spirit. I had become virtually unrecognizable at home. I had become the beloved stranger, at home. I was beloved due to the memories we shared of life together in a microcosm born right out of an episode of *In the Heat of the Night*. I was a stranger because of the alien nature of the call of God upon my life. I was now a preaching woman, a preacher lady, a pleasant anomaly for some, an amusement for others, and an abomination for a die-hard few. I believe that this crisis, this dilemma of loneliness in ministry becomes one of those *"go ye therefore experiences[4]"* whereby we are commissioned to abandon all, l*et the dead bury their dead[5]* and ask this question of all who seek to

84

impede the work of Christ in our lives, *"Who is my mother[6]?"* I was alone in ministry.

In that situation and in all situations, I am on theologically solid ground when I posit a resolute surety that God is in all things. He is with us when we meet that spiritual crisis of loneliness face-to-face. In times of isolation and abandonment, God is real. Though not physically visible, God is the Divine Driver: leading and guiding our lives through the deepest, most isolative times. In the darkness of loneliness, it is God who steers us directly into the center of his will. John the Baptist and his disciples, Jesus and his disciples, Paul and his followers all abandoned family, friends, professions, material possessions, the opinions of men and the ridicule of the public just to be in the center of God's will. This writer, Ruth and Naomi are guilty of this same typology of abandonment. Let us now explore the typological cycle through the life of Jesus as revealed in the words of the Apostle Paul.

The Abandonment Cycle
"...no man stood with me, all men abandoned me..." II Timothy 4:16

The Abandonment Cycle
2 Timothy 4: 16

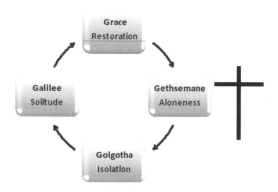

85

To abandon is to forsake or to be forsaken. Abandoned people are forsaken and forgotten people. If one has been abandoned, one has been rejected, left behind and many times left in danger at the worst possible moment. To be abandoned means to be deserted, to be given up on, or walked out on, leaving an individual without that familiar stance of support to which one has become accustomed. Forsaken people are often lonely. Abandoned people more often than not can become defeated people, if only for a season. These same people frequently may become depressed and easily discouraged. Abandoned people more often than not become angry[1], resentful and bitter people. For one to have been abandoned and to know the stings of abandonment there has to have been *a band* of people who stood with them. They trusted and relied upon them. Before the abandonment, there was *a band*, a group, a family, a church, an organization, a network, a niche of people with whom they were used to breaking bread, and quite possibly held close to their breast.

To be abandoned means that an individual has been left without protection. I would venture to say that all of us have been abandoned by someone at some point. Along other lines, we have abandoned someone somewhere at some time in our lives. How many of us as pastors and preachers, ministers and evangelists, scholars and leaders have abandoned a past that hindered us from seeking the will of God, to pursue and walk in the call of God upon our lives? Many of us are at home with wives and husbands we have not physically abandoned with "for better or for worse" covenant relationships. But we have emotionally, however unintentionally, checked out of loving families with patient spouses and confused children who suffer through a living abandonment: we are here, but we are over there. We are over there, yet we are over here, while actually we are totally devoted and committed nowhere. We are not totally at home, we are not totally with the parish or the church and we live this bifurcated existence that leaves us isolated and detached from the people who love us most-our families.

From a ministerial perspective, I have discovered that if we are going to do the will of God and survive the stings and arrows of the those who seek to render us powerless before God, we must realize that we are to always be aware of our position within cycle of abandonment stages that threaten to alienate those who support us. Congregations, deacons, trustees, budget committees and choirs abandon us when we are less obligatory, less apologetic and less self-effacing than the church powers that be think we should be.

The cycle of abandonment always begins with grace as an act of God's goodness, and grace as the ultimate gift in the person of our Lord Jesus Christ. The beautiful thing about grace is that it is freely given anywhere within the cycle. The abandonment cycle has no specific starting place other than at the place of grace; that is our point of entry. At anytime we may be afforded the opportunity to be alone with God or to experience our own personal Gethsemane whereby we go back to the garden and get in touch with the one who first loved us, called us, anointed us, equipped us, appointed us and assigned us to the awesome task of bringing Him glory through our service to His children.

The Apostle Paul, in the fourth chapter and the sixteenth verse of the book of Second Timothy (II Timothy4:16), makes it clear that at one of the lowest points in his life, in one of the times in his life when he needed someone the most and needed not to be alone, he said, *"At my first defense no one was with me to support me, but all abandoned me. May it not be counted against them. But the Lord stood with me and empowered me that through me the proclamation of the gospel might be fully accomplished and all the Gentiles might hear, and I was delivered out of the lion's mouth[7]"*.

The Apostle Paul, or resident "super-saint" makes an appearance in this chapter right out of the pages of biblical antiquity to tell us that he had been abandoned by his friends. Yet, he stands firm in his place within the abandonment cycle always, in view of the cross of Christ, to remind us that even when everyone else walked away and he stood to face his trial alone he says, "...but the Lord stood with me..."

This is the refrain of the lonely minister, the lonely pastor; that when the trustees don't trust you, the elders don't encourage you, the saints don't support you, the congregation doesn't come together anymore, the choir won't count it all joy and the money is at a minimum because folk are withholding tithes and offerings to "punish the pastor", the Apostle Paul gives us a sweet refrain, "...but, the Lord stood with me." Wherever you find yourself in the abandonment cycle, be reminded, the Lord will stand with you. Though you might be facing and fighting loneliness with your whole heart and with all of your might, remember that the Lord will stand with you.

Jesus was no stranger to loneliness. He stood and withstood the solitude of Gethsemane, the lonely isolation of Golgotha, the solitude of a post resurrection respite at the seashore of Galilee and the gift of God's Grace through it all. For the called among us, as it was with Jesus, loneliness is about missing God, missing the presence of God even when you are surrounded by people. It is about missing the very presence, the voice, the guidance and the nearness of God. Whether in Gethsemane's garden or on Golgotha's hill, Jesus was missing his Father. He was missing God because he could not feel the presence of his "Abba." In the abandonment cycle, as it was experienced by Jesus, He had spent three years repairing broken lives. Jesus was abused, mistreated, wounded, mutilated and abandoned.

I have discovered that we are all people who have answered God's call through cracked vessels. Life has wounded us. People have dropped us. The churches we pastor have not appreciated us. Our families have not understood us. The world has done its best to discredit us. And yet we are still giving it all up and laying it all down for the sake of the call of God upon our lives. I have listened to fellow parishioners preach through cracked voices and cracked vessels. I have listened with my whole heart and have put myself in the shoes of others. I have silently wrestled with my own pain, my own disappointments and shortcomings and have counted myself unworthy over and over again. I have been moved and touched by the strength and the depth of conviction my fellow parishioners have shown. And I know that only God could have brought us through the valley situations, the dry places, the hard spaces, the tough terrain and over the rough roads of life as called servants of God.

If there's one thing I've learned about Jesus it is, that even on the cross in the height of his suffering and his agony, his passion and his pain; he still found one more chance to live out his role as a servant and a healer. Even on a bloody cross, Jesus said to the thief, *"Verily I say unto thee, today shalt thou be with me in paradise."*[8] In other words, I am bringing you into a place where you never have to be lonely again. No more isolation; no more loneliness. This is the resounding hope and clarity of the words of Jesus; that immediately after this death, this painful isolative death, there he stood in the resurrection power of God the Father Almighty. There is available to all of us a supernatural super-imposition of the Holy Spirit of the Living God to aid us in enduring the loneliness of our own personal crosses. When our families don't understand us, our co-workers merely tolerate us, our children loathe us, our spouses give up on us, our friends stand back and wonder about us, our enemies gloat over us and our church members stop supporting us, the Lord will superimpose the landscape of our lives with a Galilean experience, that still begs the question, "Children, have ye any meat?"

Right on the other side of loneliness, God will give you the experience of the refreshing, cleansing, life sustaining beauty; the restorative beauty Jesus discovered at the seashore of Galilee. After Golgotha, post Calvary, Jesus made his wounds a source of healing to those for whom he suffered, bled and died. With Jesus as our example, how can we bring our wounds into the service of others without causing them undue harm or injury? With Jesus as our example, how do we minister through isolative places? With Jesus as our example, how do we minister through our own grief? We do so by realizing that we are products of every lonely place we have been, every isolative moment we have endured, every life we have touched and everything we have experienced. We realize that the places of healing within us move boundaries and parameters so that we as shepherds can feed the sheep and take care of the lambs, with care, compassion, love, understanding and forgiveness within the holy context of fellowship and a sense of the beloved community.

In Gethsemane Jesus prayed. In our own personal Gethsemanes we pray and reconnect with our Creator. Yet, I wonder if when coming out of loneliness and isolation, we recognize that our wounds, many of them, are still open. We must be careful not to cover them with the bandages of self-reliance, self-denial and loneliness. Do we as clergy bandage our wounds only to find out that when the artificial coverings were lifted, our wounded places were still open and still sensitive to the irritants of light and heat? What emotional antiseptics do we use to mask and dull the pain and give us temporary relief from the wounds that go deep beneath the surface and the epidermis of our preaching, teaching, counseling, building, capital campaigning lives?

Maybe the wounds inflicted by loneliness were never meant to heal. Maybe we preach our best sermons from wounded places. Sometimes it is the saltiness of our own tears, the saltiest of our sermons that others who find themselves abandoned will be healed and find true liberation in the call. With grace as the restoration place after the journey, we can survive the abandonment cycle because God's grace is our joy.

At the end of each cycle, I returned to the thing that was there at the beginning of my loneliness; I found grace. There in the shadow of his wing I was in pain, but I was protected by grace and accepted by grace. Grace was always seeing me through my tough times. I returned to grace not just for a moment or for a season, but for a lifetime. I found my refuge, my strength and myself in God's grace. At each stage, I found my Lord Jesus Christ, the Son of God and the personification of the gift and the act of grace.

Grace is about the rescue and the restoration of the human spirit. As I came into the grace stage of the abandonment cycle, God reassured me of a few things. It was as if He was saying, "It's alright my daughter. Because you scarched for me with all of your heart, you found me. Because you pursued me and endured hardship for me, I will restore you! I will renew you! I will revive you once again and refill you with fresh oil. I only ask of you that in this season of restoration that you rededicate yourself to me. In my restoration of your soul and even in your having been abandoned by the very people I sent you to shepherd, don't worry about it. Even as I restore you, I will rename you. They may call you crazy, but I'll just call you faithful! They may label you strange, but I will call you holy! They may call you a fanatic, but I will call you 100% sold out. They may call you a fool for Christ, but I will simply call you my friend."

Metaphorically speaking, it is through the generation of new cells that the body produces coverings (natural coverings) that begin to form over open wounds. These scabs remain in place until a new layer of skin covers the wounds underneath. Removal of the wound's natural scab too early or before it is time will cause the wound to reopen and feel as painful as when the old wound was new. Stepping into the cycle makes us recognize, examine and seal our wounds with the spiritual healing agents of faith, love, hope, joy, peace, longsuffering, patience and kindness. Therefore, even if we must be alone, we must stay connected and committed. Stay committed in service to God's people; looking ever to the Author and the Finisher of our faith, Jesus Christ, to teach us how to apply the balm of compassion for healing the vestiges and wounds in us all. Because, you see, in whatever state we find ourselves, in the final analysis, it really isn't about how others treat you, but how you treat them. My fellow puppeteers, pastors and ministers of the Gospel of Jesus Christ, that is all we are responsible for nothing more and nothing less.

---

[1] Psalm 27: 4 King James Version
[2] Romans 12:2 King James Version

[3] Ruth 1:16 King James Version
[4] Matthew 28:19 King James Version
[5] Luke 9:60 King James Version
[6] Mark 3:33 King James Version

[7] 2 Timothy 4: 16-18
[8] Luke 23:43 King James Version

How Much Is Enough Transparency?
Charles E. Booth

The issue of transparency is a precarious one, especially for those of us in ministry. Every week as we stand before the people of God we seek not only to make the Word of God incarnate, but often, without realizing it, we give conscious or unconscious clues as to who we really are. Let's face it – there is always curiosity and intrigue when it comes to the preacher. While one should always seek to be authentic, one must be cautious so as to not cross a boundary that will expose that which should remain private and personal. The preacher must prayerfully consider his or her remarks especially in this day when exposure appears to be the norm in the culture. One need only to listen to the music of our young people and the obvious becomes apparent – they think nothing of letting it "all hang out" with no thought of propriety. When considering the issue of transparency the preacher must always keep in clear focus that it is the Christ and not self who is to be lifted and emulated.

No one has better defined preaching than Phillips Brooks in his Beecher Lectures at Yale. Very succinctly put, Brooks defined preaching as "truth through personality". The essential question one must raise when considering this definition is – "How does the truth of the Gospel, which is changeless, remain so when the personality proclaiming it is always in a state of evolving and becoming?" All of us are ever developing as a personality and in that process we change. The changes we go through must in no way negate the truth of the Gospel we proclaim. We are the vessels through which the Gospel flows, and as the filter we must always be authentic, but never to the extent that we turn the truth of scripture in the direction of personal bias. Ultimately, the place of transparency and everything the preacher propagates must stand firmly on biblical ground. Transparency, like illustrations, should seek to accentuate the point being made and not be the point itself! If the transparent illustration becomes the point, then Christ has been homiletically eclipsed and this must always be avoided.

I wish to get at the issue of transparency first by using two biblical illustrations. Old Testament scholarship ascribes Psalm 51 to the authorship of David. It is undeniably a lamentation, for David writes of his estrangement from God as a result of his adulterous relationship with Bathsheba and his subsequent responsibility for the death of Uriah. David is amazingly transparent without ever mentioning the actual incidents of personal adultery and second-degree murder.

"Wash me thoroughly from my iniquity, and cleanse me from my sin. For I acknowledge my transgressions, and my sin is always before me. Against You, You only, have I sinned, and done this end in Your sight ..."   *(Psalm 51:2-4) KJV*

David conveys in this public expression the pain of his inner travail. Notice how carefully he crafts his transparency. He mentions no names. He simply languishes beneath the guilt of his own transgressions. While David exposes a personal failure, the larger issue is his recognition that he has sinned against God, feels alienated from God and pleads for God's forgiveness and reconciliation. David exposes himself without being specific and he leaves no doubt as to the point he wishes to make. David's exposed transparency leaves the reader with only one conclusion – David is pained because of a now sundered relationship with the God he so dearly loves and his sole intent is that of restoration.

All of us can identify with this psalm because of its emphasis on sin, alienation, forgiveness and reconciliation. We may not be guilty of a sexual indiscretion as David was, but we have thought, said and done things that have estranged us from God and with Israel's sweet singer we plead –
"Hide your face from my sins, and blot out all of my iniquities. Create in me a clean heart, O God, and renew a steadfast spirit within me. Do not cast me away from Your presence, and do not take Your Holy Spirit from me. Restore to me the joy of Your salvation . . ."
(Psalm 51:9-12) KJV
I recall a conversation between two ladies in the aftermath of a revival worship service in which I preached. I happened to be in a city where a pastor had been caught in a sexual indiscretion and these two Christian ladies were discussing him as they stood in line to speak to me following the worship. I was not eavesdropping on their conversation because they were speaking so loudly that one could not help but overhear their dialogue. I distinctly remember one lady declaring she would never listen to this local pastor again to which I replied when she spoke to me - "Then you should never again recite Psalm 23 for its author was also caught in a sexual indiscretion and was responsible for the woman's husband's murder."

In St. Matthew 26:38 our Lord says to his disciples – *"My soul is exceedingly sorrowful, even to death . . ."* Jesus the Christ has a transparent moment in which he reveals and unmasks how vulnerable he feels as he approaches the moment of his death. The Master does not hide his inner feelings. He is willingly

95

open in sharing his authentic feelings. He chooses to be transparent among those closest to Him during his earthly journey. However, the point Jesus seeks to make is not so much his personal sorrow, but how destiny must be fulfilled even at the expense of personal pain. It's all about what the Father has ascribed and what He as Son must accept.

The life and ministry Dr. Harry Emerson Fosdick is rich fodder as we further plough the issue of transparency. His great ministry at the Riverside Church in New York City is legendary. However, Dr. Fosdick in his mature years did not hesitate to preach and write about that dark season in his life when as a seminary student he contemplated suicide. Dr. Fosdick was involved in ministry in the Bowery section of New York as a part of his fieldwork as a seminarian. It was exceedingly difficult for him to reconcile his middle class lifestyle with the harsh realities he witnessed in the Bowery. This harsh contradiction created for him inner turmoil. When he visited his parent's home in upstate New York the stress and strain of his struggle pushed him to a suicidal moment. One morning while shaving Dr. Fosdick reported that he put the razor to his throat and at that moment his father happened to pass by the open door of the bathroom and shouted, "Harry!" It was Dr. Fosdick's father's exclamation that put a halt to that moment of deep, dark mental and emotional despair. His behavior necessitated his being confined to a mental institution in Elmira, New York and, by his own admission; he would have never written The Power of Prayer had he not sojourned through that dark season of mental and emotional anguish.

How much is enough when it comes to being transparent in the preaching moment? I have already suggested that one's transparent inclusion is not the point, but seeks only to *clarify* the point. I would suggest, secondly, that the preacher seeks to be instructive by being transparent and does not take an egotistical flight so that he or she becomes the center of attention. I would suggest a third consideration. Transparent sermonic inclusion should never be injurious, that is, such presentations should not intentionally seek to embarrass, humiliate or shame individuals.

There are three experiences in my life that are immensely personal and private. These issues had been totally off limits in the past. There was a time when I would never have considered any discussion of these in public proclamation. I never had any inclination to be that transparent. In many ways I felt embarrassed and ashamed. However, as I have matured in life and ministry, I have come to realize that when properly appropriated all three transparencies could be instructive to others who, like me, seek their footing on the slippery slopes of this uneven journey called life. The discovery I have made in my pastoral vineyard is that many have gravitated closer to me because of these existential similarities.

The first of these experiences can be traced back to my early childhood. I lost my eye as a child due to a congenital cataract. While cataract surgery is fairly common in this day and time, this was not the case in the 1950's. When the discovery of the cataract was made, my mother sought medical expertise and the concluding thought on the part of the physicians was that the total eye had to be removed. In later years when talking with ophthalmologists I was told that my eye should not have been removed and the only conclusion I have reached is that a little African-American boy, whose mother bowed to what she thought was the expertise of physicians, was taken advantage of. The surgery occurred at John Hopkins Hospital in Baltimore, Maryland – one of the premier medical institutions in the world. Across these years I have seriously entertained the notion of racism as well as perhaps being used as a research instrument. Whatever the truth one salient fact remains – I have had to live with this reality for at least fifty-five years. I was taunted, laughed at and made fun of as lad and I must confess that I still carry residues from those early years of my youth. All of us have had experiences as children when we were teased and taunted. However, for me, the psychological and emotional wounds were deep. When fitted with my first prosthesis I was called "ugly" and "cyclops".

As I look back on these years, I can truly say that the love of my mother and sister coupled with my early discovery of Jesus Christ has sustained and kept me. I shall never forget when I lectured on biblical hermeneutics in June 1999 at the Hampton Ministers Conference that I became transparent and shared this experience in my lecture-sermon entitled, "When God Deals You An Uneven Hand." The lecture-sermon was based on the parable of the talents in St. Matthew 25:14-30. While I had shared this experience *sermonically* with my congregation this was the first time I shared it on a national platform. I have been amazed and astonished over the years as to how many verbal and written responses I have received as to how helpful this sharing has been to many, who like me, have had to live with a "limp." I am reminded of a remark made by Dr. Gardner C. Taylor in his Lyman Beecher Lectures on Preaching at the Yale Divinity School in 1976. I paraphrase – "Our struggles and hurts become our passports into the lives of those to whom we preach." I have made this discovery over and over again. I am certain there are preachers who can, likewise, echo this claim.

Allow me to speak of a second experience that has found its way into my public proclamation – the absence of my biological father. I have no memorable recollection of my father in our family home. He and my mother divorced when I was a child. I am now in my forty-sixth year as a Gospel preacher and I make the sad report that my father has never heard me preach. It is not so much that I have been embarrassed by my father's absence in my life as it is the powerful impact of his absence. We take for granted the sociological truth as unveiled by Daniel Patrick Moynihan in the 1960's that the African-American family is largely matriarchal. However, for African-American males who have had to live with this reality, we know that as tremendous as a mother's love might be, there is a woeful void in the life of a boy who yearns for the guiding influence of a father. John Eldridge is quite poignant about this in his wonderful book on masculinity entitled Wild at Heart. He says, and correctly so, that every man must one day face his wound – *"Every man carries a wound. I have never met a man without one. No matter how good your life may have seemed to you, you live in a broken world full of broken people." (p.72)*

When this powerful element of my past began to creep into my preaching it became increasingly apparent to me that there are multitudes of men and boys who share my story and so many are in our congregations. This transparent unveiling has allowed me to minister to so many young men in my pastoral setting who struggle with the absence of a father. I remain grateful to the Holy Spirit whose prompting is always appropriate and timely. It is a blessing that such transparency creates a gravitational pull, of sorts, with young men who come within the orbit of my experience not only to seek counsel, but to share their story.

The third and final experience that I have come now to share in my preaching and teaching is my divorce. Even though we live in a generation where divorce is as common as reading a daily newspaper, one must admit, particularly in the life of the church, that there is still something of a stigma attached to the breakup of a marriage. When this occurred for me in 1989, I must confess that I lived and ministered for a season under a cloud of paranoia. It's one thing for laity to travel this path, but for the pastor to divorce – this is almost anathema to many within our ecclesiastical ranks. I can vividly recall walking to the pulpit on Sunday mornings with a lowered head feeling a sense of shame and humiliation. There was no scandal or public spectacle, but pain and paranoia for me nonetheless. There were a myriad of questions that crossed the horizon of my thinking – "What are the people saying?" "Have I lost the respect of my congregation?" "Will anyone want to hear me preach and teach again?" These were serious interrogations that created great stress and struggle for me. I shall never forget the Sunday morning when I garnered the courage to address the issue as an illustration in my sermon. This occurred several years later. Much to my surprise my marital counseling load increased as people saw my experience as one that identified with their marital struggles. I have, also, found it quite helpful to relate facets of my marital discoveries with those preparing to make matrimonial covenant with one another.

The issue of transparency is a marvelous tool in demythologizing the preacher. There are many who sit in the pew Sunday after Sunday and view the preacher with something of a stellar glance not realizing that the preacher is a flesh and blood creature who struggles daily with his or her own issues. It is my contention that transparent illustrations, when properly preached, can usher people into the presence of God with a freshness that has the capacity to deepen their discipleship. It must be stated that the pulpit is no place for cheap histrionics. One must never be transparent in order to draw an emotional response or demonstrate a flare for the dramatic. Both are totally unacceptable! The pain and pathos of transparency are to be used for one purpose only – to gain a clear vision of Jesus Christ so that the glean of His power and presence can navigate us through the most heinous of circumstances.

It is quite obvious that one cannot be transparent about everything. There are some experiences that remain forever locked in the sanctity of one's mind and heart. Not everyone in the pew, and for that matter the pulpit as well, can handle certain issues. One has to rely on the Holy Spirit and discern whether or not a transcript out of one's experience is relevant and useful for sharing. We must allow for the Holy Spirit to give us the green light when we seek to be transparent. The preacher must remember that the preaching event is a highly emotional and volatile moment. This is especially true in the African-American worship experience. In the height of pulpit discourse the preacher must reign in emotion and make truth paramount so that hope, help, healing and deliverance will come to those who hunger and thirst for the abundant life. Never allow the horse of transparency to get out of the corral before its time. Always seek to be instructive and not injurious. Every wise preacher knows that there are certain utterances that can only come forth after one, under the aegis of the Holy Spirit, has intentionally dealt with an issue so that its presentation is meticulously thought out and fastidiously delivered.

How much is enough transparency? This is ultimately a question settled by the preacher in consultation with the Holy Spirit.

"But when he, the Spirit of truth, comes, he will guide you into all truth!" (St. John 16:13)

DOING CHURCH:
building the foundation

The Challenge of Freedom in the Pulpit?
Carolyn Ann Knight

Several years ago now, while teaching an *Introduction to Preaching* class, I had an epiphany of sorts. I noticed one, that my students were getting younger and younger and two, they were becoming more informal, not disrespectful, not irreverent just more informal in their sermonic presentations. Needless to say, this was most noticeable in their dress. On the days that they stood before the class to preach they wore earrings, tattoos, jeans, sneakers, statement t-shirts and so on. These young people certainly would have had problems with my homiletics professor, Dr. John D. Mangram at Bishop College in Dallas,

Texas who required that we "dress up" on preaching days. Oddly enough this dress code change did not send me into a nervous convulsion. I was not trying to demonstrate that I was just as cool as the next person or anything like that. I guess I have always believed that what the preacher is or is not wearing should have no bearing on ones ability to hear a good sermon. But in addition to this relaxing of the dress code on preaching days, there was another shift taking place, one I could ill afford to ignore.

Not only was the dress of these young people becoming less formal than preachers of a few decades ago, but more and more the language that they used to shape and deliver their sermons was becoming more and more informal as well. This new generation of preachers was comfortable using language in the pulpit that was a part of everyday discourse. Not only that, they were also designing their sermons in ways that had greater appeal to persons beyond the church walls. Whereas, I could overlook in most cases informal or casual dress, as it is now widely called, I could not ignore the change that was taking place within the sermon.

This article will attempt to define, describe, and discuss what we mean by "Freedom in the Pulpit." I will attempt to discuss what freedom in the pulpit is and whether or not there is such a thing as too much freedom in the pulpit. I am honored to have been asked to reflect on this subject in writing after having participated in the 2008 Joshua Conference sponsored by the St. James AME Church in Newark, New Jersey. I do so from the vantage point of over thirty years in the preaching ministry and sixteen years of teaching homiletics in both European and African American seminaries. Further, I do so from a lifetime commitment of studying the art and the science of preaching. Having said this, I do not consider myself an expert on the subject of preaching, just a student of this high and holy work. Further, I do not claim to be writing anything new or original about preaching. I am however stating what I have found to be helpful in our work of preparing and preaching sermons. I make no apologies for the fact that I love the preaching enterprise and am grateful everyday to be a preacher. This is in no way to minimize all of the other ministries of the church; it just affirms that God chose "the foolishness of preaching" to save and transform the world.

Preaching is the port of entry that engages and involves the rural, local, community, and the mega-church and their members in active participation in the world. The preaching ministry of the church equips the saints for the work of ministry. I know that as the mega-church ministry has mushroomed in the mind and mentality of the members there has been a *dumbing down* of the sermon and the preaching ministry. But this is not to be encouraged.

Early on in my ministry I decided I would make preaching a priority. This decision was easy because of the fact that I was exposed to gifted preachers as a young child who valued the text and the context in their preaching. I was four or five years old when I first heard the narrative preaching of Dr. John T. Walker, pastor of the Union Baptist Church in Denver, Colorado. He baptized me at the age of eight and until he died when I was fifteen, I sat on the first pew of the church captivated by the way he told the biblical story. I was eight years old when M. C. Williams of the New Hope Baptist Church came into my life. Ernest Lewis of the Pilgrim Rest Church was perhaps the most gifted orator of my childhood days. I was devastated by his tragic and sudden death while I was in Junior High. At sixteen, I heard Frederick G. Sampson of Detroit, Michigan quote Shakespeare in a sermon and it absolutely changed everything for me regarding preaching.

Fortunately, I was influenced by the voices of women as well... one who was not a preacher. When I first heard Barbara Jordan, I was convinced that there was a place for my voice that for some reason had become deeper than most of my girlfriends at that time. Prathia Hall Wynn was the preacher that impressed upon me the importance of an informed head and an inspired heart. I mention these preachers here because they were gifted pulpiteers, but also because they were masters in the use of sermonic language. There was a loftiness and seriousness to the language that they used when they preached that impressed upon me the distinction between pulpit speech and regular speech. Having now said this, I hope I have not revealed too early on in this article any personal bias. I am concerned about preaching in the 21st century. I am concerned about the shape and direction of preaching being done in some churches and some places today. In the following pages I will detail why I believe too much freedom in the pulpit is dangerous and damages pulpit discourse. Again I do not presume that everyone will agree with what I have to say here. That is not my concern. I want to simply weigh in on the conversation about this subject. For that reason, I am grateful for the opportunity to express my views on this subject. I am always interested in writing about preaching.

Webster's New World College Dictionary defines freedom in the broadest sense as the "absence of hindrance, restraint, confinement or repression, as in freedom of speech."[1] Dictionary.com defines freedom as the "power to determine action without restraint."[2] Given these definitions for the purpose of this article I want to define freedom in the pulpit as the ability to create and deliver a sermon using language and action that is free of traditional understandings of pulpit discourse. In my own thinking, I do not believe that it is ever appropriate to suspend the rules of proper sermon preparation. Like every discipline, preaching has rules and guidelines that lend themselves to proper sermonic presentation. Just as there are limits to what we mean by freedom of speech (you cannot yell fire in a crowded theatre if there is no fire), there are likewise limits to freedom in the pulpit. Whatever a preacher's exegetical, hermeneutical, and homiletic approach to preaching, I strongly believe that it should be adhered to at all times. Freedom in the pulpit then for the purposes of this article has to do with a preacher's method of delivery.

---

[1] Webster's New World College Dictionary, Fourth Edition.
Webster's New World, Cleveland, Ohio 2000.

[2] Internet Source.

Historically, the African American preacher has always had a unique understanding of freedom in the pulpit. Because of our history in this nation of slavery, segregation, and second-class citizenship, the pulpit in the church has always been considered free space and the preacher was considered the person in the community with the most freedom. Because of the perilous predicament of the African American in America, the pulpit and the sermon became the major method of communication with a marginalized people. Because the pulpit was considered "free" the preacher was often considered the most independent person in the African American community. "The proclamation of the Black pulpit survives likewise because, in its isolation from the mainstream, it spoke and it speaks peculiarly to the needs of blacks."[3] The preacher could say things from the pulpit that no other professional of that era could say. Therefore, the pulpit became more than just a place where the gospel and cute bible stories could be heard. The pulpit became an agent for social change in the church and in the community. The preacher in the African American pulpit was always free to say what needed to be said when it needed saying.

Further, the Sunday morning service was the place where the preacher not only inspired but also informed and ignited the church members when and if necessary. Coming to church on Sunday was and is much more than a worship service. It is a communal gathering of persons from all walks of life. For that reason, announcements are made about what events and activities are going on in the community and when they are taking place. From the pulpits of the African American church, rallies were planned, voters were registered, marches organized, and monies were raised. From the pulpit, listeners were sent out with their marching orders for conduct and decorum on the job and around "the man." From the pulpits, the African American listeners learned what was "going down" and when. Since the pulpit was in the church and the Bible was interspersed with these instructions, the listeners were unable to make a noticeable distinction between the preacher's word and God's word. For

---

[3] Henry H. Mitchell, Black Preaching: *The recovery of a Powerful Art.* Nashville: Abingdon Press, 1990, 23.

the most part they were one. The preacher used the Bible to convince the listener that this is what God would have them to do and how God would have them to behave in the world. This was so different than what they had heard just a few years ago in slavery. In this regard preachers talked about political campaigns, picnics, and sporting events. Young persons were brought into the pulpit and celebrated and/or disciplined as the situation warranted. All of this took place in the "free" space of the pulpit.

But as the saying goes, that was then, this is now. In almost every generation those who study the progression of preaching have always made grand and sweeping claims regarding the state or condition of the preaching ministry. The majority of those persons would argue that preaching is in crisis. In 1928, in a lengthy article, written for Harper's Magazine, Harry Emerson Fosdick one of the foremost preachers of his or any generation and Senior Pastor of the historic Riverside Church in New York City raised the question: "What's the Matter with Preaching?" Using Fosdick's article as a point of reflection that question has been raised again in our time in a book entitled: "What's the Matter with Preaching Today?" I personally believe that people are quite capable of making their own determination about the state of the preaching ministry. Certainly the persons who listen to sermons from the pew and on other venues do. However, for the purposes of this article I want not so much to address the issue as to the health of preaching, suffice it to say that I believe that preaching is not as bad as it could be nor is it as good as it should be. There is always room for improvement. There is always work to be done. Thanks be to God. Preaching is God's business. Preaching matters to God and it should matter to those of us who are engaged in the business of preaching.

There is no question that there has been a tremendous shift in the way that preaching has been done over the last twenty or thirty years. But there has also been a tremendous change in the way preaching is heard. Just as preachers do not preach the way they used to, people do not listen the way they used to. We live and preach in a sound bite, media looped, reality-TV world. As we move forward into this third millennium, we have witnessed a tremendous shift in the way preachers approach the preaching moment and the way that we do church. But to say this does not go far enough.

There is also a tremendous shift in the way that persons listen to, hear, and respond to sermons. Attempts to compare preaching in this generation to preaching in other generations can only go so far because of the cultural climate in which we now find ourselves. John Wesley, Charles Surgeon, and Jarena Lee did not preach under the circumstances of our day. All of these preachers preached before the birth of the technological and media explosion in which we now live. No telephone, television or Internet. No blackberry, iPod or PDA . No automobiles or airplanes. Even Martin Luther King Jr., Richard Allen, and Pauli Murray did not preach with the 24/7 bombardment of noise that saturates our day. These preachers spoke to audiences that were captivated by the spoken word. These preachers preached in era when words mattered and had the ability to move people.

We live in a world full of noise. From the moment we wake up in the morning and all throughout the day; we are inundated with voices that attempt to shape us spiritually, emotionally, and psychologically. Consciously or unconsciously, voices move across our visual, oral, and aural landscape and leave an imprint upon our psyche. Where is the voice of the preacher? How is the preacher to be heard in the world today? How is the preacher to be relevant in a world of competing communications genres? How is the preacher to be heard in the midst of this cacophony of voices? The preaching ministry must situate itself not in the midst of other genres of communication, but the sermon must find a way to rise above all other genres of communication. To be relevant in the 21st century, we will have to preach Christ in a more relational way. We must help the listener understand how the ancient world of the bible intersects with the life of the listener and contemporary experience.

Many years ago I read the statement, "Wherever there is a strong pulpit, there is a strong society." Even though the name of the person who made that statement has escaped my memory, it still impacts the very high view that I hold of preaching. I am greatly encouraged by the revival of biblical preaching that is sweeping this country. We are encouraged by return of persons to houses of worship in this land. They are returning to houses of worship and synagogues expecting to hear something, a word from the rabbi, priest or minister that will speak specifically and concretely to their circumstances. They want to know what God is doing in their world and how they should respond. There is a greater need now and in the future for men and women who preach to deliver relevant sermons from their pulpits. In addition to providing a way of salvation, wholeness, and a personal relationship with Jesus Christ, the sermon must hold some social significance if it is to be relevant to the listener.

Preaching is essentially a redemptive activity. In the very act of preaching, God encounters, probes, and challenges the human spirit. Preaching is one of God's methods of saving the world. But preaching is also a transformative activity. God uses preaching as an avenue through which lives, and thereby the world, can be changed for the better. Preaching is also a theological act. In this way, preaching is an activity that involves God in the day-to-day affairs of humanity. All of this is to say, that preaching is an activity that links the divine to the human and Christianity to the concrete. Karl Barth, that great theologian of the twentieth century, is often quoted as saying that "every preacher should prepare their sermons with the bible in one hand and the newspaper in the other." I am sure that if Professor Barth were alive in this high-tech environment in which we now find ourselves, he would suggest that Cable News Network (CNN) and Headline News and other means of communication be included in every preacher's study. This suggestion would not be hard to receive because we live in an age where the rapidly changing scenario of our nation and the world make it necessary for the preacher to have almost instantaneous information at his or her disposal.

The preacher, like everyone else, is bombarded with breaking news and ongoing updates of current events that are happening in other parts of the world. As preachers sit in their study, awaiting a visitation from the Holy Spirit, the world changes right before their very eyes. On any given day, issues of global war, home foreclosures, government bailouts, homelessness, domestic and sexual violence, child abuse, homophobia, women's rights, HIV/AIDS, and racism flash across our television screens. The way these events are brought on an hourly basis into our studies make them impossible to ignore, as we prepare for Sunday's sermon. Our preaching can only make sense as the listener/audience comes to understand and know about God's involvement and investment in light of their existential reality. Is God concerned about poverty, global warming, and the environment and gang violence? Persons in the pew want to know. It is one thing for people to hear sermons that address grand themes of faith, hope, and love. It is quite a different story to hear those same themes addressed in light of an HIV/AIDS pandemic and the backdrop of racism, sexism, and an economic recession. What is God saying about the issues that face a people living in such tumultuous times? How is the preacher to give an impartial, objective exegesis of biblical texts that will help the listeners understand God's action in their world?

We preach in a 9/11, Katrina, Enron war-torn world. Ours has been called the post age. That is, we are a postmodern, post-denominational, post-gender, post-racial age. Where then is the place of the sermon? Further how is the preacher to address an audience that must daily negotiate the vagaries of the human landscape? What is most important in all of our preaching is to convince the audience/listener that God is not only concerned about them in the "sweet bye and bye" but that God is also concerned and involved in their affairs right now. This element is critical for preaching because it announces God's action and demonstrates God's involvement in the world. The sermons that have the greatest and lasting impact are those sermons that are deeply biblical. To make sense of this world through the sermon, calls for a constructive engagement of the realities of this life between the biblical text and the contemporary context. In this regard, the preacher in a postmodern context must be willing to move beyond the "three points and a poem, the hoop and the holler type of sermon methodologies. What is needed and required are thorough exegesis, research, and creative delivery to communicate God's involvement in this world.

All preaching begins with God. When we preach we attempt to put into words that which must be accepted in faith. In this regard, the preacher has the awesome assignment of making clear and relevant an ancient story that must be lived out in a contemporary context. Preaching is God's word to us not our words about God. The preacher's exercise of freedom in the pulpit can never overshadow the need of the audience/listener to hear the biblical text with accuracy and clarity. Our challenge then is to make our preaching attractive enough to the listener to override the innate resistance to the sermon in the first place. This involves the work of creative imagination on the part of the preacher. Freedom in the pulpit is about the preacher's ability to design, develop, and deliver a sermon in such a fashion that it intersects with the life of the listener and the world of contemporary ideas. It is an exercise of creativity and imagination. This is what we mean by freedom in the pulpit.

Every sermon, regardless of subject matter involved, requires thorough exegesis, adequate preparation, and much prayer. Simply put, sermon preparation is hard work. The use of creativity and imagination is a part of the preparation process. The Bible is the primary tool of the Christian church and of preaching. The Bible is a collection of books that we turn to again and again to discern God's action in the world, and our response to all God has done in the life, death, and resurrection of Jesus Christ. But the Bible is also a book of particularity in that it was written in a particular time and place, for a particular people, living in a particular culture. This has been and is the most critical task and challenge of the contemporary Christian church—to understand and interpret those ancient texts in light of their present reality. How the preacher links ancient Biblical texts with the contemporary context is the most important task of creativity and imagination. An accurate understanding and interpretation of the Biblical text reveals God's will for the community of faith.

An inaccurate understanding and interpretation raises more questions than it answers and confuses rather than enlightens. The preacher's use of imagination can never conflict with an accurate interpretation of the Biblical text. One of the problems with the preacher's freedom and use of imagination is that the preacher usually already knows what he or she wants to talk about before finding an appropriate Biblical text. Many times the preacher will already have the sermon roughly outlined in his or her head then begin searching the Bible for a text that will fit the subject of the sermon. As long as there is consistency between the text and the sermonic idea, the preacher is on solid homiletic ground. But when there are inconsistencies between text and sermonic idea, the Biblical text must always supersede any creative ideas that the preacher has for the sermon. For this reason, the preacher must rely on careful exegesis of whatever passage is selected for the sermon. If after reading the passage, doing an exegetical outline and arriving at an exegetical idea, if the scripture passage selected is not suited for what the preacher has in mind for preaching, either the scripture or the idea must be abandoned and the entire process must begin again.

Preaching does not take place in a vacuum. The preacher is not coming to the Biblical texts as one who is preaching this text for the very first time. The truth of the matter is that all of the texts in the Bible have been preached many times before. In this way, the preacher is not plowing fresh ground or turning new soil. Someone has been this way before. Knowing this should eliminate the preacher's sitting before Biblical texts trying to invent an original thought. There are none. It is not necessary that the preacher be original, it is important that the preacher be fresh and relevant to their specific preaching context. The preacher who is committed to the use of creative imagination or freedom in the pulpit will make proper use of the Biblical texts by doing thorough exegesis and homiletic work.

Another consideration of the preacher's freedom is the preaching context. The preacher can only be as free as the context in which the sermon will be preached will allow. Freedom in the pulpit requires that the preacher be sensitive to the language of the culture. Biblical texts are difficult enough to understand. There are words in scripture that we do not use in everyday discourse. On any given Sunday, these words must be translated for the listener/audience. Further, when you consider the educational, economic, political, and generational composition of the average congregation, there is the possibility of another language or communication barrier. The preacher must be aware of the conversations that are taking placing in the "marketplace of ideas." He or she must be attuned to the discourse of diverse people who are influencing the attitudes of the culture.

How is the preacher then to be heard amidst the many diverse conversations that are transported over a variety of media and communication vehicles? Fortunately, the preacher can make use of these same vehicles of communication. We have already seen the impact of television, cyberspace, and digital sound devices on the preaching enterprise. The preacher is certainly free to employ all of these venues in preaching, but we must be aware of the dangers that are inherent in doing so. Truthfully, it could be argued that the preacher and the church must make use of these mediums in order to be relevant in this age. The case could and is to be made that these venues are forms of evangelism and are assisting the church in carrying out a modern-day interpretation of what Jesus Christ meant when he told His disciples to "go into all of the world and preach the Gospel." How is this to be done in a global world that can be reached with the simple click of a mouse? All one has to do is log on to their computer and within seconds one is connected to any number of religious networks that allow for the carrying out of the Great Commission. Certainly Facebook and MySpace and other social networking sites are being modified to accommodate the need to have access to potential disciples and devotees 24/7. What does this mean for the sermon? How is the sermon to be designed and delivered in such a way that it will appeal to this emerging audience?

114

One could argue that the Christian preacher should be concerned with the place of the sermon in this communication-saturated age in which we live. We preach in interesting times. Our sermons are heard alongside a plethora of talk shows and other television talking heads. I am often intrigued when I turn on TBN and other religious programming and listen to popular preachers mimicking the talk-show format. A live band warms the audience up before the show begins, special guests are invited to talk about specific issues while seated on a couch or behind a desk, and then there is the appeal and attraction of a special musical guest. The use and the popularity of this format make it clear that we in the church believe this is a road we need to go down. When preachers are invited to actually preach in these formats, the ones who have the most appeal are the ones that can keep the audience on their feet and the viewers calling in. Certainly, this is not your parents' type of preaching. The whole preaching moment must be designed in such a way as to give the preacher the freedom of movement and speech that will keep this "congregation" engaged for eyes and ears. The danger here is the Biblical text is often overshadowed by the need of the preacher to appeal to this particular audience.

Why should the preacher be concerned that persons in our time would prefer to watch music videos or MTV all day, but can only endure a sermon for twenty minutes once or twice a week? Why should preachers be concerned about the role of the sermon in the midst of a new brand of "preacher" that sits behind a judicial bench in a black robe on television preaching, counseling, and mediating between opposing parties while the cameras roll and the "congregation" applauds? Why should the preacher be concerned that he or she now preaches to an entire generation that defines themselves from clothing to music to culture to worldview and spirituality as a Hip Hop nation?

I want to suggest that our concerns should be many and varied because all of these matters have to do with freedom in the pulpit. To ignore these shifts in the times and culture in which we live is simply to risk preaching in a way that cannot and will not be heard. How then can the preacher preach relevant, liberating and transformative sermons without violating exegetical and homiletic protocol? How can the preacher be true to the Biblical text and the contemporary context? How can the preacher preach with authenticity and attractiveness without *"dumbing-down"* the sermon? This is the challenge of sound Biblical preaching and freedom in the pulpit. The challenge of the preacher is to negotiate a delicate balance between the need to be relevant, creative, and authentic during the preaching moment.

The modern-day church attendee faces many challenges just by entering the sanctuary of the church. First, many of them have little or no knowledge of the Biblical text. Although the Bible is the best selling book of all time, it is not the most read book of all time. Further, we know that people who carry the Bible, do not often read the Bible. Even those that do read it read only the "good parts." The most seasoned church member is not always that familiar with the world of the Bible.

For many persons in attendance on Sunday morning or Saturday night, the first encounter that they have with the text is when they are instructed by someone to "turn in your Bibles to...." I do not want to seem overly critical here, we all know that there are persons in the pews and throughout our congregations that are better students of the Bible and theology than most seminary graduates and pastors. We thank God for that. But we also know that these persons are the exception not the norm. For this reason, the preacher must be careful how he or she uses the Bible in the preaching moment. The Bible must be engaged in the preaching event to demonstrate that God is actively involved in the affairs of humankind. That God was very active in the ancient world of the Bible and that God is very involved in our contemporary context is the point of all preaching. Its purpose is to prove that the God who spoke and acted in the Bible is acting and speaking to this present generation. The Bible should always be used in preaching to point to a God who is involved in a very personal way in our lives and our affairs. Preaching should use the Bible to point the world of the ancient culture to the contemporary world.

In every age where preaching has been taken seriously, good preachers have realized that they have had to be sensitive to the cultural winds and ecclesiastical trends that are taking place and preach in ways that persons who are being impacted by these trends cannot only hear the sermons, but also appreciate the intersection of the sermon with the world of ideas and contemporary experience. In other words, sermons have to make sense in the world where people live or they make no sense at all. This is what brings most people to church. They want to know what God has to say to me, and my situation. What does God have to say about the real issues that I am dealing with? The persons in our pews today are reluctant to suspend the drama of their lives while the preacher takes them on a journey of Biblical archaeology or ancient Biblical languages. The listener today, for good or ill is attracted to the preacher that uses the Bible to address the real issues that confront their chaotic and confused circumstance. Persons who make their way to church gather in retreat and solace; retreat from the harsh realities of this life and solace that at some point in the worship service, something will be said that will get them through the week, on their jobs in the classrooms and at home. What does the Bible say about my finances, divorce, sex without marriage, and playing the lottery? The listener expects that the preacher will creatively connect this Biblical text their real world. But the preacher has the greater responsibility of addressing these issues while focusing on the grand Biblical themes of salvation, love, hope, redemption, grace, and mercy. Further, the preacher must do all of this in a way that will move the listener to behave in a more responsible way as a result of hearing the sermon.

There were times when preachers felt the need in their preaching, to be pastoral and priestly, preaching sermons in a more therapeutic way. The sermon was used to diagnose the needs of the listener and then use the Biblical texts as a prescriptive remedy for their condition or circumstance. At other times, preachers felt the need to speak to the issues of their day.

In this way, preachers used the sermon as a prophetic sword to challenge individuals, nations, and leaders to "do justly, love mercy, and to walk humbly with their God"(Micah 6:8). More importantly, the preacher is challenged in every era to remind those who hear them preach as well as ourselves that the church is not a hospital for the sick, it is a clinic. The difference between a hospital and a clinic is the length of stay.

Our task, our assignment as preachers, is to preach in such a way that persons get spiritually, emotionally, mentally, psychologically, and financially healthy as quickly as possible and return them to the larger mission of being the church in the world. Among the problems with many of the sermons we hear today is that they focus too much on the individual and not enough on the larger mission of the church in the world. Our greater responsibility is moving the people of God towards the kingdom of God, which is already and not yet. The church and the preacher must never lose sight of its most important vision of bringing the Kingdom of God here on earth. This is the primary task of all preaching.

In any age preaching is a complicated task and a risky undertaking. We live in an era where the Gospel as we know it is being rejected by persons inside and outside of the church. Until the Gospel intersects with the real life situation of the listener, persons simply tune the preacher out. But this is not new to this generation of church attendee, this has always been the case. However, preaching in our age is an extremely complicated task. Again, ours is an age saturated with words. In previous generations, there were periods of the day when individuals could have long moments of silence, reflection, and meditation. This is no longer the case. For this, we have only ourselves to blame. I will use myself as the illustration for the point that I am making here. On most mornings when I leave my house, this is what I have in my possession: the latest in cell phone technology, my blackberry, my iPhone, and my Bluetooth. In addition to this, all of these devices are synced with two laptop computers in my home. In the automobile I drive, there is a premium sound system. I live alone but I have four TV's and three CD players. We are surrounded by words. Need I mention that I daily attempt to read the New York Times, the Atlanta Journal Constitution, USA Today, and the Wall Street Journal, all online editions.

We live and preach in these times. Thomas G. Long and Edward Farley writing in the Foreword of *A Captive Voice*, a book of essays honoring Dr. David A. Buttrick, a former professor of homiletics at Vanderbilt University in Nashville, TN believes that the preacher in the 21st century must be willing to preach beyond the walls of the church:

"Once more we will have to turn and converse with the secular world. Once more we will have to preach the gospel beyond church walls. Sermons will be more evangelical and, above all, more apologetic. For fifty years…there has been some tendency to regard the secular world 'out there' as the enemy of biblical faith…if nothing else, the adversary position lacks courtesy. Once more we must learn to converse with the mind of our age and we must do so with genuine love and respect."[1]

Buttrick says that the focus of preaching must always be on the negotiation of the Biblical text and the contemporary situation: "The focus must be on helping preaching to move from the biblical text to the contemporary situation, and on recasting theology in the present."[2]

Preaching that is relevant, transforming, and empowering in the 21st century must link the ancient world of the Bible with the contemporary context with the goal of practical application for the life of the listener. While there have been radical shifts in the way preaching is being done in our day, we need not panic. There will always be a place for sound Biblical preaching. Preaching is God's way. It is God's chosen methodology for the salvation, liberation, and transformation of individuals and

---

[1] Preaching as a Theological Task: World, Gospel, Scripture; In Honor of David A. Buttrick. Thomas G. Long and Edward Farley, editors. Westminster/John Knox Press, 1996. From the Foreword.
[2] Ibid., 137.

institutions: *"For since, in the wisdom of God the world did not know God through wisdom, God decided through the foolishness of our proclamation to save those who believe" (1 Cor. 1:21 NRSV).* So until Jesus Christ returns for the church there will always be a need for preachers and preaching. And the good news is there is a place for freedom in the pulpit. That is, there will always be a need for the Biblical preacher to make use of creation and imagination to make biblical stories come alive in the hearts and heads of the listener. Whenever the preacher exercises freedom as a means to make the sermon clear, relevant, and practical, there is room for the imagination to have its way. As long the preacher understands the difference between freedom and recklessness, between words that transform and words that merely shock, then the preacher can speak without hindrance, constriction or restraint. It is never permissible to be insulting or offensive in the preaching moment. It is never necessary to be vulgar or obscene to make a point in preaching.

The technological inventions and advances of this day are available to those of us who preach to fulfill the Biblical mandate to *take the gospel into all the world.* We need not avoid or divorce these venues from our preaching. The arrival of the twenty-first century was a moment of swift and sweeping change; we find ourselves living in interesting times. Church and how we do church is changing and will continue to change. The church must meet the demands of change.

The churches that maintain a hard dogmatic line of doing church will see a dwindling of their memberships and offerings. There is a whole generation of young adults who have never known a world without computers, iPhones, and MP3s. They are at home in the world of Youtube, Streaming Faith, and the Word Network. The twenty-first century, the third millennium, has thrust us catastrophically into a different and often frightening new world of mystery and wonder, chaos and confusion. We can never lose sight of the world in which we now preach, a 9/11, Enron, Katrina, Virginia Tech, and economically depressed world. But, we also live in a world that elects an African American to the highest office in the land. These are occasions that demonstrate God's mercy and grace. It is that grace and mercy that we are called to preach. Our preaching cannot fail to witness to this New World Order and God's involvement in it. The preaching and theological wisdom of fifty years ago is no longer sure; the language that we speak is changing. This language has invaded the church and the pulpit. But the Church's evangelical and prophetic mandate is still compelling, the Gospel must always be preached. It is our task to discover how.

Preaching is an exercise of power. God calls the preacher to be faithful to the task of preaching and the congregation calls the preacher to be faithful to the task of exegesis, hermeneutics, and homiletic presentation. To this end, the preacher is free to express and experience the authority that comes from being twice called to the preaching ministry. But there are limits. The goal of preaching is not to focus on the words of the preacher. Whenever the people focus too much on anything the preacher does and the manner in which something is said, that is a problem for preaching. Preaching should always point persons to the new life and relationship Jesus Christ is inviting them to enjoy. The freedom, the license that we take in the pulpit, is only to serve as an instrument for getting this done.

As a practitioner and theoretician of the art and science of preaching, I believe these are exciting times to be a preacher. Ours can indeed be a Golden Era in the history of preaching. There is good news for those of us who preach in these times: preaching and the church are on the minds of the people. God is out of the proverbial closet and even Jesus Christ is back in vogue. Persons inside and outside of the church are no longer ashamed to mention the name of Jesus Christ in public places. The dynamic and rapid growth of the mega-church and televangelism is evidence that there is a renewed interest in matters of religion and faith. Popular preachers fill up football arenas and basketball coliseums with the same frequency as today's chart topping performing musical artists. Some have suggested that we live in the day of the homiletic hero and the sermonic superstar. Today, thanks to television and the Internet, the popularity and also the scrutiny of the preacher and the pulpit

121

is greater than it has ever been. In this postmodern, high-tech, digitized information age in which we now find ourselves, the church is keeping pace with all other genres of communication in its efforts to get the message of the Gospel heard. Everywhere and through everything the voice of the preacher can be seen and heard. This is the future if preaching is the twenty-first century.

Freedom in the Pulpit then, means being responsible when engaging the Biblical text and creative and imaginative in presenting the Biblical text to a contemporary context. It means allowing the sermon to dictate what are the proper movements, language, and gestures to incorporate in sermonic delivery. Freedom in the pulpit means to be sensitive to the community, the culture and the context. Understanding that the preacher can only be as free as the context will allow. Remembering that to preach is to take a risk. Freedom in the pulpit is taking a risk, to be sure. But ultimately it is not the credibility or the integrity of the preacher that is at stake, it is God's message. It is God's action. It is God who has spoken into existence the possibility of a better world and a better future for all of humankind. Therefore, it is always God's word and credibility that is on the line. But it is through the preacher that the integrity and credibility of God is manifested. The preacher's use of imagination, the preacher's need to be free in the pulpit must always be tempered with the need of the people to see God moving in the sermon and working in their lives. The preacher who understands that this is what freedom in the pulpit really means will enable those who hear them preach to come to a mature understanding of God in the world and a relationship with Jesus Christ that will empower them to live with hope and assurance as they move forward into their future.

NOT SAUL, NOT ABSOLOM, BUT DAVID
Fostering a Productive Senior
Pastor/Executive Minister Relationship
Lee Washington

The Senior Pastors Perspective...

Introduction
Leadership and administrative skills are critical for the pastor to manage even the smallest congregation. Traditionally, administrators, both laypersons and professional, have assisted pastors in leading and managing the financial, facility, and related administrative functions in many churches.

The growth of a church usually includes an increase in giving, members, staff, and volunteer ministers. With this growth, the role of the pastor becomes more complex in order to meet not only the spiritual needs of the congregation but also the strategic, operational, and personnel functions

Pastors are called upon regularly to preach, visit, counsel, console, and provide spiritual leadership. Pastors are also expected to set the vision for the church, develop the strategy, communicate clearly the purpose and direction of the local congregation, manage and lead change, build and maintain the team of lay leaders, and shepherd people in the church including the ministry staff. The pastor is called on to accomplish this while balancing his/her spiritual relationship with God and maintaining healthy relationships with the family.

The expectation of success in each of these areas by the pastor, the congregation, or his family is unrealistic for most ministers. In managing the challenge of balancing both the managing and shepherding of the church, a new position entitled "executive minister" is evolving.

When a church moves from one staff member to two or three, there are obvious significant changes in the way the church is administered. However, such changes are usually not the changes that are at the point where a church has a staff of seven or eight or more full time program people and several part time staff members. At this point the coordination, supervision, and management of the staff so that all are contributing toward the larger goal, pulling in the same direction, doing their share of the work, having access to their share of the resources, experiencing a sense of being cared for and important, and given the opportunity to use their gifts in the most effective manner, becomes a very large and necessary task.

SENIOR PASTOR READINESS
At the point in the life of the congregation when it is both evident and advisable to add an Executive Minster, the Senior Pastor must be ready for it. The Senior Pastor must be aware of her/his own sense of being overwhelmed and needing help. I call this "Senior Pastor readiness." If the senior pastor is

reluctant to show public support for the need and addition of the Executive Minister position or demonstrates a spirit of half-heartedness when working with the Executive Minister, the results will be less then beneficial.

The Senior Pastors who have large denominational responsibilities or who have a national reputation and sizeable ministry through conferences or outside speaking engagements will come to recognize more quickly their need for an Executive Minister because of the necessity of having someone to be in charge during their frequent absences from their local office. The spread of this administrative arrangement has been promoted by contacts between Senior Pastors in formal and informal networks.

FUNCTIONAL CLARITY

The Executive Minister position is a new phenomenon in many churches of varying sizes across the United States. The function is a pastoral role that is focused primarily on the development and maintenance of the staff and the church organization. Some may consider the Executive Minister position to be the church administrator, while others may understand the position to be an extension of the role of the minister of education. One may conclude that this position is similar to the chief operating officer (COO) in for-profit or not-for-profit organizations. Bringing clarity and understanding to the necessary leadership and management practices common to Executive Ministers lays the groundwork for developing the next generation of Executive Ministers and supporting those currently in place.

One misconception is using the Executive Minister and Church Administrator titles interchangeably. A church business administrator may be defined as one who manages the finances, data processing, personnel, physical plant, strategic planning, and church protocol. The basic skills needed for church business administrators include administrative, personnel management, a commitment for professional development, and growth in one's faith. The administrative skills include knowledge of fund accounting and budgeting, governmental reporting, planning, and data processing.

An Executive Minister has a similar function but a different focus. Executive Ministers are men and women who oversee the ministries of the church, but report to someone. The Executive Minister usually reports to the Senior Pastor as his only direct report. While leadership and management take place in this function, the administrator has a more procedural and legal focus with some attention to strategy. The Executive Minister focuses more on strategy implementation and overall staff leadership and coordination. The Executive Minister is actually in more of a team role regarding strategy.

EXECUTIVE MINISTER QUALITIES
It would be possible to list the qualities that such a person would need as Executive Minister in much the same way one would describe the appropriate qualities for any leader or any pastor. I have listed a few of the qualities I looked for in the establishment of the Executive Minister position where I pastor.

Loyalty: The first set of qualities that need to be considered in the relationship between the Senior Pastor and Executive Minister is loyalty. I listed this first because more than any other of the qualities, loyalty will determine whether or not the association between the two will have a chance to work. The leadership of the Senior Pastor must be recognized, supported, and implemented. One way of picturing this quality is to say the Executive Minister needs a John the Baptist attitude. His posture towards the Senior Pastor should be, "He must increase, and I must decrease." The latter part "I must decrease," is primarily applicable to public leadership. Executive Ministers use phrases such as "behind the scenes" or "low profile."

Confidentiality: This is a vital quality. It is imperative that the Executive Minister deal with knowledge shared by the Senior Pastor in the strictest confidence. It is a courtesy that should be reciprocated toward the Executive Minister by the Senior Pastor. This principle is necessarily suspended when dealing with immoral or unethical behavior. One of the tasks of the Executive

Minister is interpreting the Senior Pastor to the rest of the staff. That interpretation ought to be done in a way that will enhance the standing and stature of the Senior Pastor to the degree which honesty and integrity prevails.

Shared Philosophy: Some would put the theological argument before the shared philosophy. However, it is possible for both to work together having some theological differences but not if there are differences in the way ministry should be approached. When this shared philosophy has had some time to be tested and known, the Executive Minister will develop a quality of compatibility or knowing the mind of what the Senior Pastor wants without talking to him. Without a shared philosophy such identification will surely create a crisis of conscience or integrity.

Leadership: This is another crucial quality for the Executive Minister. The Executive Minister needs to be able to act as though s/he is the Senior Pastor, while knowing that s/he is the Executive Minister. There must be sensitivity to the "when" and the "how much" of leadership. The Executive Minister can be free to exercise leadership if it is very clear that s/he doesn't covet the senior job or any of that turf.

There is a wide range of styles of leadership among Executive Ministers, but if there is a preference, I believe it is for a pastoral leadership, "a leader's head and a servant's heart." It is the kind of leadership that will serve Christ and the Church best.

Entrepreneur: The Executive Minister needs to be an enterpriser, an initiator. S/he must be able to recognize needs and opportunities and respond to them. S/he must be ready to make decisions and take risks.

A final set of qualities may be categorized as personal qualities. The person in the Executive Minister position must be teachable. If they are not teachable they will not make it. They need a strong ego with maturity. The Executive Minister must be able to maintain his/her own conscience, integrity, and identity. Finally, an Executive Minister must be a real person; a phony will not last very long.

AUTHORITY: SHARING and GIVING UP

The Executive Minister must be assertive enough to work at shaping the job description to reflect his/her own gifts and interests and according to their own vision of what the job can be. They must not presume to do this autonomously or in a manipulative way but in cooperation and consultation, and sometimes in conflict with the Senior Pastor and others in authority.

The Senior Pastor must be willing to give up some things, including some authority if they expect to find the potential benefits in working with an Executive Minister. They need to be in touch enough to recognize his/her own reluctance to do so and be open enough to acknowledge that reluctance to others particularly the Executive Minister.

Included under the issue of authority is the Executive Minister's relationship with the rest of the staff. Some Executive Ministers who were promoted from within the staff experience resistance to their leadership by their former peers who are now their subordinates. Where a pattern of reporting to and being supervised by an Executive Minister has been established there is less of a problem.

THE REID TEMPLE SENIOR PASTOR -EXECUTIVE MINISTRY MODEL

As Senior Pastor of a ten thousand plus member congregation, there are insights and practical advice I have gained from the Senior Pastor and Executive Minister relationship. Rev. Matthew Watley serves as the Executive Minister and reports directly to myself as Senior Pastor. Together we have witnessed numerous positive results as we have sought to move the congregation from where they are to where God wants the congregation to go.

The Senior Pastor and Executive Minister model has become

more of an evolving faith journey. The relational process has helped to build the body of Christ called Reid Temple AME Church. It has helped the overall membership to discover and define the purpose of the Church. The Senior Pastor and Executive Minister relationship has helped to enlarge the vision and expand the ministry.

SPIRITUAL LEADERSHIP MODELS
The Senior Pastor and Executive Ministry model can provides a clear image of a healthy spiritual leadership model. The Bible provides several spiritual leadership models. There is the apprenticeship model between Moses and Joshua. The apprenticeship model is also found in the relationship between Elijah and Elisha.

It seems that persons God singled out for service or leadership find themselves being paired up with people who provide spiritual leadership. These are friends, mentors, spiritual partners, or those who helped nurture them along their journey. Abraham brought his nephew Lot along with him. Samuel followed Eli around step by step. Elisha shadowed Elijah, Ruth clung to Naomi. Timothy blossomed under Paul and Jesus had the motley crew called disciples.

The Saul and David leadership model is particularly interesting because of the unhealthy dynamic we observe between the two. Often times what we witness between Saul and David's leadership interactions all prevalent in local ministry.

Saul was the first King and David was the second king of Israel. David's life was intertwined with the life of Saul at the beginning. Early in Saul's leadership, he was Holy Spirit inspired. Saul led Israel to resounding victories and a number of worthy accomplishments. He was a good commander, leader, and successful in his early day. But Saul made a foolish mistake. He just could not avoid presumptuousness. He assumed the prerogative of a priest. God had made him a king, not a priest.

Saul's mental stability began to deteriorate. He became more and more self-willed and focused on the gifted life of David. Saul began to suffer from bouts of depression. Over time, Saul grew jealous. He became suspicious, distrustful, and envious. He regarded David as a competitor. Subsequently, Saul gave himself over to demonic influence.

Unfortunately, Saul never came to appreciate David's anointing and gifting. What resulted was an ungodly leadership model dominated by competitiveness, undermining, and subversive tactics that created division and ongoing dissension. This is not a good model of leadership for ministry. However, you are likely to see this unhealthy image reflected between Senior Pastors, Executive Ministers, Assistant Pastors, Bishops, Elders, and officers in many of our congregations.

MINISTRY IMAGE
We live in a society obsessed with image. We worry about having the right image. We work to improve our image and work to protect or promote our image. Both the Senior Pastor and Executive Minister must be intentional about presenting a godly image in ministry so that the people of God can move forward in faith. Reflecting a Godly image in ministry is not an easy thing for free will-wielding sin prone humans like us preachers. It requires us to struggle with the idea of Godliness and faith as we also struggle with life. The Senior Pastor and Executive Minister function with a single philosophy towards ministry.

Our central objective is to help people to move forward in faith. This requires a highly relational approach to programmatic concepts related to the objectives and goals of the Church.

SENIOR PASTOR AND EXECUTIVE MINISTER LINK
The Executive Minister position necessitates a clear understanding of tasks and actions to move the Church to the next level. The Senior Pastor has to articulate what kind of actions specifically will accomplish the desired goals. The meaningful actions are not simply one more thing to do. Instead they are the right things to do or things to stop doing to get where God

desires the Church to be.

Each year, the Senior Pastor presents a set of clear objectives covering the areas of Evangelism, Education, Economics Empowerment, and Expansion. These objectives are quantified and shared with the Commissioners who are tasked to manage the designated ministries and their budgets to reach specified goals.

The Executive Minister is responsible for the oversight of the infrastructure and day-to-day operations. The Executive Minister reports directly to the Senior Pastor. The activities for the Executive Minister in the area of economics involve coordination of the Church Federal Credit Union and Bookstore. For education, it requires the oversight of the Reid Temple Church Academy and Education Board. In expansion, the Executive Minister was responsible for navigating the building construction meetings for the planning of the present 120,000 square foot campus and has recently completed the development of architectural plans and design for the second site 40,000 square foot ministry location.

Evangelism and Discipleship formation is paramount in the life of the Church. Preaching is essential and the Executive Minister preaches at the second location each Sunday morning and returns to the main campus for the evening service. This service is structured toward the college students from the neighboring universities. Reid Temple AME Church provides transportation from their respective universities, students receive a meal when they arrive, and after eating are required to attend the worship experience.

The Senior Pastor has to be intentional about what s/he is hoping to accomplish. The Senior Pastor must first have a devotional life, hear from God, and have a God given vision for the people. It takes nothing short of a Godly relationship with the Holy Spirit in order to get real results.

The Senior Pastor and Executive Minister paradigm is a creative process that inspires both positions to maximize their personal and professional potential. The Executive Minister is trained to observe, listen and customize his/her approach to solutions and strategies that work in the ministry context. The Senior Pastor seeks to unlock the wisdom in the Executive Minister so that s/he can find their path of success. This means that the Senior Pastor must be mature and secure enough to allow the boundaries of growth for the Executive Minister not to be limited by the experience or expertise of the Senior Pastor.

The Senior Pastor speaks truth into the life of the Executive Minister and guides him/her in what they should and should not do. To be healthy the Senior Pastor and Executive Minister's relationship journey should be one that embraces a curious mind over against a closed mind. There should be openness for dialogue versus debate, asking as opposed to telling.

FROM THE EXECUTIVE MINISTER PERSPECTIVE
Matthew Lawrence Watley

Two Questions
Whenever I attend church conferences and conventions, there are two questions that people ask me without fail: 1) "When are you going to get your own church and start pastoring?" and 2) "How can I get somebody like you on my staff?" Each of these questions say more about the speaker's perspective on ministry and leadership, than serve as reflection of my own experiences or views. Because of the frequency of these questions, I have developed standard responses, which reframe the speaker's point and addresses the real issues being raised. My interpretation of the question, "When are you going to start pastoring?" reflects the traditional belief that the only legitimate and laudable ministry in the Black Church is pastoral ministry. This tradition, however, is being met with a new paradigm where full-time ministry opportunities abound in many forms. Youth Ministers, Preaching Assistants, Pastoral Care Ministers, Counselors, Researchers, Ministers of Christian Education, and

132

Executive Ministers are all viable career opportunities that are tied to parish ministry. It is not uncommon that persons may serve their entire career in one of these vocations or choose to perform the same ministry function at another church. The need for education in the areas of specialized ministry has been recognized in the academy. Targeted instruction is now provided in seminary, ministry tools and resources have been developed, and professional associations have emerged to support these roles. The idea that legitimate ministry does not exist beyond the Senior Pastor is somewhat old thinking, and may unintentionally cause persons, not called or gifted as Senior Pastors, to take on this leadership role to their personal detriment and that of the church where they serve.

My response to the question is simple because I take this opportunity to express my contentment and fulfillment with my role as Executive Minister. This, *"if it ain't broke don't fix it"* response is meant to legitimize the role of the Executive Minister. My motive is to redirect the questioner, not to compare one role to another, but to create space for both in the mind of the asker.

Opportunity: The most successful Executive Ministers I know have the skill set necessary to be effective Senior Pastors, but they have all felt called to work under a Senior Pastor instead. This may seem counterintuitive at first glance, so I have identified a few drivers to clarify this point of view. To begin, Executive Ministers generally are employed by large and growing churches, which tend to be more progressive in worship style and have more of a corporate culture. As a result, the Executive Minister has the ability to join a winning team as opposed to trying to start a church with no base of support or restoring a floundering institution to its former glory. Of course, churches that may be in decline deserve strong leadership, but these should not be the only options made available to ministers. Secondly, the Executive Minister handles a host of issues, including preaching, managing staffs, budgets, risk, capital projects, worship, organizing conferences, interacting with public officials, and other duties assigned depending on the particular ministry context. Lastly, Executive Ministers are not exposed to the same kinds of threats and challenges that are aimed at the Senior Pastor. The Executive Minister carries some of the burden of ministry for sure, but there is also a weight reserved solely for the shoulders of the Senior Pastor, which many Executive Ministers are not inclined to bear.

Security: There will always be songs sung within the hearing of the senior leader about the exploits of the junior leader. Saul had to hear about David's accomplishments and achievements and became immediately insecure and sought opportunities to undermine and destroy David. David provided Saul with essential personal support, helped to ensure the protection of Saul's kingdom, and created a new mood of excitement within the kingdom. All of these actions worked to Saul's benefit, but he could not see it. In my view, every Senior Pastor must do a personal assessment as to his/her comfort level with the role of an Executive Minister. Every senior leader should conduct a self-examination – a Saul test – to see if she or he can handle attention and affirmation being given to the junior leader without being threatened.

We should underscore one of the sources of Saul's insecurity, which was the people's comparison between he and David. Both Senior Pastors and Executive Ministers must be wary of the tendency of congregations to pit them against one another. The Senior Pastor will no doubt hear whispers of Executive Ministers defying their authority, planning to "split" the church, and other forms of disloyalty. Likewise, Executive Ministers will be told of how their gifts are being stifled, how they could start their own church with great support, and how they really are preferred to the Senior Pastor. Each person must be careful not to give way to these contrary winds, which are designed to cause disruption and disunity. Dr. Washington often says that people reveal their true motivation over time. Rather then feeding into character assassinations, one should remain consistent in his role, and supportive of the position of the other minister while keeping the age-old axiom – trust but verify.

Loyalty: While Senior Pastors must be secure, Executive Ministers must be loyal. After David assumed the throne, he became victim of a coup from his own house. His son Absalom, out of naked ambition, hatched a plan to steal the throne out from under his father. Absalom positioned himself in a manner that ingratiated him to the people, while casting a negative light on his father's leadership. While his authority and resources were not equal to the king, he leveraged them to effectively oust David from his position before his father realized what was taking place. Absalom literally took what the senior leader had given him, and used it for his own agenda. Ministers who desire to become Senior Pastors should do so by following the official processes of pastoral appointment or candidacy available in his or her denomination. To attempt to steal or split a church is a mark against that person's character and ministry. Before serving as an Executive Minister, s/he should perform an "Absalom test" to ensure that their true motivation is to assist in the building of someone else's church and not the formation of their own.

Vision: While Executive Ministers can do a lot, vision must come from the Senior Pastor. S/he must be sure to provide the picture and the parameters for where the Lord is taking the congregation. The role of the Executive Minister is to help execute that vision, which means buying into the vision as if it was his/her own. This does not mean that the Executive Minister cannot or should not have vision for ministry, but that vision must be approved and supported by the Senior Pastor if it is to be fulfilled. This means the Executive Minister must be prepared to have their vision delayed or denied without internalizing or harboring resentment. To the extent that a pattern of incongruent vision exists between Senior Pastor and Executive Minister, then the process of transition should begin to both assist the church in finding a suitable replacement, and help the Executive Minister find ministry opportunities outside of the church where he or she may fulfill their vision. In this way, each vision may be fulfilled with the net result of the kingdom's expansion versus division.

Support: This component is crucial and comes along side the issue of security. If every decision that the Executive Minister makes has to be approved by the Senior Pastor, then the Senior Pastor's workload has not been lightened. Internecine rivalry exists in all churches both within the staff and the laity. If the congregation senses a lack of support for the Executive Minister's role or initiatives, they will seize upon this perception and use it to limit his/her effectiveness. The Executive Minister must know that his/her decisions are in line with the overall vision of the Senior Pastor, and that the Senior Pastor will support him/her.

Complimentary Strengths: While both of us are effective preachers, Dr. Washington is also an accomplished musician, adept in organizational leadership specifically in the area of conflict resolution, and a master pastor. His leadership style draws high capacity workers, both volunteer and paid, to serve in the ministry because of his big tent approach to leadership. My skills are more detailed in areas of strategy, corporate governance, and development. The combination of our skill yields a greater sum and depth of skills than either of us could muster on our own. This allows us to operate in our respective areas of strength and interests.

Self-Legitimization: Ultimately titles and even conferred authority and support from the Senior Pastor will not make the Executive Minister automatically effective. There must be some measure of value added that the Executive Minister brings to the table such as their seniority and standing based, their personal character and reputation, or their educational and vocational background which allows them to speak authoritatively in relevant areas. It may be a track record of success in former positions within or outside of the church or strong gifts in preaching, teaching, pastoral care or counseling, which raise their image in the eyes of the congregation. At some point, the Executive Minister must be able to prove their salt beyond the endorsement of the Senior Pastor or their effectiveness will be severely limited.

My role at Reid Temple, under the leadership of Dr. Lee P. Washington, has been an ever evolving one. I was originally hired as the Youth Minister with the added responsibility of preaching at the 6PM service each Sunday. Dr. Washington, from the beginning, modeled all of the attributes of a great Senior Pastor and helped facilitate my effectiveness. He lent his support to a number of revolutionary (read non-traditional) programs we were embarking on in youth ministry. He endorsed my leadership at the 6PM service, which he communicated to me, and others in the church as "Rev. Watley's service." As a result, I had all of the institutional support necessary to accomplish my vision, which was in line with his vision.

As the church began to move forward in building the Glenn Dale campus, he promoted me to the Executive Minister position to oversee all aspects of the project, to manage the ancillary corporations of the church, and provide leadership to the other executive positions that were created. After one year of having moved into our Glenn Dale Campus, Dr. Washington authorized me to start a second location in nearby Silver Spring, MD. Unlike many multi-site models where the Senior Pastor either preaches at each campus live or via video, Pastor Washington extended me the opportunity to be the main preacher for our North location and with leading its growth and development. By the Lord's favor, as we complete our 4th year, we are also renovating a 40,000 square foot facility which will house a sanctuary with seating for over 1000 to accommodate the rapid growth of this congregation.

Congregational Confidence: When we came up with the vision to begin the new location, we experienced the usual mix of skepticism, opposition, and support that any kingdom minded idea elicits in church. Since I would be preaching at the new location every Sunday and effectively leading a completely different congregation, a couple of things had to evident in the minds of the people. First, my loyalty to Dr. Washington had to be apparent so that everyone would clearly understand this was not an attempt, on my part, to usurp authority, or steal members. Second, my own gifts had to be confirmed through my prior activities in preaching the evening service and leading the congregation and other endeavors.

Dr. Washington provided the same kind of support in this effort that he did when I first arrived at Reid Temple over 11 years ago. He cast the vision to the church, affirmed my leadership, provided personnel and budget, and the freedom for my gifts to operate. The result has been a congregation that has added to the membership roles, the budget, and expanded the churches footprint into another country.

Counting the Costs: My response to the second question, "How can I get someone like you on my staff?" may seem a bit abrupt at first. Generally the person making this statement sees the benefits without the costs. They see a person to lighten their workload by dealing with issues in ministry and administration from which they are either overwhelmed or uninterested. They often do not realize all the ramifications that go along with hiring an Executive Minister. If they are a micro-manager the idea of not knowing every detail of a given enterprise may result in frustration. Or they may risk losing the individual who has been hired but effectively kept from doing his job. For the Senior Pastor in need of constant attention, this means stepping out of the spot light or at least expanding the light to afford the Executive Minister his/her opportunity to shine.

In my experience, many Senior Pastors are rarely comfortable with creating this kind of shared space. My response about 90 percent of the time to the question, "How can I get somebody like you?" is, "You probably don't want someone like me." Perhaps what they are looking for is a Church Administrator who can deal with internal systems, a pastoral care minister that can handle congregational interaction, or some other specialized field of ministry. When one says he/she wants to employ an Executive Minister, they are effectively saying they are willing to make space for someone to be as successful as their gifts will allow. My view is that a number of ministers are not naturally built nor have they been trained to affirm and allow someone else's gifts to flourish.

Davidic Leadership Model: I have lifted up two Biblical characters as examples of how not to conduct ones self. Senior Pastors should not act like Saul, and Executive Ministers should not act like Absalom. The right model to follow is difficult to embrace because at first glance it seems to be unsuccessful. David is the right model for both positions to embrace. David's leadership orientation was exactly right both as the junior leader and as the senior leader. If there is one word that summarizes David's tenure under Saul it was loyalty. David, although seemingly more popular then Saul and having had several opportunities to kill Saul, chose not to touch God's anointed. The closest he got was cutting off the corner of his cloak. The end result of his trustworthiness was that the throne came to David in God's own time, by God's means, and the kingdom was expanded.

The word that best characterizes David's leadership in Absalom's case is freedom. David unwittingly provided sufficient resources for Absalom to mount and win a successful coup d'état. He did not limit Absalom's authority out of an abundance of caution and it temporarily cost him the kingdom. Yet, Absalom's abuse of power did not invalidate David's leadership approach anymore than Saul's. In each case, David had to flee for his life, risking the throne, but ultimately God protected him and his throne, vindicating his leadership. In other words, leadership within the senior or junior position is not an enterprise that should be entered into by those that are risk averse. Of course, risk should be considered, and one should not lay hands on any person quickly. Ultimately, one's faith must abide in God that they are being sent to serve under the right leader, or the right leader will serve under them, and if not, God will preserve and protect God's people and God's kingdom will continue to be expanded

Our relationship even expressed itself in the writing of this article. Rather then our sitting with each other, going through potential thoughts and formats, we simply wrote our own sections independently and shared them with the other as a matter of course.

The Need for Flesh and Blood Mentors and How To Select Them
Cecelia E. Greene Barr

Like newly licensed doctors entering the field of medicine, and newly barred attorneys entering the field of law, each year thousands of women and men are ordained to serve in the Christian ministry. Additionally, there are vast amounts of persons, primarily women, who engage in Christian ministry without the validation of ecclesiastical bodies. With and sometimes without ecclesiastical credentials, persons are emerging onto the field simply to "Do Church." Their destination church, or as referred to in culturally popular vernacular ministry, is like unto a territory to be explored, developed, and sadly, exploited much like the wild west during the early stages of American history. Without flesh and blood mentors on post in this territory called church, the body of Christ has seen clashes between the clergy and congregation, the minister and the ministry, that resemble the 30 second shoot out known famously as the Gunfight at OK Corral.

Conflict In Ministry

"For all of us make many mistakes..." James 3:2 (NRSV)
Conflict in ministry is inherently due to the assembling of personalities, organizations, and time lines. This is a reality that not even one who is being guided by a sound mentoring relationship can completely escape. Whereas mentoring does not provide an impenetrable shield against conflict arising in ministry, it does provide the wise mentee with a safe haven while navigating through difficult waters. Mentors well acquainted with the nuances of church life are able to help their mentee keep the dynamics of the situation in perspective. Consider the experience of a new pastor as an example.

Pastor Springfield (name has been changed) had served as a full time assistant in a mega-church as the Director of Education for many years. Now he is the pastor of a congregation sized, like most American churches, with less than 250 members. The church was located in a part of the inner city that seemed long since forgotten and hard hit by years of a down turn in the economy. It did not take long for Pastor Springfield to realize that he would not be able to follow his former pastor's example of working full time in ministry. If he were to survive financially, it would be necessary for Pastor Springfield to become bi-vocational. An opportunity outside of the church became available for which Pastor Springfield was well suited in demeanor and skills, but the position proved to consume far more of his time than the growth of his ministry could afford.

With the equilibrium of employment, ministry, and family floating increasingly out of balance, Pastor Springfield was not able to calculate the impending course he was on. While others in ministry watched without warning, and sometimes jokingly critiquing behind his back, Pastor Springfield was aided by a mentor who helped him see the need to redirect his energy so the priorities of his life would not be ruined or depleted. His mentor had been like a lighthouse that helped avert inner conflict that would have ultimately erupted into great ministry disappointment.

Church life is more than a series of conflicts needing management. The church is the bride of Christ and with it comes the unexpected. An event occurs in town that causes news reporters to search for the prophetic voice of the church. For the minister who has held to a strong opposition towards social and political activism this becomes a litmus test for whether the church is seen as relevant or just another piece of property on a city street. A mentor who has experience in the pulpit and the public square would be invaluable during unexpected moments like these. A mentor willing to share their experience and provide insight could help the mentee search their own heart for the subtle inspirations that bring life to a new social position. The words "I remember when..." begins to sound like a prelude to a much-needed answer.

Staying Connected To The People
"When he has brought out all his own, he goes ahead of them, and the sheep follow him because they know his voice. They will not follow a stranger, but they will run from him because they do not know the voice of strangers".   John 10:5-6 (NRSV)

Persons living out God's divine purpose in a Kingdom reality will notice very quickly the distant side of "Doing Church". Experiences of isolation, vulnerability, and separation are unavoidable. Some leaders have even confessed that once the church membership has increased beyond a few hundred, their interaction became more restricted to a few key leaders on their staff. The more the leader takes steps to isolate him/herself from the membership the more vulnerable the leader becomes to a type of disconnection that makes even their voice unrecognizable. The people who once seem to connect so easily to the voice of their leader slowly fail to recognize the leader's voice. Someone has to help the leader to remember the need for staying connected. Flesh and blood mentors, who themselves face heavy administrative and ministry demands, show by example the importance of nurturing connection with the people God has sent them to serve.

A wonderful example of a leader doing what he could to avoid separation is seen in President Barack Obama. After President Barack Obama was elected a news report was released about his desire to keep his Blackberry Smartphone®. For those who are not so enthralled with Smartphones like the Blackberry, this device helps the owner stay connected instantly via text messages, email, and of course phone calls. The device helps bypass gatekeepers, like secretaries, who may not assess your inquiry as relevant for the moment. President Barack Obama knew that loosing this Smartphone was in a step towards true disconnection with the lives he was sent to serve.

A Safe Place To Unburden Yourself
"Bear one another's burdens, and in this way you will fulfill the law of Christ".   Galatians 6:2 (NRSV)

Church structure has experienced new alignments in some pockets of Christendom. Organizational structures, which were once very vertical, are becoming flat. Vertical leadership invests authority and primary wisdom in one person, i.e. Pastor or Senior Pastor. With that comes a certain mystique around the top official that allows those under their influence to share their personal concerns, ministry quests, and life issues with them. But this same mystique has been known to work against the top official when those under their influence are not able to accept their need to share their personal concerns, ministry quests, and life issues. Who will listen when the only ears are those under your influence?

In a vertical ministry structure where can the leader unburden him/herself without the fear of no longer being respected? This is not to imply that a leader's burdens are sensational. Sometimes the burdens are run of the mill like wrestling with personal doubt about a decision, the occasional visitation of depression or dissatisfaction with performance. A flat organizational structure may help to give leaders a safe haven among peers, but these structures are more acceptable in some cultures than in others. For those who live in cultures not open to flat organizational structures, a mentor becomes that safe haven.

Transference And Training
"For this reason I remind you to rekindle the gift of God that is within you through the laying on of my hands".   2Timothy 1:6 NRSV

Something happened when Paul laid his hands on Timothy. This was not a mere pat on the back but something far more substantial and spiritual in nature. The gift of God upon Paul's life and ministry was transferred to Timothy through this act of laying on of his hands. In the denomination for which God has called me to fulfill my Kingdom assignment, when we are ordained, seven elders lay hands on our head. Observers may think this practice to be ritualistic, but as Paul reminds Timothy there is a spiritual reality-taking place in this action. Flesh and blood mentors are needed in the church so that the gift of God within them may be transferred to their spiritual sons and daughters. Paul was keenly aware that God had invested spiritual gifting within him. Paul was further aware that Timothy's ministry would benefit greatly if he were also endowed with the gifts that were manifesting in his life. Mentors are not selfish leaders, but generous even in their gifting. Timothy's ministry was confronted with heresy from within and attacks from outside. As his mentor, Paul understood the need to transfer the spiritual reality of God's presence that had so effective accompanied him since his first encounter on the road to Damascus.

Flesh and blood mentors not only transfer the spiritual reality of *giftings*, they also serve as on the job trainers. Paul had to remind Timothy to rekindle the gift of God. Having played sports for many years, I learned how to value trainers. As an athlete, I was gifted with speed but it took a trainer to teach me how to round a base or slide to keep from being tagged out or avoid broken bones. Trainers not only teach you what you do not know, they also watch you perform what it is you think you already know. A

144

batting coach will watch you swing for several throws before walking up to remind you how to hold the bat or where to place your feet when trying to pull the ball to the opposite side of the field. Likewise, mentors are in the experience with you, often watching you perform and at critical times they speak words of remembrance.

Psychological Undergirding

"But as for you, continue in what you have learned and firmly believed, knowing from whom you learned it, and how from childhood you have known the sacred writings that are able to instruct you for salvation through faith in Christ Jesus".   2Timothy 3:14-15 (NRSV)

Behind the facade of every leader is a person in need of psychological support. I say this not to allude to the notion that Christian leaders suffer from psychological instability, but to call attention to the occasions when our soul needs comfort. Doing church is as much a mind game as it is a spiritual battle for eternity. Mentors are able to teach their mentee that their minds cannot afford to be blank canvasses for which anyone can craft the latest theological trends. Our minds are pulled upon all of the time to see how the news from the White House and news from the local drug house will speak theologically to the people we have been called to serve.

Our minds seldom enjoy void moments, for even rainbows and leaves blowing across an overgrown lawn are able to speak revelation from God. Our mind is a battleground where spiritual images are formed into words and ideas palatable for a cross section of members. Our minds grow weary when doing ministry and during those times when the light of inspiration is barely flickering mentors are there to help us think afresh. For all of the reasons I have shared in this conversation about the need for flesh and blood mentors, perhaps this need is one that is most critical in application.

It is critical in application because the mentor must be sensitive to how men and women differ in their response to the psychological demands of ministry. There are those who respond to the fatigue of psychological demands by engaging others in lots of dialogue, while others may respond by brooding. Flesh and blood mentors invest themselves in their mentee to the point that they are able to accurately interpret behavior patterns. They genuinely care about you and this love causing them to watch your life. They watch your methods. They measure your standards. They discern irregularities because they know you well enough to pinpoint the difference between one night's lack of sleep verses an emotionally frazzled servant. Paul psychologically supported Timothy by taking him back to his foundation, his childhood lessons. As his mentor, he loved him enough and knew him well enough to be able to provide the precise support that fit Timothy's need.

Flesh and Blood Verses Distant Observation
"But she came and knelt before him, saying, "Lord, help me." He answered, "it is not fair to take the children's food and throw it to the dogs." She said, "Yes, Lord, yet even the dogs eat the crumbs that fall from their master's table".   Matthew 15:25-27 (NRSV)

Wisdom can be gained by distant observation just like crumbs that fall on the floor can still feed an empty belly. When a person is determined to learn and no one is willing to give of him or herself in a personal way, a degree of knowledge can be obtained from afar. Yet this is not the best that mentors should bequeath to the church. Flesh and blood mentors bequeath to the church a well thought out plan of succession. They provide a systematic way to develop with the mentee's needs in mind. The process crosses generations and forces the mentor to turn their attention away from themselves. Personal expansion is built into the process for both the mentor and the mentee. None of which is available when the church is only left with learning strictly through distant observation. Reading books about how gifted preachers prepare and deliver their sermons is not the same skill sharpening as having a mentor read or listen to how you have prepared and delivered sermons. Preaching vicariously through someone else's method and style opens the door for a lack of personal authenticity. The church deserves more than second hand imitations because first hand guidance was not available.

Selecting Flesh and Blood Mentors

The method of selecting flesh and blood mentors is not like applying a mathematical algorithm. The process is very organic because it is relational. Lives are converging. Schedules are intermingling. Sensibilities are being challenged and the raw truth is that both persons need to like one another. Persons seeking mentors are often drawn out of admiration. But admiration fades quickly when professional accountability is demanded and the mentee is not willing to comply. Before offering wisdom in selecting a mentor, I caution you to remember that the mentoring relationship is a living organism and should be approached with appropriate care.

Begin with a look in God's direction. Like all other relationships, the mentoring relationship needs prayer to find life and prayer to maintain a healthy life. Ask God for a flesh and blood mentor to help you in ministry. The nation of Israel erred with God when they demanded that God provide for them a king because they were unwilling to trust the Lordship of God and they wanted to be like other nations (1Samuel 8:19-22). Mentors do not take the seat of lordship in your life and ministry. Therefore, asking God to provide a mentor is not akin to the mistake made by Israel. Asking God to provide a flesh and blood mentor also signals that you understand that all that you have comes from the Lord. Getting someone to agree to place your ministerial needs on their agenda should be accomplished by the unction of the Holy Spirit and not political manipulation or any other methodology.

Secure Leadership

There are qualities that mentors should exhibit which make it easier to identify the person God has chosen for your development. Secure leadership is an absolutely necessary quality. Mentors share their influence, resources and tricks of the trade. Mentoring creates replacements and only secure leaders are able to give unselfishly, knowing full well that they are looking into the eyes of one who will potentially take over for them one day. Secure leadership will not relegate their mentee to warming up a cold car after the mentor has preached a revival, but will invite them into the room along with other ministers for purposes of observation and networking.

Mastery in Ministry

Mentors are more than persons willing to give advice or who are available to give you a shoulder to cry on. The church has persons who have demonstrated mastery in ministry. The focus of those seeking a mentor is to find the ministry leader who has demonstrated mastery in the area for which they are seeking development. An example is found in Elijah and Elisha's relationship. Elijah demonstrated mastery in the prophetic ministry. The anointing on his life resulted in students sitting at his feet to be molded for God's service. Elijah's spiritual ranking was evident when encountering the enemies of God's Kingdom. The preponderance of evidence that Elijah was a master prophet caused Elisha to follow him constantly in order to receive a double portion of his mantle. Do your research and look for the fruit of their ministry.

Your Potential Is a Priority

Potential takes time and lots of effort to transform into life purpose or tangible results, and time is a leader's precious commodity. The more mastery they exhibit in their given area of anointing, the more the body of Christ will make demands of their time. Family relationships and the church are all competitors of a leader's time. Therefore, when looking for a mentor, identify someone who is able to make your potential a priority. Otherwise your need for guidance can become quickly overshadowed and you are reduced merely to a resource for helping the mentor's priorities become reality.

Tolerant of Mistakes

One can only remain in the laboratory but for so long. At some point, they must try out what they have been observing and learning. With trial there comes error and mistakes will be made. Discerning whether a leader will be able to provide mentoring can be seen in the way the leader responds to your errors. Is the leader so embarrassed by your error that they deny the relationship when in the presence of their peers? Or is the leader so intolerant with even minor infractions that the mentee is subjected to verbal scolding? Ask yourself this question: If I spread my wings and break something in the process, will that be the end for me? Trying to learn under the pressure of perfection or intolerance for mistakes creates a hostile environment. People become nervous and often reluctant to ever try new ideas. Ministry breeds creativity and even outrageous ideas that call upon courage. When leaders are intolerant of mistakes it dampens the boldness that a courageous spirit needs in order to thrive. Do yourself a favor and do not simply look for great moments of victory in the leader's life, but also analyze moments of defeat. It is there that you will gain insight into how you may possibly be treated when you make a mistake on their watch.

Gift of Wisdom
Lastly, when expecting God to provide a mentor in your life, look for the spiritual gift of wisdom to manifest through the leader. In the church, everyone is full of advice and are quick to tell you what you should be doing in every situation. There is always a deacon, trustee or steward who thinks they know how you should handle the particulars of ministry. You simply can not do ministry by listening to every speaking spirit. A mentor's voice rises above the white noise of all the other voices. It is able to do so because they speak by the spiritual gift of wisdom. Their words are timely and insights are uncommonly accurate. Just as Moses became as God to Aaron, the gift of wisdom makes the mentor just as prophetic in the mentee's journey.

I am reminded of an experience when I was presented with a small window of time to make a major ministry decision. I called a leader who had in times past provided mentoring to me, but I was unable to make contact. Time had expired and my decision was being requested. With the peace of God dwelling in my spirit, I answered in the affirmative. Shortly afterwards my phone rang and the first words I heard were; "Cecelia, I listened to your message... what did you decide?" At this point, I had very little to offer in conversation for I was in listening mode. What I needed to hear was a word of wisdom that would bring

149

affirmation to the decision I had just made. I was not disappointed, for a bounty of wisdom was spoken into my spirit. The mentoring moment crystallized for me when I heard the concluding statement, which began with, "Cecelia, and when you pull this off..." I sat there holding the phone and feeling light covering my countenance. I was living the truest form of mentoring because the words spoken to me were not empty phrases of encouragement, but a God message that had the Lord's purpose for my life clearly in view. A few times every month, when I quiet my soul, I hear afresh those words; "Cecelia, and when you pull this off..." Those moments of mediation remind me to thank God for answering my prayer through the relationship that exists.

The church of Jesus Christ deserves competent leaders in every generation. The flaws of the apostles are examined thoroughly, but the Bible proves that they give solid leadership to the first century church. Twenty-one centuries later the bride of Christ is still able to examine the fruit of ministry leaders and see an abundance of effectiveness. The practice must continue where the church and ministries of God's Kingdom continue to move forward in the right path, guided by exceptional leaders. Mentoring aides in the accomplishment of this task. To those who demonstrate mastery in ministry, I appeal to your sense of spiritual stewardship. Take the time to become a flesh and blood mentor to a few whom God is preparing for the next mantle in ministry. Let's pray together.

Holy Spirit, just as you have empowered me to do great exploits in the Kingdom for your glory, use me now to transfer this anointing to another one of your servants. I submit myself to this new level of service as an act of spiritual worship and stewardship. May I have eyes to see another servant not by their earthly status as a new minister, but allow me to see them according to their spiritual rank and order. I release my influence, resources, and wisdom for the development of their potential. In Jesus name I pray. AMEN.

Developing and Maintaining a Strong and Visible Music Ministry

James Abbington, D.M.A.

In his enduring classic *The Souls of Black Folk*, published in 1903, W. E. B. DuBois declared that "[t]hree things characterized this religion of the slave- the Preacher, the Music, and the Frenzy. The Preacher is the most unique personality developed by the Negro on American Soil." He continues, "The Music of Negro religion is that plaintive, rhythmic melody, with its touching minor cadences, which, despite caricature and defilement, still remains the most original and beautiful expression of human life and longing yet born on American soil." And finally, "the Frenzy or 'Shouting,' when the Spirit of the Lord passed by, and seizing the devotee, made him mad with supernatural joy, was the last essential of Negro religion and the more devoutly believed in than all the rest."[9] One need only visit

151

a worshiping African American church today to witness the significance and reality of DuBois' statement in the twenty-first century.

The sermon, or more accurately the *preaching*, and the music, or more accurately the *singing,* are the focal points of worship in the Black church as the magnets of attraction and the primary vehicles of spiritual transport. C. Eric Lincoln and Lawrence Mamiya concluded "In the Black Church, good preaching and good singing are almost invariably the minimum conditions of a successful ministry. Both activities trace their roots back to Africa where music and religion and life itself were all one holistic enterprise."[10]

Since the seventeenth century, Black Americans have participated in two culturally distinct religious traditions. According to Portia Maultsby, "The first tradition represents that associated with White Protestant denominations. Blacks, utilizing the concepts and practices retained from their West African heritage, independently developed the second. These two traditions are easily distinguished by ideology, worship style, and musical practices."[11] The musical repertoire of Black congregations that adhered to White Protestant doctrines is derived from official hymnals that include psalms, hymns, and spiritual songs. Conversely, the repertoire of churches whose religious ideology is uniquely and indigenously Black consists of Black folk spirituals and gospels. Maultsby concludes "Songs of these two idioms are derived from several sources: (1) West African musical traditions; (2) Black secular idioms; (3) original Black compositions; and (4) White Protestant psalms, hymns, and spiritual songs."[12]

For many years, Black churches were defined and associated by their specific musical styles and traditions, which brought them national fame and reputation. In the writer's personal experience, the St. James Missionary Baptist Church in Detroit, formerly pastored by the late Reverend Charles H. Nicks, Jr., was known for its great gospel choirs and recordings. On the other hand, the Abyssinian Baptist Church in Harlem, New York, was known for its performance of great oratorios, anthems, concert spirituals, and concerts with the New York Philharmonic Orchestra.

One of the most quintessential factors for pastors, worship leaders, and music directors who desire to develop and maintain a strong and viable ministry is *knowing* and *respecting* the history, theology, mission, stories, traditions, customs, and values of the congregation that they have been called to serve. Linda J. Clark says, "At the center of a successful music program is a vital connection between music and the life of faith of a particular congregation. In worship, music and faith are inextricably linked: the purpose of a church music program is to manifest and make articulate the faith of the people. There are two major facets to this process: expression and formation."[13] She explains that "[m]usic expresses faith; that is, it is a vehicle through which the faith within a person and a community comes forth. People's favorite hymns or anthems have this function.[14] Music also forms faith. If the hymn or anthem is new and unfamiliar, it confronts a person and a community with a reality they must come to terms in order to be faithful. This process of formation can also take place in the midst of very familiar music – one that the listener or performer hears anew in a very different way".[15] Therefore a successful music ministry is one that both expresses and forms the faith of the community.

Music is integral to worship. It sets the tone of worship more than any other aspect. "Our identity as a people – what our values are, our culture, our theology, our mission – is often signaled to people by music before they ever hear it described in words"[16] says William Roberts. He continues, "Much of our worship is word-oriented, and Christianity needs its rational, discursive presentation. What people in our culture seem to crave, however, is a sense of wonder, mystery, holiness, and transcendence. For those churches that value liturgy, even the words alone, of course, can carry a sense of transcendence, but music can undergird, amplify, and illuminate the language of praise and prayer. Music gives wings to worship".[17]

Musical Styles

One of the most critical issues confronting the Black church, and the Christian church in general, is the explosive issue of musical styles. Many churches are fighting and buzzing with anxious, fevered discussions, and mediated meetings on the subjects. Others have divided in order to meet the differing preferences of the congregations, some by scheduling contrasting services at different times and days, and others by establishing new churches. The greatest cause of segregation, competition, discord, and quarreling in our churches is not evangelism, outreach, sacramental understanding, denominational creeds and doctrines, Scripture, or mission, but whether or not there is a praise and worship team, traditional hymnody is sung, Holy Hip-Hop or contemporary gospel should dominate, which choir can out-sing the others, and who can get the house with what song and with what soloist leading the song! Even more, choir directors, musicians, pastors, and congregations are more concerned about the style of music rather than the substance, the charisma rather than the content, and the tempo rather than the theology.

The Reverend Dr. Otis Moss, III says, "We're arguing whether we should sing this hymn or sing this anthem. We're arguing about if it's all right to praise God. Don't stand up; it doesn't take all of that. Meanwhile, our children are going to hell in a hand basket."[18] I strongly concur with Reverend Moss and add that many of our adults and seasoned-citizens are going with the children in the same "hand basket".

In his book *I Don't Like That Music*, Robert Mitchell raises six essential questions of any style or genre of sacred music: "Is it scriptural? Is it traditional? Is it good music? Is it comfortable? Are they good texts and tunes? Are they comfortable?"[19] These questions should always be present in evaluating and selecting music to be sung in the worship of God's people. Brian Wren declares: "Whether classical or popular, [music in the church] should aim to be one or more of the following:

(1) *Formative*, shaping and modeling our faith as it tells a story within the whole story of God in Christ and draw us into the drama of God's saving love;

(2) *Transformative*, moving us from isolation to belonging, indifference to interest, interest to conviction, and conviction to commitment;

(3) *Cognitive*, giving us something to ponder and think about;

(4) *Educational*, teaching us something we didn't know about the Bible, the Church, and Christian faith, and

(5) *Inspirational*, lifting us out of ourselves into hope, joy, and peace."[20]

The "music wars," as the furiously raging battle has been labeled, with all of its casualties, seems to be fueled and perpetuated by personalities, personal preferences, and a commercial music industry that has little or no concern for what is pleasing to God, what honors God, what is Biblically based, theologically sound, or culturally relevant, and what helps to form, transform, illuminate, educate, and inspires the people of God. Music in our churches has become a device of complacency, self-possession, self-gratification, self-aggrandizing, and preference with no regard to our neighbors. I am troubled by the thought that we have successfully reduced the entire discussion of worship in the Black church to preaching and music, and it all has to do with what we prefer, what we like, and what we know.

The rich and diverse musical styles and diversity that have long characterized the Black church heritage and tradition are seriously in danger of extinction. By neglecting and discarding the historical congregational, or folk spirituals, arranged spirituals, traditional Christian hymnody, hymns, and pioneering gospel music by Black composers, the Black church stands to lose its rich musical legacy that has sustained, uplifted, formed, and defined it. This music has been the scaffolding for which new generations may now enter and become a part of a rich tradition. The Black church cannot afford to abandon its Christian *tradition*, even though it certainly must critically and

155

responsibly abandon useless and unjustifiable *traditionalism*! And there is a great difference.

Struggle and resistance over the influence of new music styles and popular culture are not at all new to the Black church. The church wrestled with Thomas A Dorsey, considered the "Father of Black Gospel Music," who took the blues and jazz and coupled them with religious texts. The church opposed the advent of the Reverend James Cleveland, known as the "King of Gospel Music," and his new gospel recordings and founding of the Gospel Music Workshop of America. In 1969, Edwin Hawkins' "Oh Happy Day" created such an uproar in many churches that people said the devil had been brought into the church. Then came the gospel music icon of my generation, Andrae Crouch, whose music was considered too worldly and forbidden by many churches. In 1997, when the single "Stomp" was released and debuted on MTV, controversy loomed over the heads of Kirk Franklin and God's Property, the then Texas-based young adult gospel choir. It inspired a new and youthful Christian audience and sold close to 3 million records. Many Black churches labeled Kirk Franklin as a radical and criticized him by saying that he had gone too far by performing and blending church music with the slick, funky innovations of hip-hop and rap. He performed in casual and athletic apparel popularized by hip-hop culture. He and his music were strongly resisted because Franklin's break dancing did not belong in the sanctuary, and the struggles and resistance continues today.

Writing in 1979, The Reverend Dr. Wyatt Tee Walker made this profound observation and declaration: "...There is no way, generally or specifically, that the Black Church can function in the real world of the American nightmare without the instruments of the struggle: [1] *a theology grounded in liberation,* [2] *a contemporary sense of historical context,* [3] *a God-ordained sense of destiny in this land, and* [4] *the determination to endure.* Each of the above could require an inquiry in the context of the Black experience in America. They are listed here as ingredients which are contained in the music of the Black religious tradition. It is a very short step to conclude

156

that maximizing the potential of the Black Church enterprise can be facilitated best through the use of its primary vehicle – Black sacred music!"[21]

Developing and maintaining a strong and viable music ministry should never be reduced to an *either-or* program but *both-and* program which celebrates the rich and unique diversity of the historic Black church **and** the creative musical gifts and offerings of the contemporary composers and artists. We need not place our foot on Europe to raise Africa, nor visa-versa, but rejoice and grow in the beauty of all of God's creation.

In a discussion about the use of Euro-American music in the Black Church, The Reverend Dr. Charles G. Adams exclaimed, "The rationality of European music is sanctified and beautified by the startling spontaneity of African and African American artistic ingenuity and fervor... The aim of all church choirs is to sing with the intensity of conviction that can move the souls of people who feel jaded, empty, and defeated by the deadening oppressions, dynamics, and confusion of post modern culture. Even the strictest of music can be made spiritually dynamic and convincing if it is sung with enthusiasm and ecstasy. On the other hand, conviction that is not informed and enthusiasm that is not controlled will not be edifying. Undisciplined enthusiasm repels rather than attracts. Uncontrolled light blinds rather than illumines."[22]

Developing and Organizing the Ministry
Several years ago the word "ministry" became a buzzword around Black Christian churches, especially for those who were very corporate and institutional-minded and felt that this new label brought with it a sense of purpose and would somehow add a new dimension to an old title and position. The word "ministry" (which sounded more ecclesial and "purpose-driven") began to replace "department." Therefore, those who ushered at the doors were called the Ministry of Hospitality; those who prepared food were called the Culinary Arts Ministry; those who taught or worked with Sunday School, Vacation Bible School, and weekly Bible study became the Ministry of Christian

Education; those who witnessed in the community, invited people to church and talked with them about the church and Word of God became the Evangelistic Ministry, and so on. Other labels include: Men's Ministry, Women's Ministry, Singles' Ministry, Children and Youth Ministry, and Seniors' Ministry. For those who sang, danced or played instruments, the new title became the Music Ministry or the Ministry of Worship Arts.

In order to develop of sense and meaning of ministry, those who are involved must understand the dichotomy of servitude and leadership in effective ministry. It is easy enough to lead, but to minister means placing oneself at the disposal of others. The meaning of ministry must become incarnate in the mind, life, and activities of each member. They must see themselves as an integral part of the total church ministry. The music ministry must see themselves as the musical extension of the preacher and the spoken Word – in effect, musical servants of the Word. In many cases, it is because the members have simply not been taught nor have a real understanding of the labels and titles that they bare that they get all twisted and tangled in everything except *ministry*. This is particularly true when examining some of the names that Black churches have given choirs (e.g. Senior Choir, Inspirational Chorus, Anointed Voices of Praise, and Youth and Young Adult Choir, etc.). Are we saying, you must be at least 65 to become a member of the "Senior Choir"? Does this mean that an "Inspirational Choir" has exclusive "inspirational" music and all the other choirs and music is not inspirational"? Are only anointed, saved, and sanctified voices of the church permitted to sing in the "Anointed Voices of Praise" and all others must find other refuge in the "Joyful Noise Chorus"? While it is not my intention here to dismantle or poke fun at our historic names and titles, I do think that it is worth visiting the meaning of them and re-evaluate them for the future.

The truth is much of what we referred to as the "music department" was a group of choirs that sing in the church on designated Sundays but seldom have anything to do with the other known as the "war department." In the African American

158

church, no group or organization is more visible and audible than the choir. Its history reaches into the nineteenth century: "as black churches began to emerge after the Civil War, church choirs were organized," writes J. Wendell Mapson Jr. "However, this development was not without conflict. These choirs represented a wide spectrum of music, from choirs steeped in the tradition of the Fisk Jubilee Singers to note-singing (using do-re-mi) choirs and quartets in the deep South. It is essential to understand that among the black masses particularly, the black church became the center of community activity. Music became an important function and the church became, among other things, a kind of entertainment center. To some extent, the congregation became the audience, the pulpit a stage, and the folk preacher and choir, the entertainers."

"[C]hoirs have elected officers, purchased music and robes, conducted special events, and participated in visits and exchanges too numerous to count," according to Floyd Massey Jr. and Samuel B. McKinney. "These activities have not only enriched the church but also have created another arena for participatory growth for its constituents."[23] In the black church, one typically will find at least five or six choirs, even if the church only has one hundred members. Probably no other church boasts about the number of its choirs.

Graded choir programs usually include preschool children (ages 3-5), primary (ages 6-8), junior (ages 9-11), middle school or junior high (ages 12-14, which music educators agree present the greatest challenge), high school (ages 15-18), an adult choir, and senior or seasoned adults. By contrast, most Black churches have a choir for children and/or youth, a male chorus, a women's chorus, at least two additional gospel choirs, a senior choir, and the mass choir that sings on the first or fifth Sunday and for special events. The mass choir is usually made of delegates, a few faithful willing to work with other choirs, from all of the choirs and usually totals fewer members than any one choir.

It is understandable that churches that have two and three services each Sunday need choirs and singers for these services.

However, the norm is one choir sings on the first and third Sundays, one choir sings on the second Sunday, and the children and youth sing on the fourth or fifth Sunday. Unfortunately, this means there will be a different congregation depending on the choir and singers participating in the service. The congregations from the first and third Sunday rarely interacts will the congregations from the second and fourth Sunday, except on special occasions when their favorite choir or guest preacher is in town.

One might expect each of the aforementioned choirs to sing different styles or genres of music, but in most cases they all sing some type of gospel music. One choir may sing traditional gospel, while the other choir sings contemporary gospel. One choir sings the fast gospel, while the other sings slow gospel. One choir has to sing whatever the musician can play and teach, while the other choir has several musicians and directors who teach what they like, what they know, and what is on the top charts list.

What is lacking in most situations is a well-balanced group of singers. That is, Senior Choir No. 1 may have twelve sopranos, sixteen altos, three tenors, and one bass, a man who sings the melody two octaves lower. The Male Chorus has eight, first tenors; four, second tenors; two, baritones, and seven basses who sing in two-and-a-half part harmony. And that is not to say that all of the singers have strong, reliable voices. One would think that it would be logical for two groups to combine to form a better group, but this is unlikely. The men enjoy doing everything else with the women but singing with them in church! Many choir directors cannot get men to join the mixed chorus, and unfortunately, contemporary gospel has no part for baritones or basses. Contemporary gospel music is characterized by three-part harmony (e.g. sopranos, altos, and tenors,) and the ranges are very high and a man with a bass or baritone range need not consider joining the group. This is very unfortunate for young and older men who have very beautiful and rich, God-given deep voices.

Historically, Senior Choir No. 1, the Chancel Choir, or the Sanctuary Choir has sung the anthems, hymns, and arranged concert spirituals, with some gospel. Senior Choir No. 2, the Gospel Chorus, or the Inspirational Chorus has sung gospel. Many people disagree, and I respect their position, but I find that assigning and designating genres to certain choir creates dissension and competition. This circumstance violates the apostle Paul's mandate: "Let the word of Christ dwell in you richly as you teach and admonish one another with all wisdom, and as you sing psalms, hymns, and spiritual songs with gratitude in your hearts to God" (Colossians 3:16, NIV). This exhortation does not suggest that one organize a choir for each genre.

A strong and visible music ministry – specifically the choir - is one that takes first and foremost the role of the choir. The role of the choir is to lead the congregation in worship, to represent the congregation in worship, and to instruct the congregation in worship through song. Another way to consider the choir's role is that it sings to, for, and with the congregation in worship. The first task of the choir is to lead the congregation in worship, and this leadership begins with the choir's first audible or visible activity at the beginning of worship and continues as long as the choir can be seen or heard, Noticeably wandering minds, talking, walking, chewing gum, passing notes, texting, roving eyes, wiggling bodies, and sleeping will at best distract the congregation and draw more attention to them than to God. The choir should not be the focus or center of worship, but it should help bring focus to the worship experience. When this role is not clearly understood and accepted by choir members, the church will experience singing without commitment, music without meaning, religious entertainment without reverence and anointing. The choir sings *to* the congregation with its anthems, arranged spirituals, contemporary and traditional gospel music, or even Christian hip-hop that teaches, instructs, admonishes, and even challenges the congregation. The choir sings *for* the congregation in that prepared choral music, introits, prayer and benediction responses that it cannot sing for itself, and finally, the choir sings *with* the congregations in the hymns, praise and worship music, and any music sung by the congregation.

The choir and entire music ministry must lead by example, and not only musically. The choir should lead the congregation in tithing, Bible study, and prayer. How can they lead where you do not go? How can they sing what you do not know? First Corinthians 14:15 (KJV) says, "I will pray with the spirit, and I will pray with the understanding also: I will sing with the spirit, and I will sing with the understanding also." Many choirs sing texts that they do not understand or texts with which they have had no personal experience. Many choirs sit in the loft swaying and singing "What Shall I Render?" as the tithers come forward but at best tip God with a token from time to time and shout on credit! Malachi 3:8 (KJV) states, *"Will a man rob God?* But the text also means, "Will a choir, or any ministry rob God?" And choir members are not exempt from Malachi 3:10 because they are tithing their musical talents.

Choir members also need to be in prayer meeting and in Bible study so they not only sing God's Word but also know God's Word and therefore, are better equipped to sing it with power, understanding, and anointing that comes through prayer and fasting.

Austin C. Lovelace and William C. Rice describe the essential characteristics of a choir as:

(1) A dedicated group of people who have joyfully accepted the opportunities provided by the choir for advancing the kingdom of God.

(2) A leadership group in hymn singing and worship, functioning always as a part of the worshiping congregation.

(3) A priestly group, whose primary purpose is to strengthen the act of worship by singing portions of the service that the congregation is unable to do quite so effectively.

(4) An organization of people who consider that regular attendance at all choir activities is a vital part of their service to God.

(5) A crusading force, striving always to make the worship service more beautiful and more valid.

(6) A unifying force in the whole life of the church.

A choir is not:

(1) A concert organization established for the purpose of displaying individually or collectively the operatic abilities of its members. Neither is it a display for the director or organist with concert ambitions.

(2) Maintained as an entertainment and social organization to which everyone who is anyone must belong. While the social life is important, it must never interfere with the real function of the choir.

(3) A part-time group, holding the allegiance of its members on a basis of personal convenience, and accepting various flimsy excuses for their occasional attendance.

(4) A group which one condescends to serve, thereby "laying up treasures in heaven."

(5) An organization of persons who are pleased to help the director out on special occasions..

(6) An organization that increases in size, improves its attendance, and works with concentrated interest just before Christmas, Easter, and other "special" events, leaving the remaining services to get along as best they can.

(7) A group of people who may attend rehearsal, and probably the morning service if an anthem is to be sung, or the choir featured in some other fashion.

(8) An organization that offers opportunities for any kind of personal aggrandizement or for the display of temperament or jealousy.[24]

There are those who use the expression "volunteer choir" as a justification for these habits, lack of commitment, and addiction

163

to mediocrity. But one does not volunteer to attend church, to contribute to the budget, or to perform any act that is less than a just return to God. In the parable of the talents, Jesus was making a statement of cause and effect. If we fail to use our talents and by so doing fail to glorify him, we have sinned.[25] It follows then that "in the musically mature church, the ministry of choir singing is now regarded as a privilege and a trust."[26]

"Volunteer" has an additional implication that is indeed unfortunate, as Joseph Ashton aptly describes: "The shortcomings and deficiencies of the choir are many times excused on the plea that it is volunteer and that therefore a respectable standard of excellence and efficiency for its purpose is not required. That its music is distressing and the service is rendered vapid is not duly regarded. Such a plea is a matter of fact, totally unworthy of the high function of a service of divine worship."[27]

Six useful recommendations for moving toward more effective choir ministry are offered by The Reverend Dr. J. Wendell Mapson, Jr. in his book *The Ministry of Music in the Black Church*:

(1) For the health and well being of the total church, it may be advisable to limit membership in the choir to those persons who are members of the church. The church is a whole made up of many parts, and because of the interdependent nature of the body of Christ, to limit choir membership may reduce potential friction from those who may not be sensitive to the purposes and goals of the church and its ministry.

(2) One of the ways to improve the quality of music in the church is to reduce the number of choirs. Most churches have too many choirs, many of which are unnecessary....To encourage the formation of more choirs in a church is to invite as well as promote competition and confusion.

(3) One of the perennial problems in many choirs is the problem of the soloist, which in reality is the

problem of the choir. Again, the gift of the individual must be weighed against the needs of the choir as a whole. The soloist does not "own" a song, nor should one or two persons render all of the solos. However, it is also helpful to recognize that not all choir members are soloists.

(4) Church should provide money in the budget for the operation of the choir since the choir belongs to the church. It is suggested that the church, not the individual choir members, own the choirs robes, for the choir robes are church property, just as the choir is church property in the sense of accountability. Choir robes should not be faddish or profane. Their colors should reflect the symbols of the Christian faith….the aim of the choir member is not to show itself but to engage in collective worship.

(5) Choir members must guard against the temptation to exhibit self. There are manifestations of excess in the Black church. One of the most disturbing is the tendency of many choirs to become exhibitionists and performers. Many soloists thrive on attention reccived as they parade from front door to back door. Much of this is contrived and artificial.

(6) The choirs in the Black church of the masses spend much of their time and energy participating in choir anniversaries. The usual format for these annual events is for choirs from local churches to render two or more selections. These choir festivals are frequently in black churches, especially in those whose members feel a greater sense of social and economic disenfranchisement. Such events are entertaining and tend to be competitive as each choir seeks to out-sing and perform other participants.[28]

I certainly underscore all of Dr. Mapson's recommendations for moving toward more effective choir ministry, but I would hasten to add the following:

(7) Choir members must clearly understand and take

seriously the meaning of *ministry* and be equallycommitted as a servant and a leader in worship. Each member must see him or herself as in individual "minister of music."

(8) The choir director, choir members, and musicians must establish and maintain a personal commitment to Bible study and devotional periods in their lives, as well as committing to active involvement in the cooperate Bible study, prayer meeting, Sunday school, and even tithing! The choir should lead the congregation by example and not by singing.

(9) Occasionally, the choir, in conjunction with thepastor and ministerial staff, seek to deepen their understanding of the texts and meaning of what it is they are really singing. Many choirs sing the "top forties" on the charts but have no real understanding of what it is they are singing. Two questions should be paramount for every musical selection: First, does it honor God? and second, Is it biblically based, theologically sound, and culturally relevant? Choir members must understand what they are doing what and why they are singing.

(10) All rehearsals and meetings of the choir should be well planned by the director and should begin and end *on time*! People appreciate the fact that you respect their time and don't waste it after they have come to rehearse or meet. Rehearsals should move with a sense of urgency and direction. When rehearsals lag, attention is lost, boredom sets in, and discipline problems may even arise. **Where there is no discipline, there can be no serious learning.** Don't waste valuable time in rehearsal.

(11) Music ministries should have a well-defined mission statement that complements and supports the overall mission of the church. That mission statement should answer the questions, Why do we sing? For whom do we sing? What do we sing? What is the ultimate purpose for our existence as a choir or instrumental

ensemble? Every choir member should be able to recite that statement on the sport.

(12) Finally, a music ministry must have a sincere desire to grow and develop. "Getting the house," stirring up a shout, applause, and standing ovation from the congregation, and getting a record deal is not what singing is all about in the church. A serious strategic plan for choir growth and development – spiritually, musically, and socially will bring to the group a more serious commitment among existing members and attract others in the congregation to a thriving and mature music ministry. Whether the choir's goals are to increase the members hop, to broaden the repertoire to include more diverse musical offerings, to develop sight-reading and basic music fundamental competencies, or to provide retreats that address that musicianship, spirituality, and purpose, a short-and long-term plan should always be before the group. The choir should have measurable objective and should be able to clearly assess their progress.

In today's churches, music ministry is not limited to choirs, but to instrumental ensembles, orchestras, and praise teams. An orchestra or instrumental ensemble, well prepared and rehearsed, adds a new dimension to a worship service – whether playing by itself, with the choir, or accompanying congregational singing. Instrumental music is most effective in worship when the music brings to mind the text of the song or provides a background suitable for Scripture meditation. It is a great blessing to instrumentalists to minister with their gifts and skill in worship. Not all members of the congregation are singers. Many adults have instrumental backgrounds having played instruments throughout their secondary school and college years. They continue to play for recreational purposes or just for the pure enjoyment of playing and seek a place to put them to use. It is important that the pastor and church leaders are in full support of beginning and perpetuating an instrumental group. A pastor's support in and out of the pulpit is effective and vital. Quintessential to the success of an endeavor demands a gifted, talented, skilled, God-loving, patient instrumental director. The players must enjoy and respect their conductor, enjoy the rehearsal, and know that they are accomplishing something. They are giving their time to God, not to the director, and the director must be prepared to make maximum use of it.

Jeff Cranfill offers these helpful ideas for beginning an instrumental program:

(1) Pray that God would bring the players necessary, as well as meet the schedule and budget needs.

(2) Select a date to begin rehearsals and a date for the group to play in a service. A goal for a certain worship service is important to get players motivated.

(3) Advertise church-wide and in the community for interested players.

(4) Have players call in advance to register to help determine what music can be played.

(5) Select, purchase, and distribute music before the first rehearsal. Select music that glorifies God, ministers to your congregation, and suits your group.

(6) Love and encourage the players in rehearsals; make them feel welcome.

(7) In the service, the orchestra can play solo pieces (preludes, offertories, and postludes) or accompany congregational singing. There are several instrumental hymnals available.

(8) Have an all-church orchestra. Invite everyone who plays or has played an instrument in the past to come for a one-time event on a Sunday afternoon. Make the music available ahead of time for those who want to practice. Rehearse together that afternoon, have dinner together, then play during the evening service.[29]

In many churches Handbell choirs have enriched the worship services and have created opportunities for more congregational participation and involvement. "Over the years," says Tracy

Wilson "the outstanding educational value of a Handbell program has been demonstrated in the arena of music education, especially when used with children….As the ringers perform in services, they learn about worship and what it means to lead in worship."[30] There is an outstanding fellowship value for all age groups in the Handbell ministry. Many adults will join a bell choir who would never join a vocal ensemble. Do not underestimate the power of bell choirs for your church.

Ideally a music ministry of the church should have a mission statement that supports and harmonizes the church's mission statement. This has to be more than just well chosen rhetoric on paper but a genuine commitment in perpetual practice. One church developed the following mission statement: "The purpose of this church shall be as revealed in the New Testament, to win people to faith in Jesus Christ and commit them actively to the church, to help them grow in the grace and knowledge of Christ, that increasingly they may know and do his will, and to work for the unity of all Christians and with them engage in the common task of building the Kingdom of God."

Once the mission statement is defined, a ministry can write corresponding goals and objectives that support that mission statement. Church members are effectively assimilated into the life of the church when they feel a sense of purpose, direction, and value. Bill Owens provides this helpful insight: "Develop at least a five-year strategic plan that shows the present operating status of the church and what the church hopes to accomplish at the end of five years. Include information such as: Mission Statement, Values, Vision, Who We Serve, Long-range Goals, Assumptions, Strengths, Weaknesses, Challenges, Opportunities, Critical Issues, Strategies, and Future View".[31] Once there is a plan, the intermediate steps and daily tasks must be accomplished. The, "Plan your work and work your plan!"

When the mission is clear, it is easy to evaluate the strengths, weaknesses, and growth opportunities of the music ministry. On an annual basis, a more detailed evaluation should take place and may be part of the "Music Ministry Summit" or "Music Ministry

Retreat or Workshop". As it relates to the perpetuation and use of Black sacred music, in conjunction with European American music, Wyatt Tee Walker strongly declares:

"...[A]t the individual church level at least and, one would hope, at denominational and educational levels as well, a conscious decision must be made to preserve the musical idiom of the Black religious experience. It will not suffice for any such program to move on the charisma of the pastor, who may be gone next week. An unsympathetic successor can undo in five months what a predecessor has labored five years to develop. The conscious decision might well take the form of a church resolution of policy, acted upon by the entire body that says in substance, 'We will be true to our heritage and preserve the musical idiom of our forefathers, whose faith has brought us as far as we have come.' This step is buttressed by conveying to musicians employed by the congregation that the use of Black sacred music in all of it traditional forms (in conjunction with European American music) is a matter of church policy."[32]

An old preacher once said, "Every Sunday I try to find *new* ways to tell the *old* story." As a music ministry, we must too find *new* and creative ways to tell the *old* story in song so that it is formative, transformative, educational, cognitive, inspiring, uplifting, and palatable to the congregation. Several years ago I was invited to a consultation with the Mormon Tabernacle Choir in Salt Lake City, Utah. As I waited in the office for the director and associate director of the choir, I noticed a sign on the wall that hung above the administrative offices, which read "Organized for Excellence". It caught my attention and certainly justified what I had observed and heard from that outstanding choir for many years. Excellence honors God and should be the goal and expectation **every** Sunday and not just for "special" occasions and events such as: Christmas, Easter, Church Anniversary, choir concerts, or for a CD or DVD project. Excellence in music ministry strives to be consistent therefore avoiding the beating-into- shape and panic-mode teaching and preparation for the special occasions. A well-organized and vital music ministry must have goals, standards, and objectives, which are the scaffolding on which great music is created and the foundation on which a strong and visible ministry stands.

Recruiting, Hiring, and Retaining Staff
Once the church has established a mission statement, effective church ministries, departments, and committees develop corresponding goals and objectives. These guidelines give direction for ministry style, staff hiring, and program development. Without a clear mission statement, church leaders and laypersons become polarized and divided. Many attempt to implement their own desires rather than serve the needs of others. Since preferences vary, this issue is especially relevant when acquiring church music staff.

"The church is becoming what the church staff is!"[33] This statement bears out the importance of positive church staff relationships. There may be no greater challenge facing ministries today than maintaining a positive staff relationship with colleagues. Bo Presser says "If the church of today is going to enjoy a healthy congregational life, the church staff must learn how to relate positively with one another."[34] Lyle Schaller in *The Multiple Staff and the Larger Church* outlines the "7 C's of Staff Relationship": compatibility, continuity, competence, confidence, coherence, complementary relationships, and conceptualization of the role in regards to the particular congregation.[35] A closer looks at each of these may provide a positive model of the characteristics for productive staff relationships.

(1) *Compatibility* – Compatibility speaks to how well the staff ministers work together. This trait speaks to the passion, harmony, and unity of the staff.

(2) *Continuity* – The staff that stays together grows closer and more comfortable with one another. According to George Barna in his "Research Trends" (2001), the average length of service for ministers is now less than four years. Longevity of service allows ministers to understand the inner workings of the congregation. Longevity allows the minister time to build relationships and put in place procedures for getting things done.

171

(3) *Competence* – Obviously, hiring competent and professional staff is crucial. Ministers must operate with a high degree of professionalism. Congregations have high expectations of their staff ministers. They pay us good money to do good work. Our work is a reflection of the congregation.

(4) *Confidence* – Professional behavior elicits trust and confidence from the congregation. As you work hard and work smart, the confidence in your leadership grows. In doing the right thing, and doing things right, you exhibit professionalism and build confidence. Working with confidence also instills confidence in those with whom you work. Confidence breeds confidence.

(5) *Coherence* – Staff ministers spend a tremendous amount of time making sure all the ministries of the church flow together. Staff ministers have to share in a team approach to ministry. All the ministries must flow toward the same goal.

(6) *Complimentary Relationships* – This area describes how we fit together as a staff. Each brings gifts and abilities to our ministry. If all staff ministers have the same strengths, we are not complementary; we are one-dimensional. Churches should call staff ministers who complement one another.

(7) *Conceptualization* – This speaks to a congruence of ministry to the individual congregation. Too often, ministers come to a church, put in play a set of ministry programs, and when they run out of programs, they simply go to the next church and work through their "bag of tricks" again. This approach to ministry does not show much congruence to a particular congregation, nor does it show professional growth. While all ministers have a basic set of programs and approaches, these must be tailored to reflect an understanding of the particular church setting in which the minister serves.[36]

While Lyle Schaller refers to the ministerial staff in his book, his "7 C's" are most appropriate and applicable to the staff of a music ministry. When hiring and compensating the music staff, the church must understand the value of skilled and trained music leaders. According to Kennon Callahan, after a pastor is employed, the part-time or full-time director should be the second staff person hired, regardless of church size.[37] This opinion correlates to the principal music ministry role of enhancing corporate worship and thereby moving persons into a closer relationship with God. Callahan states: "If only one thing can go well in a given local church, it is important that worship go extraordinarily well."[38]

Music staff employment should be based upon education, experience, a variety of skills, and most important, leadership. Since music is extremely influential in the Black church and in reaching baby boomers, salary priorities and long-term employment should be given to highly skilled leaders. Whether hiring a choir director, an organist, a pianist, bass or leader guitarist, percussionist, or a paid soloist, successful music ministries require talented leadership, not prima donnas and divas. Bill Owens asserts "Musical aptitude and talent will not transfer from church musician to the layperson. Leadership, theology, knowledge, and skill development do."[39]

It actually cost less to compensate a gifted music person competitively than to hire several part-time or full-time persons with inadequate salaries over a period of years.[40] Higher turn over requires additional training and negatively affects church growth and other staff. Also, other churches will always consider underpaid gifted music leaders "fair game." **Talented staff positively affects church growth and justify their own salaries through their effectiveness.**

In 1985 Wendell P. Whalum identified five categories of problematic music personnel who were serving in many churches at that time.

The talented but untrained musicians. These musicians often cannot read music, have no knowledge of choir organization or directing, and have no knowledge of a study of hymns, liturgy, or religion in history.

The untrained and untalented, but willing musicians. This group, larger in number than one would suspect, is made up of those who usually have had one or two years of piano, not music, and are willing because no one in the church will (or can) assume the music responsibility.

Those musicians with basic music training who accept church duties without understanding what the program should be about and how it should be conducted. The result is that much of what is offered is out of focus with the needs and understanding of the congregation.

Those musicians with good training and excellent exposition who shut their eyes to what the level of their congregation actually is and, instead of educating them, operate on a plane always too sophisticated. It is this group that will frequently impose oratorios, cantatas, and pageants on people not yet fully educated in hymns and anthems and who are, therefore not ready for extended works.

Those musicians with excellent training who, unfortunately, take an attitude of superiority and make no attempt to lift the level of musical awareness upward except by chance. This kind of musician is usually organist-director and is so "important" until he will only officiate at Sunday morning services, funerals, and weddings of families of prominent citizens in the community.[41]

Since that time at least three new "problematic" categories of musical personnel can be found in our churches. One is **the** *artist in residence.* This person often has received national or international acclaim and has recorded CDs with one or two popular songs. The artist in residence appears for a limited number of rehearsals and the Sunday morning worship services. He or she may perform only two or three Sundays a month; this leaving the other Sundays to the youth and children, seasoned saints, and another musician.

The second new category is the *minister for youth and music, the minister of Christian education and music,* **or the** *church administrator and music director.* This person serves the church part-time as a youth minister, Christian education director, or

174

church administrator, or any combination of the aforementioned. From 9:00 am to 5:00 pm Monday through Friday, this person answers the phone, tends to clerical details, runs errands, and administers other aspects of the church's ministries. This employee is overworked, tired, and unable to do either job well because of the overwhelming responsibilities related to each position. However, the church feels that they can better justify a full-time salary if one person has all of these duties and responsibilities and spends that many hours at the church.

The third new category is **the *gifted and talented gospel musician*,** who can perform only contemporary gospel music but is given the title "Minister of Music" or "Director of Music Ministry" and placed in charge of the music program. This music does not read music, and often does not work with the youth or children. If hymns are used in the service, they are all *gospelized.* The choir is trained by rote, and all music is learned by CDs, even in rehearsals. What is popular on the radio, television, and *Billboard* charts determines the selection of music for the choir and congregation.

James Robert Davidson defines a minister of music as "the person who combines the tasks of ministry and music leadership...and is often ordained to the ministry with music as the tool of his calling. This role includes the gathering of the people, the teaching of them, and the caring for them through a musical dimension within the total redemptive-creative activity." He explains that the term "is relatively recent to church music having appeared around the mid-twentieth century among evangelical Protestant churches in America. A real impetus toward its use came from the Southern Baptist Convention with its establishment of the Department of Church Music in 1941 as a part of the Sunday School Board and its implantation of Schools of Church Music in the various seminaries."

An even more important difference, says Davidson, is that unlike the director of music, the minister of music is involved with more than simply choral and instrumental ensembles and leading the congregational singing. He is concerned with the total

175

congregation, what the needs are of the congregation as individuals, and what music will best meet the needs, and effect a desired response. Through his choice and use of music, he is involved in the process of instilling theological concepts as well as a devotional vocabulary. His ability to know his congregation and individual attitudes, to identify with these, and to provide the catalyst for a feeling of community in the proclamation of Christian truth through music comprise the discipline and limits of his work.[42]

Although this definition does not reflect what many minister of music do, it is a model to which we can aspire. Some churches refer to this person as the director of music, director of music and worship, the music coordinator, or director of choirs. The main issue is the specific role of that musician for that congregation. The title assigned to the musician should be accompanied by a comprehensive, explicit job description for the position. It must be clear what is expected, what is required, and what method of evaluation will be used to assess those expectations and requirements often referred to as duties and responsibilities. They will not be the same for every church![43]

Before earthshaking forces began to transform the church during the 1960s, there was an acknowledged right way to fulfill the role of church musician. However, there is no longer a generic right way but rather *many* right ways. The role now requires that musicians seek to determine what is appropriate for the particular occasion in which a particular congregation gathers to worship.[44] This decision involves interrelated and sometimes conflicting needs, including the church's tradition, the ever-expanding repertoire of congregational songs, what resources are available, current history, acoustics, liturgical developments within the denomination, the state of the relationship with the pastor and worship committee, the pastoral needs of the community, and the kind of musical leadership that is available among the people.[45]

"Good musicians cost money" says Wyatt Tee Walker. "The effective development of a musical program with a pronounced

176

bicultural stance will not proceed with a church policy statement alone. It must have the parallel *budget* commitment. Church musicians generally received short shrift for any number of reasons too varied to list here." Walker believes, "The primary reason is low-budget priority. It will become the responsibility of church leadership to see to it that companion budget commitment is made attendant to the policy commitment."[46]

The music ministry is not only for those members who are involved in it as direct participants, but also for the entire congregation. Therefore, investing a substantial portion of the budget in the music ministry can have dramatic and revitalizing results that invigorate the whole church. Nevertheless, there will be frequent opposition to adequate funding of the music ministry, and wise pastors will prepare themselves in advance for its support. Such opposition usually comes from the church financial leaders, staff, or volunteers, and from people who are advocates of other areas of the church's ministry. In his book *Music and Vital Congregations: A Practical Guide for Clergy*, William Bradley Roberts observes that "When parish finances leaders, staff or volunteers, look for ways to trim the budget, they often look quickly over the figures and target what looks like an excessive amount for music. For reasons that a psychologist could explain better than I, financial people – church treasures, budget committees, others charged with fiscal responsibility – often seem unsympathetic to funding music."[47] He continues, "Perhaps the analytical nature of accounting contrasts with the expressive, emotionally charged nature of music. Indeed, in looking for a good accountant, you want someone who approaches the work objectivity rather than with feeling. There are blessed exceptions, but the tendency to discount music is apparent in the behavior and value system of many financial folks."[48]

A standard rule of thumb is that the music budget, including salaries should be about a tenth of the overall church budget. This can be explained as a tithe of our resources for worship, since every aspect of music ministry leads to that goal. Some of the things that are needed to be included in a music budget

177

include: (1) salaries (which is likely to be the largest item), (2) staff musicians/singers, (3) instrumentalists, (4) instrument maintenance and tunings, (5) sheet music and CD recordings, (6) copyright licenses, (7) professional growth and development for the ministry – e.g. workshops, conferences, guest artists, and (8) robe maintenance. Even in the smaller churches, these are items that should be included to insure a strong and visible music ministry. There are many excellent resources that can assist pastors and music leaders with music ministry budgets.[49] However, when planning a budget, one must keep in mind the needs and financial ability of the local congregation as opposed to the budgets in these resources.

Finally, the supply-and-demand for good church musicians seems to be on the side of the musicians now. Therefore, the recruiting and hiring of a good musician can be complicated and discouraging. There is a not a week that goes by that I do not receive a call, email, or letter from a church or pastor looking for a musician. Ideally, our colleges and universities should be the obvious place to contact when searching for a musician, but many of them do not have students interested or preparing for church music ministry or program in church music that are sensitive to the unique needs and preparation for the Black church, unfortunately that includes many of our Historically Black Colleges and Universities (HBCUs). There are students that are very competent in performance areas but lack people-skills, a commitment to the church, and a love for the Lord.

The first and foremost requirement for a church music should be to Lord God with all one's heart and one's entire mind and to treat their neighbor as themselves. In addition to possessing natural gifts and talents, and skills, musicians must love the Word of God so much so that they become lifelong students of the Word. Musicians must also love the church and its people. Too often, churches are held hostage to a musician with great skills and talents but no love for people or the church. Quite simply, it is about the check!. The "pastoral" aspect of their ability is seriously wanting. A musician that cannot work with people, love people, care for people, and be considerate of their circumstances will not be effective and will, at best, frustrate the members that remain and ultimately, lead to decreased participation.

One of the finest books that I have found very useful in hiring and negotiating salaries for musicians, written with the Black church in mind, is *Excellence in Worship: Should Church Musicians Be Paid?* by Darrell R. Alexander. Alexander offers these "Seven Suggested Principles When Hiring a Church Musician":

(1) The musician has a personal relationship with God.

(2) The musician is anointed, skilled, and educated; possesses administrative and communication skills; and can teach all genres of Christian and gospel music.

(3) The musician demonstrates leadership qualities and works well with the pastor and others.

(4) The musician plays either piano and/or organ, can read music, is familiar with traditional hymns, and can conduct an entire worship service.

(5) The musician returns tithes and offerings to the church of their choice. (Some musicians are members of churches other than those they work for.)

(6) The musician's compensation package should be commensurate with their duties – including time required for rehearsals, preparation, and travel – education, and years of experiences. All are vital.

(7) The musician respects the leadership of the church and has knowledge of and experience in budget management.[50]

Another very helpful resource written specifically for the African American church musicians by Roland W. Perry II is entitled *The African American Church Musician's Compensation & Salary Handbook*. It is a must-have for pastors, church personnel committees, ministers of music, deacons, and trustee boards. It is written in two sections and provides sample job descriptions, pay scales, evaluations, and other helpful information. Prior to the resources of Perry and Alexander, we did not have resources specifically for the African American church and churches often referred to the American Guild of Organists and other charts and guidelines that were not relevant or applicable to the majority of African American churches.

Again, while colleges and universities are appropriate places to look for musicians, it is wise to consult with music professors, current music ministers of successful music ministries, and other musicians who network and travel on a larger scale for references. Occasionally, there are musicians who want to make a change, but have not been able to make connections. Recently, websites have emerged that post church announcements for employment and musicians' resumes. The annual Hampton University Ministers and Musicians Conference have instituted an Academy of Church Music for graduate and undergraduate students who are seeking employment and opportunities in church music. Most of them are currently working in churches while they are pursuing their degrees but have expressed interest in new opportunities.

The never-ceasing question, "Where can we find a musician?" will need to be addressed *proactively* instead of continuing in our current situation which has *reactively* responding, hiring, and promoting anyone who plays in C, F, G, and Bb on Easter. We must identify talented young people in our churches as well as "nontraditional" students who are willing to submit to the discipline and training needed to become proficient in ministering church music. Scholarships for quality training programs must be provided in this regard. However, specific criteria must define how and where these scholarships will be paid. These scholarships should be for students who have an expressed interest and demonstrated commitment to the music of the church, who will serve the church while completing their training, and who will make a commitment to return and serve the sponsoring congregation for a specified number of years.

One of the most neglected areas that pastors and church leaders tend to overlook is in their own backyard! God has placed in their church adult members and gifted and talented young people who need to be encouraged and supported into further developing and utilizing their gifts in the church. The members are often overlooked and will eventually find other places where their gifts will be utilized.

When developing, recruiting, hiring, and maintaining vital staff for the music ministry, do not neglect the most important ingredients and essentials – prayer and fasting!

Pastor and Musician: Forging a Partnership
"It will remain bad theology so long as the theologian and artist refuse to communicate with one another, as long as the theologian regards the artist as fundamentally a temperamental trifler, and the theologian as an obstinate and ignorant theorist, the best we shall get is patronage from church to music, together with tentative moralisms from musicians to musicians," Eric Routley wrote in his classic *Church Music and Theology.* "At worst it will be, as it often in practice is, a wicked waste of an opportunity for glorifying God through fruitful partnership."[51] If we substitute the word *pastor, minister,* or *priest* for "theologian" and the term *musician,* or *choir director* for "artist," these words are still relevant in the twenty-first century Christian church.

In the ideal situation, the pastor will select the music director or minister of music. While it is true that the congregation serves the congregation and needs to be able to work with a variety of people (including the music committee, choir, deacons, trustees, stewards, etc.), it is the pastor with whom the musician must work closely on a weekly basis. Although music committees or human resources representatives may present candidates, the final decision should rest with the pastor who has carefully examined and screened the candidate for musicianship, spirituality, sociability, integrity, and their ability to work with others.

It is unfortunate that pastors and musicians in so many churches give little to any time in developing a strong and fruitful partnership. In some worship services, the pastor takes one path and the musician takes another, and there is little evidence of communication about the service. Sunday after Sunday, the congregation must endure liturgical collisions and digest casseroles of unrelated topics and elements in worship. The worshipers wonder, "What in the world are we doing?" "Why did they not talk about this before now?" It is distracting, disengaging, and confusing when the sermon, scriptures, and music are not related. It is devastating when, after a wonderful sermon, a musician selects an invitational hymn, choir selection, or solo that is unrelated and destroys the message or puts out the fire! This happens so frequently that most Sundays the congregation expects "Just As I Am," "I Surrender All," "Come to Jesus," "Amazing Grace," "Softly and Tenderly," or "I Have Decided to Follow Jesus" regardless of what the minister has preached.

Although the pastor is the chief shepherd and executive officer of the church, he or she must be willing "to abdicate an autocratic attitude, open up to dialogue, and move from pride to partnership," a phrase coined by Don Wardlaw. Successful partnerships begin with understanding, and productive partnerships rely on quality communication.

Many people confuse talking with communicating! People think the more they talk, the better they are communicating, but good communication begins when we stop talking and listen. Much of the time we can improve our communication skills by listening more. Talking at people means we not only miss what they are saying but always risk misunderstanding their point of view. We then leave the encounter further convinced of how right we are, which hardens our position.[52] It is no wonder that the other person in not enthusiastic or optimistic about future dialogue.

"Four ways to improve communication between pastor and musician," says N. Lee Orr, are to "make no assumptions, to check out things before acting, to learn to listen, and to use reason rather than emotion."[53] This essential partnership may be strengthened by genuinely understanding each other, being dependable, and learning how to negotiate. Learning to negotiate is challenging but can be achieved by following these suggested steps:

(1) Focusing on the problem, not the person.
(2) Staying open to other ideas, not arriving with a closed mind.
(3) Listening genuinely, not simply waiting until it your turn to speak.
(4) Remaining flexible, not stating things in absolute terms.
(5) Staying committed to the process, not retreating when things become difficult.[54]

Successful partnerships require more than following the suggestions in this chapter or any other book. Affirming a partnership needs broader participation than enacting correctly and avoiding mistakes. Working partnerships between ministers and musicians are the result when both parties actively support the other, avoid public criticism of the other, ignore minor irritants, and work toward building a friendship.[55]

Pastor and musician need to possess a rudimentary knowledge of the suppositions, skills, and vocabulary of each other's discipline. Without this knowledge communication and partnership become difficult or even impossible, and even the best-intentioned efforts at collaborative ministry become strained. "Clergy who have had excellent instruction in pastoral care often lack in sense of how to converse in a professional way with one of the single most colleague in their ministry: the church musician." [56] Carol Doran and Thomas Troeger continue, "The story works in reverse as well: the musician, inexperienced in discussing theology and often feeling powerless, is fearless of beginning a conversation about the way music functions in the liturgy. Sometimes musicians view their contribution entirely from the perspective of performance without considering how it fits with the liturgical and pastoral needs of the congregation."[57]

The quintessential pastor and musician possess a common vision of their task and a sufficient understanding of each other's vocabulary and perspective. If the two lack a common vocabulary and vision, the church's worship life suffers, and it is a rare Sunday when people experience unity and being on one accord. Then, the finest preaching and the most polished and spirited singing and playing cannot redeem the situation. The first redemptive means to expand our thinking about theology and music, Doran and Troeger believe, is to develop a more positive appreciation for the non-verbal dimensions of the Word (Logos) and to understand music as a pastoral art.

Wyatt Tee Walker declares, "[P]astor and choir director/minister of music/organist must be partners for Christ sake!....Pastors and musical directors must face the reality that when we approach the task of preparing to lead the Lord's people in worship, we need to check out egos at the door. This idea of turf...is counter productive to that which is our central mission – leading folks to Christ."[58]   The musician ought to be able to take the minister's subject and sermon text and provide music that will complement, reinforce, and support the message. A general knowledge of Scripture is a must, as is knowledge of a repertoire that will enhance the message. When the musician does this, the congregation is inspired, educated, and lifted through both the sermon and the music, which serves as handmaiden or servant of the spoken Word. When the minister and music work together, worship can be a glorious experience. Their fruitful, harmonious collaboration blesses the congregation. Musicians commonly complain that ministers do not know what the sermon will be until late that week and sometimes not until Sunday morning. If this is case, it is not likely that the sermon and music will correspond.

Although weekly meetings are ideal, a monthly meeting of the music staff with the pastor and other worship leaders is the minimum. Regular meetings allow staff to evaluate the past and plan for future worship experiences. Candler School of Theology's associate dean of chapel developed a worship planning model called the POW'R Model which stands for – planning, organizing, worshiping, and reflecting. It is a very successful model, which I highly recommend for these meetings. Coming together allows interaction, critique, compliments, and opportunities to be present in an environment that provides for growth. The meetings should always begin with the positive aspects of the worship service, more to constructive evaluation, and then review the negative aspects. Pastors and musicians owe it to the congregation – the people who pay their salaries – to meet regularly and plan for the gathering on the Lord's Day. As people are invited to the Table, the pastor and musician are responsible for preparing for that meal!

One of the questions from my dissertation was, "What can be done to improve the relationship between the minister and musician?" "Three things: commitment, communication, and consecration," replied The Reverend Dr. Frank Madison Reid, Pastor of the Bethel AME Church in Baltimore. "I think that the relationship at best should be that of a good marriage…Constant communication fosters the partnership….Finally, prayer and fasting should be a part of the spiritual life of both the minister and musician and should be shared as an ongoing part of the partnership – consecration, that is."[59]

Pastors and musician must purpose in their hearts to have a genuine, consistent partnership for the sake of the mission that is much bigger than either of the two individuals. This is easier said than done, but it **must be a priority** if a strong and visible music ministry is to be developed and maintained.

Cautions
I offer these few cautions that I hope and pray will help to develop and maintain a strong and visible music ministry and congregation. Several have already destroyed music ministries and congregations.

Church leaders often have difficulty obtaining the insights necessary to design worship music programs that meet the spiritual needs of [**all**] age ranges. Often, leaders unknowingly amputate their church's future by wall-to-wall reruns of effective church music from the 1950s or by insisting on the top 40s of the contemporary gospel music charts. While youth and young adults will not put up with what they define as bad and boring music, in order to hear good preaching, the adults and seasoned-citizens will not tolerate the loud and showy music, in order to remain in the churches that they had been members for a number of years. Unfortunately, many congregants, if forced to choose between good music and good preaching, will pick a church with what spiritually and musically re-creates them but has less effective and substantive preaching. Ideally the preaching and music should be so carefully planned and prepared that this will not become an issue.

Today many pastors, choir directors, musicians, and congregations confuse "praise-centered" and exciting worship with authentic, God-centered worship. The instrumentation, singers, ecstasy, volume, and style of music tend to define the experience that, while filled with excitement, hand capping, swaying, rocking, and dancing, can quickly become entertainment. The risk is that when pastors, worship leaders, musicians, and congregations have not been taught to worship, or even what worship is, they must be entertained and those who lead the worship must provide the entertainment. If or when this musical/religious entertainment loses it appeal, worshipers will soon seek other venues for the desired response. The late Wendell P. Whalum, Sr., once said, "As I see it, clergy and musicians are both to be blamed for what has occurred and logically, it is their responsibility to correct. [Some] of the blame, too, will inevitably point to many of use who, in addition to being practicing church musicians, also have, little by little, abdicated our responsibility of instructing those who have not had good solid training but who, for various reasons, assume the task. We are therefore guilty of standing by through the years watching music in the Black Church, to a large degree, deteriorate and, to some extent, decay."[60]

This is perhaps why the Black church is experiencing an appalling release and replacement of seasoned and trained

186

musicians with new and younger contemporary musicians, many of whom have little or no musical training, who help fill the pews with "praisers" and the offering plate with bid dollars. These aforementioned musicians who have faithfully served the church are being let go because pastors feel that they have lost their usefulness and relevance. This less-than-pastoral gesture and often unfair treatment has split churches and perpetuated even deeper tension and wars, dividing not only churches but also families. If these musicians are to be released or replaced, it is only appropriate that it is done in a dignified and amicable manner that should characterize a Christian church.

The music wars, with all of its casualties, seem to be fueled by personalities, personal preferences, and a commercial music industry that has little or not concern for what is pleasing to God, what honors God, what is biblically based, theologically sound, culturally relevant, or what brings people to know God. In our churches, music has become a device of complacency, self-possession, and preference with no regard for our neighbors. I am afraid that we have successfully reduced the discussion and subject of worship in the Black church to preaching and music, and it all has to do with what we prefer and what we like. The rich and diverse musical styles that have long characterized the Black church tradition are seriously in danger of extinction. By neglecting and casting out the historical congregation spirituals, traditional Christian hymns, and hymns by Black composers, the Black church loses the rich musical heritage and legacy that has made it possible for new generations to enter. This would not be a consideration in Judaism! The Black church cannot afford to abandon its Christian musical *tradition,* even though it certainly must critically and responsibly abandon its *traditionalism!* The Black church should not close its mind and ears to the creative sounds and texts of contemporary gospel music and Christian hip-hop. It should sing all of the music that is appropriate for cooperate worship in the church. I only caution that the biggest word in *contemporary* is "temporary" and too often what is here today is swiftly forgotten and gone tomorrow. To simply replace multi-verse hymns with "7 Elevens" is not spiritually healthy if music is to be formative, transformative, cognitive, educational, and inspiring. By "7 Elevens", I am not referring to the popular food store chain, but songs which contain 7 words that are sung 11 times and then modulated only to have the same 7 words sung 11 more times louder, faster, or slower!

While music wars continue to be, in my opinion, the greatest cause of division and segregation among generations in the Black church, there are many churches, pastors and worship leaders who are conscientiously, effectively, and diligently seeking to be relevant to all generations within their congregations. However, simply "blending" musical styles, traditional and contemporary, hymns and praise and worship, old and new substance and relevance is not the answer. My colleague Thomas G. Long, Bandy Professor of Preaching, warns that, "the bare word 'blended' tends to convey the idea of a mix-and-match approach – a dash of contemporary thrown in with a measure of traditional." Too many congregations," says Long, "have adopted this compromised –we'll do a traditional hymn, then we'll do a praise song. We'll have the classic structure, but we'll spice it up with skits. A little of this and a little of that and everybody will be happy." Long is eminently wise and acutely discerning when he concludes that congregations should "create a new thing in the earth – a service of worship completely attuned to the American cultural moment but fully congruent with the great worship tradition of the Christian church; a service that attracts young people and seekers and the curious and those who are hungry for a spiritual encounter, but that does so by beckoning people to the deep and refreshing pool of the Gospel of Jesus Christ as it has been understood historically in the church."[61]

I caution pastors and musicians to resist the temptation to simply imitate or duplicate other churches or other choir programs. Many churches are aggressively impersonating, and attempting to reproduce the music and worship of other churches, denominations, television evangelists, and mega church ministries without considering the community of worshipers in which they are ministering. I have seen church choirs buy robes that are identical to another church choirs' that had become their idols; churches that build sanctuaries to the exact specifications of their idol's building, and churches that purchase furniture, fixtures, carpet, fabrics, and draperies to duplicate their idol's facility. Many churches implement organizational structures and titles to replicate their models. Models are certainly good if they genuinely enhance, elevate, augment, and are effective for a particular congregation. There are choir directors who struggle to make sure they are singing the top-forties and latest hits like their models. Pastors redesigned their worship and music programs to imitate others – thinking the grass is greener on the other side – only to discover the coveted greenery is Astroturf!

Finally, I offer this tremendous caution and warning by A. W. Tozer in the collection *Tozer on Worship and Entertainment* for pastors, worship leaders, and musicians. He seems to have accurately diagnosed the cause of the music and worship wars that we are experiencing today in our churches:

> *Pastors and churches in our hectic times are harassed by the temptation to seek size at any cost and to secure by inflation what they cannot gain by legitimate growth. The mixed multitude cries for **quantity** and will not forgive a minister who insists upon solid values and permanence. Many a man of God is being subjected to cruel pressure; by the ill-taught members of his flock, who scorn his slow methods, and demand quick results and a popular following regardless of **quality**. These children play in the market places and cannot overlook the affront we do them by our refusal to dance when they whistle or to weep when they out of caprice pipe a sad tune. They are greedy for thrills, and since they dare no longer seek them in the theater, they demand to have them brought into the church.[62]*

It must be an unswerving and nonnegotiable commitment of the pastor and the minister of music, and worship leaders to adequately plan organize, pray, implement, and reflect on the music and worship of the church to develop and maintain a strong and visible music ministry that God may be glorified, the people edified, and the world evangelized.

[1] Psalm 27: 4 King James Version
[2] Romans 12:2 King James Version
[3] Ruth 1:16 King James Version
[4] Matthew 28:19 King James Version
[5] Luke 9:60 King James Version
[6] Mark 3:33 King James Version

[7] 2 Timothy 4: 16-18
[8] Luke 23:43 King James Version
[9] W. E. B. DuBois, *The Souls of Black Folk* (New York: Dover Publications, 1994), 116.
[10] C. Eric Lincoln and Lawrence H. Mamiya, *The Black Church in the African American Experience* (Durham, NC: Duke University Press, 1990), 346.
[11] Portia J. Maultsby, "The Use and Performance of Hymnody, Spirituals, and Gospels in the Black Church", in *Readings in African American Church Music and Worship*, edited by James Abbington (Chicago: GIA Publications, 2001), 77.
[12] Ibid. 77.
[13] Linda J. Clark, *Music in Churches: Nourishing Your Congregation's Musical Life* (Herndon, VA: The Alban Institute, 1994), 3.
[14] The terms "hymn" and "anthem" are used here to devote the music, regardless of genre or style, specifically sung by the congregation – "hymns" and music sung specifically by the choir – "anthems".
[15] Clark, *Music in Churches*, 3.
[16] William Bradley Roberts, *Music and Vital Congregations: A Practical Guide for Clergy* (New York: Church Publishing, 2009), 1.
[17] Ibid., 1.
[18] Otis B. Moss, III, "That Was Then, This is NOW," in *The African American Pulpit*, 10, no. 1 (Winter 2006-2007), 8.
[19] See Robert H. Mitchell, *I Don't Like That Music* (Carol Stream, IL: Hope Publishing Company, 1993).
[20] Brian Wren, *Praying Twice: The Music and Words of Congregational Song* (Louisville, KY: Westminster John Knox Press, 2000), 71.

[21] Floyd Massey Jr. and Samuel B. McKinney, *Church Administration in the Black Perspective* (Valley Forge, PA: Judson Press, 1976), 42.
[22] Austin C. Lovelace and William C. Rice, *Music and Worship in the Church* (Nashville: Abingdon Press, 1976), 89-90.
[23] Ibid., 88.
[24] Ruth Nininger, *Church Music Somes of Age* (New York: Carl Fischer, 1957), 13.

[25] Joseph Ashton, *Music in Worship* (Boston: Pilgrim Press, 1943), 132.

[26] J. Wendell Mapson, Jr., *The Ministry of Music in the Black Church* (Valley Forge, PA: Judson Press, 1984), 42.

[27] Jeff Cranfill, "Building a Church Instrumental Ministry" in *Music Ministry: A Guidebook* edited by Donald Clark Measels (Macon, GA: Smyth & Helwys, 2004), 130.

[28] Tracy Wilson, "The Church Handbell Program" in *Music Ministry: A Guidebook* edited by Donald Clark Measels (Macon, GA: Smyth & Helwys, 2004), 121.

[29] Bill Owens, *The Magnetic Music Ministry* (Nashville: Abingdon Press, 1996), 16.

[30] Wyatt Tee Walker, "What Lies Ahead?" in *Readings in African American Church Music and Worship* edited by James Abbington (Chicago: GIA Publications, 2001), 471.

[31] Bo Presser, Charles Qualls, *Lessons from the Cloth* (Macon, GA: Smyth & Helwys, 1999).

[32] Bo Presser, "Church Staff Relationships" in *Music Ministry: A Guidebook* (Macon, GA: Smyth & Helwys, 2004), 39.

[33] Lyle Schaller, *The Multiple Staff and the Larger Church* (Nashville: Abingdon Press, 1980).

[34] Bo Prosser, "Church Staff Relationships" in *Music Ministry*. Prosser gives an extensive discussion of Lyle Schaller's "7 C's of Staff Relationships" in *The Multiple Staff and the Larger Church* in his chapter on pp. 45-49.

[35] Kennon L. Callahan, *Twelve Keys to an Effective Church* (San Francisco: Harper, 1987), 48.

[36] Ibid.

[37] Bill Owens, *The Magnetic Music Ministry*, 26.

[38] Callahan, *Twelve Keys to an Effective Church*, 51.

[39] Wendell P. Whalum, "Church Music: A Position Paper (with special consideration of music in the Black church) in *Readings in African American Church Music and Worship* edited by James Abbington (Chicago: GIA Publications, 2001), 503-504.

[40] James Robert Davidson, *A Dictionary of Protestant Church Music* (Metuchen, NJ: Scarecrow Press, 1975), 205-206.

[41] Paul Westermeyer, *Te Deum* (Minneapolis: Fortress Press, 1998), 1-2.

[42] Carol Doran and Thomas H. Troeger, *Trouble at the Table* (Nashville: Abingdon Press, 1992), 76.

[43] Ibid;, 76-77.

[44] Wyatt Tee Walker, "What Lies Ahead?" in *Readings in African American Church Music and Worship*, 471.

[45] William Bradley Roberts, *Music and Vital Congregations: A Practical Guide for Clergy* (New York: Church Publishing, 2009), 89.

[46] Ibid., 89.

[47] I strongly suggest the following sources for a more detailed discussion of church music budgets: William Bradley Roberts, *Music and Vital Congregations* (New York, Church Publishing, 2009);Bill Owens, *The Magnetic Music Ministry* (Nashville: Abingdon Press, 1996); *Music Ministry: A Guidebook* (Macon, GA: Smyth & Helwys, 2004); and C. Randall Bradley,

From Postlude to Prelude: Music Ministry's Other Six Days (St. Louis, MO: MorningStar Music Publishers, 2004);
[48] Darrell R. Alexander, *Excellence in Worship: Should Church Musicians Be Paid?* (Victoria, BC, Canada: Trafford Publishing, 2005), Chapter 10, pp. 182-207.
[49] Eric Routley, *Church Music and Theology* (Philadelphia: Muhlenberg, 1959), 110.
[50] N. Lee Orr, *The Church Music Handbook for Pastors and Musicians* (Nashville: Abingdon Press, 1991), 54.
[51] Ibid., 55.
[52] Ibid., 59-66.
[53] Ibid., 67-70.
[54] Carol Doran and Thomas H. Troeger, *Trouble At the Table* (Nashville: Abingdon Press, 1992), 79.
[55] Ibid., 78-83.
[56] Wyatt Tee Walker, "Music in Ministry, Just as Preaching is Ministry," in *Score Magazine* (September-October 1994), 66.
[57] James Abbington, "Directions for Music and Worship in the Twentieth-first Century African American Church: Interviews with Pastors, Theologians, and Musicians" presented in partial fulfillment of the requirements for the degree Doctor of Musical Arts, Horace H. Rackham School of Graduate Studies, The University of Michigan, Ann Arbor, 1999). Unpublished.
[58] Wendell P. Whalum, "Church Music: A Position Paper (with special consideration of music in the Black Church), in Abbington, *Readings in African American Church Music and Worship* (Chicago: GIA Publications, 2001), 503.
[59] Thomas G. Long, *Beyond the Worship Wars: Building Vital and Faithful Worship* (Herndon, VA: The Alban Institute, 2001), 12.
[60] A. W. Tozer, *Tozer on Worship and Entertainment,* compiled by James L. Snyder (Camp Hill, PA: Christian Publication, 1997), 101-102

Doin' Worship: From the Perspective of Musical Leadership
Patrick Clayborn and T. J. Martin, II

Introduction

One of the most important aspects of a church's life is worship. How a church comes together to glorify God speaks volumes about that church's identity. Music – singing songs and playing instruments – is one way the church worships. In this chapter, we will delve into the nature of worship and the role of music therein. We will also discuss the responsibilities of those who shape the church's music in worship: the chief musical administrator (often referred to as the minister of music), the worship leader, and the church musician.

Approaching the Definition and Nature of Worship
The term worship is flooded with meanings. The late James White, who was one of the world's foremost scholars in the area of worship, noted that the secular lineage of the term worship could be traced to "the Old English word *weorthscipe*—literally *weorth* (worthy) and *–scipe* (-ship)—and signifies attributing worth or respect to someone."[1] In the sacred history of the word worship, a wide range of meanings appears. From the Hebrew Scriptures to the Greek New Testament, worship can mean offering a sacrifice, singing, playing a musical instrument, physically bowing, dancing, shouting, praying, paying homage, confessing one's sins, confessing Jesus as Lord, or the assembling of a group to do one or more of the previously stated activities.[2]

However, by wading through this flood of meanings for worship, a unifying factor emerges: communion between God and humanity. All of the acts of worship previously named are ways in which a person or a group of people can seek an encounter with the Creator. Therefore, *worship is the communion between God and humanity*. This communion can be either individual or corporate in nature. Corporate worship is often called liturgy since "liturgy…is a work performed by the people for the benefit of others…To call a service 'liturgical' is to indicate that it was conceived so that all worshipers take an active part in offering their worship together."[3]

Worship then is a cooperative work. Either God or humanity can initiate worship. From the previously mentioned wide range of meanings for worship and from the above definition of liturgy, one can see how humanity initiates worship. Yet, one may be led to believe that worship is always begun by humanity. Two counterexamples are Jacob's dream at Bethel (Gen. 28:10-22) and Paul's travel on the Damascus Road (Acts 9:1-9). Jacob has a dream of angels ascending and descending on a ladder in Haran (a place he later names Bethel). In the dream, God promises to bless Jacob and his family. God is responsible for both the dream and the promise. Jacob confirms this when he wakes from the dream: "Surely the Lord is in the place—and I did not know it" (Gen. 28:16). Paul, on the other hand, was interrupted by Jesus the Risen Lord while he was awake.[4] As Paul journeyed to persecute the early church, Jesus confronted him with a flash of light, blinded him, and sent him in a new and peaceful direction. In both cases, God initiated the communion with humanity. These examples suggest that every moment of worship is not joyful.

The mystery of God often enshrouds worship. As a result, worship is not constantly happy or understandable. Though Psalm 16:11 states that in God's "presence there is fullness of joy; in [God's] right hand are pleasures forevermore," one must be aware that the joy in this verse is a final result of worship. This verse does not clarify the nature of the journey preceding this pleasurable destination. Many times the "path of life" God reveals is a far cry from being joyous. God commands Abraham to sacrifice his son (Gen. 22:1-14); Job receives no answers when he faces God after his ordeals (Job 38-41); the Spirit drives Jesus into the wilderness to be tempted by the devil (Luke 4:1-13); Jesus, in facing the cross, sweats as if he is bleeding while he prays (Luke 22:39-46); and Paul's prayer to God for the removal of a thorn from his flesh is denied (2 Cor. 12:1-10). The identity of worship as both bitter and sweet posits the notion that worship is holistic – no division between joy, pain, individual, corporate, sacred, and secular. All of the pieces come together and nourish each other.

Accordingly, worship entails the totality of a person's life. Communion with God is not confined to a particular time, space, ritual, liturgy, denomination, or character trait. Instead, worship is most concerned with God communing with a whole person or a whole group of people, which involves all times, all spaces, all rituals, all liturgies, all denominations, and all character traits. Jesus told the Samaritan woman, "God is spirit, and those who worship [God] must worship in spirit and truth" (John 4:24). Jesus did not make the woman's controversial marital status, her Samaritan heritage, her preferred location for worship (the mountain), or her lack of knowledge determinants for her encounter with God. Rather, Jesus challenges her to bring all of who she is, (the truth), into communion with God. Jesus tells her that true worship engages her whole life. As a result, she gives her life in service to God.

Likewise, worship has a prophetic nature. The act of worship will stand against the powers of evil. Just as a person is transformed in the moment of worship, the person's context – particularly if it is evil – can be transformed as well. David played a lyre when an evil spirit came upon King Saul, and that moment of worship relieved Saul of the evil spirit (1 Sam. 16:23). When the people of Judah were threatened by their enemies (the Ammonites, the Moabites, and the people of Mount Seir), King Jehoshaphat of Judah worshiped God and sent the singers out to the battlefield. As they sang praise to God, "the Lord set an ambush against" Judah's enemies (2 Chron. 20:5-23). After Paul and Silas were unjustly imprisoned, they prayed and sang hymns to God. During their time of worship, an earthquake shook the jail with such force "that the foundations of the prison were shaken; and immediately all doors were opened and everyone's chains were unfastened" (Acts 16:26). In each of these victorious examples, the act of worship stands against injustice. True worship always resists the powers of evil even if the results are not always immediately favorable. The writer of Hebrews mentions men and women whose worship stood against the evils of their day; unfortunately, their earthly stories end in demise (Heb. 11:35b-39). Again, they conducted their acts of worship knowing the fatal consequences. They (and their worship) rejected the evil of their time.

Interestingly, these specific acts of worship previously mentioned involve music. Once more, the musical aspect of worship is the focus of this chapter. In the next section, we will discuss the role of music in worship.

Music in Worship
Music is a typical element of worship in ancient Judaism. Psalms 95, 96, 98, 100, 101, 147, and 149 are documents used within the worship life of ancient Judaism that invite – or

perhaps command – all to worship God through singing. Psalm 150 is a directive to worship God with any and all musical instruments (including the human voice). In Num. 10, ancient Israel is commanded to play trumpets during times of celebratory sacrifices. Consequently, singers and musicians are a natural part of the liturgical landscape (1 Chron. 9:33; 15:16, 27; 2 Chron. 29:28; Neh. 7:1).

Similarly, music is a regular component in the worship of the early church. At the conclusion of the Last Supper, Jesus and the disciples sing a hymn (Mark 14:26). The writer of Colossians directs readers to "sing psalms, hymns, and spiritual songs to God" (Col. 3:16) with grateful hearts. The apocalyptic work Revelation is filled with heavenly scenes of worship through music (Rev. 4, 5, 7, 11, 15, 19). Though these scenes are visions, they reflect – in some sense – what the writer considers worship. Thus, the writer of Revelation sees music as integral for worship.

Music plays a vital role within the life of worship. First, music helps to establish the mood for worship. For example, when David retrieves the Ark of the Covenant from Obed-edom's house, David appoints singers to play instruments "to raise loud sounds of joy" (1 Chron. 15:16). Obviously, he wants to counteract the tragic memory of leaving the ark with a festive atmosphere. Second, music "keeps the group together."[5] Music tends to unify its hearers. "Thus the ideal of early Christian singing was unity...."[6] Additionally, the early church felt that its music helped them to unite with the choruses of heaven as well as with each other.[7] Third, music is one of the primary ways in which the church praises God. The early church's strict stance on the hymn as a song that gives God praise typifies this idea.[8]

In the Black Church, the importance of music for worship comes from its African origins as well as its Christian religious heritage. John Mbiti, a renowned scholar of African traditional religions, explains that worship for African peoples is their response to the spiritual world, which can be highly systematized and formal or unregimented and informal.[9] In either case, Mbiti finds that worship for African peoples involves more than just the contemplative posture. He states, "Worship is 'uttered' rather than meditational, in the sense that it is expressed in external forms, the body 'speaking' both for itself and the spirit."[10] Music is a common expression of worship among African peoples. According to Mbiti, while sacrifices, offerings, and various types of prayers are typical acts of African traditional worship, "God is often worshipped through songs, and African peoples are very fond of singing...Music, singing and dancing reach deep into the innermost parts of African peoples, and many things come to the surface under musical inspiration which otherwise may not be readily revealed."[11]

The most important inspiration music gives in worship centers on God's proclaimed word – the sermon. Music sets the atmosphere for preaching. It encourages the congregation to become attentive. In Num. 10:10, the blowing of trumpets is a signal for ancient Israel to remember God. Music also aids the preacher's preparation. When the prophet Elisha sought a word from God, he called on a musician. "And then, while the musician was playing, the power of the Lord came upon him" (2 Kings 3:15b). In addition to giving support to the sermon, music can serve as the sermon. Paul's most celebrated view of Jesus comes from his quotation of one of the early church's hymns:

> *who, though he was in the form of God, did not regard equality with God as something to be exploited, but emptied himself, taking the form of a slave, being born in human likeness. And being found in human form, he humbled himself and became obedient to the point of death – even death on a cross. Therefore God also highly exalted him and gave him the name that is above every name, so that at the name of Jesus ever knee should bend, in heaven and on earth and under the earth, and every tongue should confess that Jesus Christ is Lord, to the glory of God... (Phil. 2:6-11).*

This should not be a surprise since the musicians of ancient Israel came out of the Levites, the families of priests. The relationship between song and sermon is intimate and requires great care to keep ambiguity from dominating worship. Therefore, those responsible for the church's music have a tremendous task. They are called to offer their skills, their gifts, and their own worship in ways that inspire an environment of worship, participation in worship, and attentiveness to God's word in worship, the utterance of God's word in worship, and their own music to become God's word in worship. As a result, the standards for musical leaders in churches are high, particularly for chief musical administrators, worship leaders, and church musicians. Let us now survey their primary responsibilities and take note of their importance to the life of the church's worship.

The Roles of Musical Leadership
Both of us serve the church with our gifts in music. Each of us has led church music departments, directed choirs and praise teams, written and performed original Christian music, and served as worship leaders and church musicians. We know very well the joys, disappointments, blessings, and burdens that follow those who are called to serve God through music. If we were to share all of the lessons we have learned, the space in this chapter would be insufficient. Hence, we will focus primarily on the responsibilities of the chief musical administrator, the worship leader, and the church musician.

The Chief Musical Administrator
"Chenaniah, leader of the Levites in music, was to direct the music, for he understood it."   1 Chron. 15:22

The chief musical administrator in a church is known by many names. Music pastor, minister of music, ministerial liaison to the music department, music director, and director of worship and arts are just a few examples. In some churches, choir director continues to be the designation of the primary musician. Regardless of the title, the job remains the same – to enhance the corporate worship of a church by giving leadership to that church's music ministry.

The musical administrator gives effective leadership to the church's music ministry through a number of practices. The first two are often overlooked but are vital to the life of music ministry. First, the minister of music must have and consistently maintain a relationship with God. While this aspect of the chief musician's life is frequently assumed or ignored due to her or his talent, the music minister's relationship with God must be primary. The gifts of the Spirit are guided by the fruit of the Spirit.[12] This means that the full consummation and manifestation of a person's gifts and talents are guided by that person's character. Thus, the music pastor must seek to positively develop her or his character through a relationship with God. Second, the music director provides worthy leadership by following the church's senior pastor. We are not suggesting that the music pastor becomes a non-critical, thoughtless automaton of the senior pastor. Rather, the musical administrator – in conversation with the senior pastor – should critically survey the senior pastor's comprehensive vision for ministry and discern how her or his gifts in musical leadership can complement that vision. In 1 Chron. 15:22, Chenaniah was chosen to be the musical director because he had understanding. The verse clearly suggests that Chenaniah has a superior understanding of music. However, the verse implies that he also understands how music fits into David's larger vision for temple worship. Hence, the minister of music must constantly cultivate and nurture connections between the music ministry and the church's overall ministry.

In order to view the other practices of the musical administrator, we will briefly delve into her or his skill set. The minister of music should have competency in the areas of music, administration, and theology. Like Chenaniah, the music pastor should posses a thorough understanding of music and worship. This is what separates a minister of music from a talented singer or musician. The minister of music's understanding serves as the foundation for her or his ability to teach other musicians and singers both musical techniques and how to successfully integrate those techniques into corporate worship. Furthermore, the effective music director presents a variety of music in such a way that the congregation (people of varied musical talents) feels free to participate in song during the worship service.

Alongside the musical gift is the minister of music's gift for administration. The idea that having organization and being Spirit led are antithetical is unproductive. The leading of the Spirit should not become an excuse for failing to organize the music ministry. The music pastor should rely on the Spirit in her or his planning and should allow those plans to be adjusted by the Spirit. Consequently, the music director should make sure that all divisions within the church's music department are prepared. This includes formulating and maintaining a schedule of rehearsals and prayer meetings for all choirs, praise teams, and musicians; meeting with the church's worship committee (which in many cases may be only the pastor) regularly to critique previous musical performances, to discuss how the upcoming music will be integrated into future worship services, and to put forth plans for special musical offerings such as seasonal concerts by the church's music ministry (for Christmas, Easter, etc.). This also includes concerts by visiting artists and choirs, or recitals by budding church musicians; periodically reviewing the musicianship and the pay of the entire music staff (musicians, choir directors, praise team leaders); maintaining the budget for the music program; allocating funds for leaders in the music department to attend workshops and seminars in music and worship; meeting often with the church's sound team to ensure that they are updated on the needs of the musicians and singers; and being in touch with the life of the congregation through regular attendance in order to keep the church's music programs relevant.

In addition to musical and administrative skill, the minister of music needs an understanding of theology. According to Graham Hughes' *Worship as Meaning*, worship has meaning for an individual when the worship event "makes sense," is "multi-sensory," and "theologically competent."[13] Therefore, the music for worship must be theologically competent. However, this requires that the musical leader chosen to select the songs have a sound theology. A sound theology for an effective music ministry is a view of God that is responsive to the move of the Spirit, sensitive to the needs of the congregations, and in harmony with the theology of the senior pastor. A theologically competent minister of music decides on songs that promote the love, grace, justice, and mercy of God; that highlight the selfless work of Jesus; that invoke the presence of the Spirit; and that explore the full range of human reactions to an encounter with God or the trials of life (praise, awe, repentance, gratitude, petition, expectancy, disappointment, grief, joy, love, hope, etc.). Further, the songs selected must be appropriate for the occasion of worship (e.g. Christmas songs during Advent). They also need to be supportive of the pastor's sermon. If the pastor is preaching a series of sermons on peace, then songs upholding images of war (e.g. "I'm on the Battlefield for My Lord") will very likely undermine the pastor's efforts. The selected songs should attempt to meet the needs of the congregants as well. For instance, if persons in worship voice a struggle with health challenges, then the music director ought to move the musicians into songs that focus on healing (e.g. "Healing" by Richard Smallwood). Additionally, the music pastor has to avoid music that is theologically destructive. This involves but is not limited to music that has no clear view of God, that paints God as a cosmic genie, that focuses on the denigration of women, that excludes any of God's children from God's grace, and that is inconsistent with message of the Gospel.

In order for the music pastor to possess these skills in music, administration, and theology, she or he needs training, intuition, and the calling. Ideally, a minister of music would have degrees in music, administration, and theology; however, that notion may not be viable. Often, musical administrators in churches have at least an undergraduate degree in music or requisite musical training and experience that gives them the capacity to read, perform, and teach music at a professional level. This standard should be maintained to keep excellence in church music departments. By having great musical proficiency, the minister of music is better able to offer a wide variety of music, to demand musical excellence from musicians and singers, and to draw those with broad skills in music.

Though the music administrator may not need degrees in administration or theology, she or he ought to develop a competency in both areas. Increased competency can be gained by taking courses in administration and theology, reading works in these fields, and apprenticing for a minister of music well versed in these areas. In addition to training, a music pastor should possess intuition – an innate ability to perform music, administrate the affairs of the music department, and make certain that the church's music is theologically sound. This kind of intuition is the gift that only God can place in the music pastor. Hence, God must call the music pastor into the service of music ministry. Training and intuition are not enough assets to give a minister of music effectiveness and stability. God's call to this special service is what leads the musical administrator to a specific church and guides her or his skills and gifts. God's call is also what opens the heart of that church to the musical administrator's ministry. Therefore, it is vital for the music director, senior pastor, and entire church to stay in close relationship with God so that they can discern God's call for the church's music ministry. As a result, the gifted and anointed minister of music enlists musicians and singers who are gifted and anointed as well and provides a pastoral presence in the music department. This helps to maintain the spiritual integrity of the church's music ministry.

Now we must touch on a subject that can be controversial but is a large concern for the minister of music: finances. Those who are asked to offer their skills, gifts, and anointing in music to lead or assist the corporate worship of the church should be paid (1 Tim. 5:18). To pay musicians and praise leaders little or to disregard there payment altogether disrespects the music ministries of these persons and dishonors God. As a result, those who are skilled, gifted, and anointed for music ministry will leave churches that do not invest in music.

After the Babylonian exile, the Levites, who provided music for the temple, left the place of worship because their pay was withheld (Neh. 13:10). These musicians did not leave due to a love of money; rather, they returned to their fields because those who controlled the distribution of their payment debased the worship of God. We acknowledge that most churches cannot afford to pay musicians and singers the kind of pay they receive from record labels and that there are those with musical gifts who seek to gouge churches out of greed. However, churches ought to pay what is reasonable for their budgets, and church musicians must be willing to work with congregations that do their best to monetarily honor the musicians' faithfulness. Here, the minister of music can educate senior pastors and congregations on the financial necessities of the music ministry.

For example, a music budget is more than musicians' salaries; salaries make up one line item in a music budget. A music budget includes but is not limited to line items for the purchase of new music and equipment (musical instruments, sound equipment for music department, choir robes, etc.), for equipment maintenance, and for continuing education for the music staff (entailing conferences and music workshops).[14] Just as the church seeks ways to invest in the pastor's salary, the salaries of other staff ministers and church employees, the upkeep of the church building, and materials for Christian education, the church should and must find ways to invest in its music ministry. This is imperative because God desires for the church – even the whole world - to "break forth in joyous song and sing praises" (Psalm 98:4b).

The Worship Leader

"[The Levites] sang praises with gladness, and they bowed down and worshipped."　　　　　　　　　　2 Chron. 29:30b

A worship leader is one who guides a congregation through a worship service. This person can be a clergyperson, a layperson, a musician, a singer, or one with no musical skill. However, we will confine our brief discussion to musically inclined worship leaders: praise team leaders, psalmists, choir directors, and musicians.

The primary objective of the worship leader is to help establish an environment in the space of worship where the congregation

204

can encounter God. The leader does this by inviting the congregation to praise God, by selecting appropriate music to under gird that praise, and by encouraging the congregation to sing along with the musicians, praise team, or choir. Further, the leader, particularly the praise team leader or the psalmist, invites the church to worship through her or his singing.

Worshipping is a way of worship leading. Worship leading is not always explicitly asking the congregation to join in song, lift up or clap hands, dance, or shout. Leading worship also involves the worship of the worship leader! Of course, the worship leader can be tempted to forget the congregation and focus solely on her or his worship, but the worship leader who desires to faithfully encourage the congregation to encounter God will find her or himself mysteriously more aware of the congregation's engagement with God's presence. We have found through our experiences of leading worship that when the worship leader worships God along with the congregation, the worship leader becomes more aware of the congregation's needs and more aware of the Spirit's movement. In that moment, the Spirit may prompt the worship leader to sing a specific, well-known song or a new song; to allow the musicians to play while the worshippers rejoice in God's presence; to still all music for a period of silent praise; or to call out certain needs in the congregation and offer a word of knowledge. This is what separates an anointed worship leader from a mere church soloist.

These prophetic gifts of the anointed worship leader are the organic outgrowth of her or his relationship with God. The worship leader is actually inviting the congregation on a journey that is familiar because she or he worships God regularly. The life of the musical worship leader has to be in line with the lyrics of her or his song in order to be effective. We are not suggesting that the worship leader is perfect; rather, she or he is striving to maintain a healthy relationship with God and neighbor. In so doing, the worship leader stays sensitive to both God and humanity. This is the primary characteristic of the anointed worship leader.

The Church Musician

"David also commanded the chiefs of the Levites to appoint their kindred as the singers to play on musical instruments, on harps and lyres and cymbals, to raise loud sounds of joy."
1 Chron. 15:16

The church musician is unlike any other finely tuned professional musician. She or he is a vessel dedicated and called to minister to and before God and God's church. This role has often been misused and misconstrued throughout church history. In the early church, many leaders banned the use of musical instruments since pagan cults used the same instruments in their religious services.[15] Therefore, we will briefly cover what it means to be a musician in "God's house."

First and foremost, a church musician – like every minister – should be called to this musical vocation. The calling is a direct reflection of the musician's relationship with God. This should be the primary factor guiding a musician to her or his particular context of ministry. The calling is vital for church musicians. For, there are times in the ministry that are less than glorious and often spiritually grueling, and it is during these times that both the nature and character of the church musician becomes apparent. The calling reminds the musician that God is faithful and that God will reward her or him – even when her or his service seems to be overlooked.

Thus, the church musician should always seek the counsel of the Holy Spirit. If she or he is attentive, the Spirit will give the musician direction in song selection during the worship service. Consequently, the church musician will be Spirit-led, and this is vital for the pivotal points of worship: the prelude, the invocation, transitional times between the different elements of worship, times of prayer, during a sermon's celebration, the invitation, and during unexpected movements of the Spirit.

Without the Spirit, the church musician can easily lead the church's worship into confusion. One of the traditional interpretations of Lucifer as the first church musician is a prime example. In Isaiah 14:12, Lucifer ("son of the morning") – who is typically viewed as Satan, the dragon, or the devil – is depicted as a fallen angel. Ezekiel 28:13 describes this fallen angel as a cherub covered in precious stones and having pipes built within his body. This covering cherub was the instrument of praise. However, according to Isaiah 14:13, Lucifer sought to place himself above God. He no longer relied on God's guidance. Ezekiel 28:17 states that he undermined the very wisdom God gave him. Revelation 12:4 depicts his fall as a dragon plummeting out of heaven with its tail taking one third of heaven's stars.

Likewise, the church musician that attempts to play without God's guidance undermines the very gifts God has given her or him. She or he also poses a threat to the church's stability. Much like the dragon in Revelation, the church musician – when trying to put her or himself above God – brings destructive division within the church's music department. We have known church musicians who have attempted to put their agendas above God's will. They have tried to usurp the pastor's authority during the preaching moment with disruptive music, to encourage choir members not to show up for worship to display their power, and to destroy worship services by leaving the church without any warning. In the end, these musicians fell in the very same manner as Lucifer.

Therefore, church musicians have a responsibility to keep themselves and their minds focused on the Spirit. This helps the musician to become a conduit for the Holy Spirit in worship. T.J. recalls this memory from his early beginnings in music ministry:

> I remember learning a valuable lesson when I was young in ministry. While I was on my way from a nice dinner to a church service, I heard a beautiful melody. I was fully aware that I would soon enter the worship service, but I didn't realize that my mind was focusing on the beauty of the chords I heard. As I traveled, other songs played, and I no longer focused on the previously described song. However, as I sat in the worship service

and began to play, a strange thing happened. I began to hear the music from that song play back again in my mind. I realized at a young age that music has a power and spirit about it. If you doubt the validity of this statement take this test: Try having a romantic conversation with a significant other as "Just as I Am" plays in the background. Then try to have a worship service while a Luther Vandross song's playing.

A musician must be on guard for anything that will disrupt her or his spirit, especially before an opportunity to minister. The church musician's gift can also become her or his burden. Her or his sensitivity to music is what separates her or him from other musicians; however, this same sensitivity leaves the church musician vulnerable to any music that she or he hears. This means that music, regardless of its nature, leaves an impression on the church musician. When this impression is made prior to worship, it can become difficult for the church musician to focus on the prepared music for the service and on the leading of the Spirit. Even disagreements can affect one's song selections if one is not careful. Consequently, musicians must also consider their conversations before going into worship. The desire to glorify God through music should always be the essence of the musician's heart. In order to actualize that desire, the church musician must stay centered on the Spirit.

The musician, in addition to being called, should be "skilled" (1 Chron. 15:22; 2 Chron. 34:12). Skill is not just an ability to improvise on a musical score. In fact, a musician's virtuosity has little importance if the Holy Spirit does not guide it. Skill, in the context of worship, is the ability to carry one's musical assignment seamlessly. The anointing of God's Spirit moves the musician to minister before God and the congregation. In this moment, the musician becomes highly sensitive to the leading of the Lord; the direction of the pastor, liturgist/worship leader, choir director, praise team leader, psalmist, or soloist; and the needs of the congregation. As a result, the church musician seeks to play in a manner that supports the flow of the service and that complements the play of the other church musicians.

To be sure, the church musician must possess musical skills. She or he should be able to play well enough to support the church's congregational singing, the performances of the church's varied musical groups (choirs, praise teams, chorales, soloists, etc.), and the overall worship of the church. This requires practice, practice, and more practice. The rudiments of musical preparation (practicing scales, transpositions, chord progressions, fingering techniques, instrument maintenance and care, etc.), which is often called the woodshed, apply to church musicians. For example, church musicians must learn songs in multiple keys and in multiple styles since various groups may sing the same song differently. Musicians must also practice how to play with music directors, singers, and other musicians. Thus, numerous rehearsals are required with the music staff in addition to a musician's private practice times. Though these times can become "tedious and tasteless," the musician's calling helps the musician remain focused during these moments.

Even though a church musician must follow his or her call and must craft his or her skill, he or she must make a living. Often, a misconception resides in churches that music is a free service. As we stated earlier, musicians should be paid adequately by churches and ought to be willing to negotiate a fair compensation package with churches that have meager resources. In each case, the church and the musicians should uphold their ends of the agreement.

Churches should pay musicians on time; give them bonuses and raises for faithfulness, longevity, and skilled service; treat them as people and not slaves; and hold them accountable for any lack of service. At the same time, musicians must be on time for rehearsals, worship services, and other church functions (revivals, mid-week services, engagements at other churches, etc.); prepared in all contexts; willing to donate some time (free of charge) to the service of the church; and should hold the church accountable for any lack of service on its part (particularly if it fails to pay in full or on time). In cases where the remuneration from church work is meager, the church musician is torn between playing solely for the church and playing for secular events. This can seem like a division in loyalty. However, in this instance, it is not. Church musicians, who only work for churches on a part-time basis, should feel free to supplement their income with other engagements.

Though these events may not appear to give God glory, the church musician takes her or his calling into those environments. In addition to these engagements helping the church musician financially, these are opportunities for the church musician to witness to others that may never come to a church. On the other hand, musicians who are compensated by the church in a full-time basis should not allow outside engagements to compromise their ministry. If she or he is able to balance outside engagements with a full load of church work, then those ventures are acceptable. However, full-time church musicians must recognize that their primary ministry resides in their church. If it is necessary to be absent from church, the musician must consult with the pastor or chief musical administrator in enough time to make the necessary adjustments.

The position of church musician requires sacrifice and dedication. The musician must know her or his limitations - what sacrifices she or he can or cannot make. In acknowledging those limitations, the church musician must be willing to press toward a higher mark. In committing her or his life to God, she or he must be open to God's calling to expand her or his service to the church. This may entail inconvenient rehearsals, busybody church officials, and "know-it-all" (but non-musical) congregants. Yet, there are some joys: experiencing God in radically new ways, watching God grow one's musical gifts, and being called to serve the church in areas other than music. To all church musicians - *Let it Rise! Let the Glory of the Lord Rise!*

Conclusion
Worship is the church's communion with God. The church enables and enhances that moment with music that gives God praise. This is a longstanding tradition of the church. Therefore, leaders of church music – chief musical administrators, worship

leaders, and church musicians – are vital to the life of the church. They ensure that the music for the church's worship is Spirit-led, skillfully played, and well sung. These persons are skilled, gifted, and anointed in music. They combine their heart for God, their calling to serve the church through their musical gifts, and their professional musical skills to create an environment that engenders an encounter between God and those who worship. The musical leaders help to create a mood in church that encourages thanksgiving for God's blessings, adoration of God's presence, and expectancy of God's movement. This is when the church is *doin' worship*! Hallelujah!

---

[1] James F. White, *An Introduction to Christian Worship*, rev. ed. (Nashville: Abingdon Press, 1990), 33.

[2] Ibid., 31-34.

[3] Ibid., 32. From its Greek origins, liturgy literally means work of the people. See Ibid., 31-32.

[4] The theological lens of this work is Trinitarian; therefore, we often refer to Jesus and the Spirit as God.

[5] Frank C. Senn, *Christian Liturgy: Catholic and Evangelical* (Minneapolis: Fortress Press, 1997), 16.

[6] Johannes Quasten, *Music and Worship in Pagan and Christian Antiquity*, trans. Boniface Ramsey, O.P. (Washington, D.C.: National Association of Pastoral Musicians, 1983), 68.

[7] Ibid., 68-72.

[8] Eric Werner, *The Sacred Bridge: The Interdependence of Liturgy and Music in Synagogue and Church during the First Millennium* (London: Dennis Dobson, 1959), 207.

[9] John S. Mbiti, *African Religions and Philosophy*, 2nd ed. (Oxford: Heinemann Publishers, 1989), 58.

[10] Ibid.

[11] Mbiti, 67.

[12] This insight was often given to us by Dr. William Watley.

[13] Graham Hughes, *Worship as Meaning: A Liturgical Theology for Late Modernity*, Cambridge Studies in Christian Doctrine, ed. Colin Gunton and Daniel W. Hardy (Cambridge: Cambridge University Press, 2003), 31.

[14] Tony McNeil, "Pastors and Musicians Working Together" presentation made at the Institute on Black Sacred Music, American Baptist College, Nashville, TN, July 2007).

[15] Quasten, 60-62.

Developing a Tithing Church
Gregory Ingram

Most people think of Christian stewardship in terms of money rather than in terms of life. The prevailing attitudes and misconceptions many have about it are all wrong. There are churches and church leaders who mistakenly believe that all their problems would be solved if they had enough money. Nothing is further from the truth. The fact of the matter is stewardship deals with people and not purses. The teachings of both the Old and New Testaments affirm this.

In light of the misconceptions and in congruencies, the principle obligation of the church today, with respect to Christian financial stewardship, is to clarify its position on a life of giving, so that its members will better understand what Christian stewardship is all about. To talk about stewardship means to talk about a way of living. It means:

1. Everything we are

2. Everything we do

3. Everything we spend

4. Every moment we consume

When many people hear the word or listen to someone talk on the subject of stewardship in some circles, much like listening to someone on the radio or watching a program on television, they turn the channel or turn it off because they do not like it. Because many people associate the word stewardship solely with money, it takes a bad rap and is a word that deserves a greater understanding and appreciation. When people view tithing and Christian stewardship as fulfillment of their covenant with God, they also view giving as lifetime pattern. A life of giving ultimately leads us into a life of faith, excitement, and commitment to the Lord that results in a person's life mirroring God's willingness to give His most precious gift to others, Jesus Christ, as a ransom for our sins (John 3:16).

When God gets us, He gets our property. For example, when Jesus got Peter, He also got Peter's boat. He got the boy's lunch with which to feed the multitude. When God gets a person with a car, He also gets a car to be used in His service. When He gets a man or woman of talent, He gets talent to be employed in the interest of His kingdom. When God gets a person with wealth, He gets wealth to be used in furthering the Christian Church. When God gets us, we realize we are not our own. We become Christ's stewards when He becomes our Lord, the authority in and ruler of our lives. To acknowledge the Lordship of Christ means we are willing to accept the principles of stewardship as the hallmark of our commitment to a life of giving. Dedicating oneself to a life of giving is serious business. It is a commitment of a person's being, body, and possessions to God. Most of us play around at being committed but a life of giving means we have stopped playing at being in God's image and truly are working to achieve that end.

A Christian who has not adopted a life of giving is a contradiction. An individual who has said he or she is committed to Christ but has not demonstrated the joy of giving in their lives is not being true to self or Savior. An individual who says, "Christ is my guide" and then refuses to develop a life of giving denies—as Peter did when Jesus needed him the most—that God is most important in his or her life.

Dedicating oneself to a life of giving is serious business. It is a commitment of a person's being, body, and possessions to God. Most of us play around at being committed but a life of giving means we have stopped playing at being in God's image and truly are working towards achieving that end.

In far too many instances, considerable time and energy are spent trying to come up with ways to raise money and elevate the stewardship of financial giving in the local church. Some ministers have done an excellent job teaching their members in this area, while others are still drifting, struggling to raise money the hard way using various strategies to raise funds, from chicken dinners, pew rallies, stay at home teas, and church bazaars to the every member canvass and annual commitments and wondering why they are not doing any better.

I realize that all churches are not alike. What works for one does not necessarily work for another. In the area of financial giving, however, all churches are on common ground because all require money to do the Lord's work according to God's way. The question, then, is "What perceptions, attitudes, and behavior are manifested by the resource pool, the members – when it comes to giving in the church? In the African American church, many social, psychological, and spiritual behaviors are exhibited during the Sunday morning worship service, particularly during collection time. These behaviors have to do with churchgoers' motives and reasons for giving, which range from a sincere desire to do God's will and aid in Kingdom building to a self-centered hope that giving will result in some form of getting to a spiritless, weekly exercise routinely done and often with reluctance if not outright hostility. Pastors need to be aware of the varied motivations for giving so that when efforts are not successful in raising money one way in the church, alternative strategies can be employed to counteract any reason or motive for holding back and thereby increase the congregation's likelihood of giving.

THE EIGHT MOTIVES OF GIVING

A few years ago, about 1992, I came across a study conducted by a church psychologist, a sociologist, a preacher, and a newspaper columnist who collaboratively analyzed the behavioral patterns of Christian givers. Their study involved more than 3,000 people from all parts of the country. What they came up with were four motives why people give. Since that time, I have added a like number of my own. Here are the eight motives for why people give to the church

1. *Avoid guilt feelings.* The rationale behind this motive is, "I ought to share in the support of the church; if I fail to do so for whatever reason, I will feel guilty." The question for those who fall into this category ought to be, "Is the quest for a guilt-free conscience sufficient motivation to give to the church?" Giving to the church should result from a duty and obligation stemming from a loving heart in response to the goodness and grace of God instead of regulated to sentiments of guilt.

2. *Fear of retribution.* This motive emanates from some people believing that not giving to the church might lead to God's punishment. This sort of giving is little more than trying to stay God's hand and not from the believer's heart.

3. *Keeping up with the Joneses.* Those who fall into this category are persons who give according to what other folks are doing. Those who try to keep up with the Joneses are people who want to be a part of the "in" crowd. Giving to the church based on what other people give completely dismisses what God has done for you. Scripture says, "Freely ye have received, freely give" (Matthew 10:8 KJV).

215

4. *Avoid excommunication.* There are those motivated to give as little as possible to the church as long as they can maintain some self-respect, keep their name on the church roll, and claim membership in the household of faith. This category represents those who want to remain in good and regular standing but whose giving is deceptive, mechanical, and joyless, making the church weak, lethargic, and ineffective. Members who give to the church fraudulently and with shallow commitment are not dependable or reliable.

5. *Seek God's favor.* Some believe it is possible to bride, coerce, force, or intimidate God into returning goodness and material possession in exchange for their giving. Jesus did not suggest that after enough is given, sufficient pressure would result in God granting your desires. What He did say was, "Seek ye first the kingdom of God and His righteousness; and it [lots of things] shall be added unto you" (Matthew 6:33 KJV). The Apostle Paul further states, "God shall supply all your needs according to His riches in glory" (Philippians 4:19 KJV).

6. *Attitude about the pastor.* There are some who would withhold God's money, refusing to give to God's work, and—in the process—restrict their blessings, simple because they do not like the preacher. Our giving to God's work and ministry has nothing to do with the preacher. Since we are the recipients of God's divine grace and God looks beyond all of our faults and sees to our needs, we should feel morally obligated to respond by giving to the church whether or not we like the preacher.

7. *Out of habit.* Some people are motivated to give but do not know why they give. These people give out of habit and have never taken the time to understand the biblical and theological correctness of giving. While giving in this manner assists the church in meeting its obligations, members falling into this category need education on tithing and stewardship to become knowledgeable, cheerful, and generous givers.

8. *Thankful heart and love for God.* Obviously, these givers are the people who make the difference in the church. They give to the Lord from the top of their income and not from what is left over.

The more I thought about some of these behaviors, the more they troubled me. I wrestled with them and then I remembered a conservation I had with Dr. Wyatt Tee Walker back in the 70's who inspired me about stewardship and tithing. Dr. Walker told me, "Ingram, if you can get your church turned on to giving God's way, you will never have a problem." I believe I was convinced but did not really pursue the idea of implementing a stewardship and tithing program until I was convicted that the eight motives were not going to prevent me from implementing a stewardship and tithing church. I started wrestling with the idea that what was needed to facilitate the development of a lifetime pattern of giving was a plain, common sense explanation of Biblically-based justification for stewardship and tithing. Armed with Biblical and theological substantiation for the practices, expressed in clearly understandable terms, pastors and church leaders will be equipped to promote stewardship and tithing as requirements, not options, for those who profess to be God-fearing, God-revering Christians.

Everyone seems to be in agreement that there are many undeniable areas of immediate concerns in the life of the church. However, the health and growth of the church's finances is a major concern and is of utmost importance. Here is something to think about.

A well thought out and implemented stewardship program would do wonders for the church. In fact, giving to God's church, God's way, will ensure that we would have "more than enough" resources for missions and ministers. Imagine how the average pastor would feel if he or she had the Moses experience as recorded in Exodus 35:4-5, "All the artisans who were at work making everything involved in constructing the Sanctuary came, one after another, to Moses saying, "The people are bringing more than enough for doing this work that God has commanded us to do!" The people had to be instructed to stop giving because they had already given "more than enough." WOW!

One of the central issues concerning money, both in Scripture and in the church, has to do with giving. After years of studying and working with people in the area of Christian giving, I came to the conclusion that implementing a tithing and stewardship program would be difficult, until my parishioners clearly understood the dynamics and effects of the antecedents, behavior, and consequences (ABCs) of giving. Essentially, the ABCs of giving can be explained as follows: **Antecedents, Behaviors and Consequences.**

Antecedents are the conditions, events, or causes that precede a subsequent action and response, e.g., the pastor's appeal to the congregation to become a tither.
 Behavior is the manner in which an individual or group responds to the antecedents, e.g., the congregation wholeheartedly accepts or strongly rejects the pastor's tithing appeal.
Consequences are the effects or results of the behavior, e.g. the church's financial health improves, remains the same, or declines, depending on the membership's reaction to the pastor's stewardship and tithing appeal.

A closer look at the ABCs of giving reveals:
1. **Antecedents** are the stimuli or conditions that set the stage for the occurrence of the behavior, or in this case, tithing. It is at the pre-tithing stage that a persuasive presentation on a life of giving and stewardship must be made to the congregation, increasing the probability of a favorable response to the impending tithing appeal.
2. The **behavior** is giving. To properly manage a stewardship and tithing program, it is necessary to maintain records on the number of givers, amount of they give, and impact of their giving is having in the church's weekly offering. Data should be collected at prescribed intervals, e.g., weekly, monthly or quarterly.
3. The **consequences**, both positive and negative, are the outcomes of any behavior. They can be influenced through positive reinforcement. The keys to understanding and controlling what happens during a tithing campaign is in making sure that the tithing and stewardship promotion is properly planned, executed, and the principles and guidelines for

implementing the program are followed. To effectively promote the ABCs of giving, stewardship and tithing must be reinforced consistently. Monthly, quarterly, and annual appeals alone will not do. In order to make it work, stewardship and tithing education must be emphasized weekly in the church bulletin and articulated by the pastor. When I served as the pastor of Oak Grove AME Church in Detroit, Michigan, each week emphasis was placed on the stewardship of giving by challenging members to review their covenant relationship with God, exercise their faith, and come to grips with the fact that tithing and the stewardship of giving is not a scheme developed by humanity. It is God's plan. The struggle of implementing a stewardship and tithing program for most churches is a matter of faith; obedience and the conviction that this is what God will have us do. To do this was not easy because, I was consciously aware that people have different motives and reasons for giving.

The stewardship and tithing program at Oak Grove reaped a phenomenal harvest and was a tremendous success. In three years over 1400 persons became tithers, a little less than half the membership, and those who were not tithers, became strong proportional givers. When people ask me how did we do it and what suggestion I would recommend to implement one at their church I immediately tell them " Don't try to do it if money is your main motive."

Stewardship is an acknowledgement of God's divine provisions and a response to the Lord Jesus Christ's redeeming grace through a life of giving and the proper management of God's given resources. It is the practice of systematic and proportionate giving of one's time, talent, and treasure, based upon the conviction that everything we have is a gift from God and as stewards we are held accountable for how we use them. Realizing that God is the giver of all good and perfect gifts of creation, resources, and humanity, it becomes our responsibility to manage them well. Stewardship encompasses how we reflect God in discharging our daily affairs and appointments; how we care for our bodies and health; the natural resources we consume and dispose; how we utilize our God-given gifts and talents for the benefit of others; and how we earn, spend, and invest our finances.

Be warned. Embracing a stewardship campaign could cost you. Implementing a stewardship program can be uncomfortable for some members. Before it gets off the ground, pastors and leaders may be faced with a thousand and one reasons from some people who will say it can't work, and other members who will try to derail the program before it gets started. That's why serious prayer and a strong committee will be needed to help guide the congregation through uncharted waters. These people will be able to help others see the benefits of allowing God to work in new ways. In addition, constant communication is vital. Once the vision is shared and owned by the members, everyone will be moving towards a common goal.

Despite widespread interest and eagerness among churches to implement a stewardship campaign, many of their attempts fail. Some reasons for this include:
• *Poor planning.* Adequate time and attention was not given to developing and executing the stewardship campaign plan. Therefore, members were skeptical in participating or altogether unaware of what was going on. Remember to "plan your work and work your plan!"
• *Miscommunication.* People do not give when they do not have a complete understanding of the program.
• *Misdirection.* While the objective of the stewardship campaign is to raise financial resources for the local church, money must not be stressed above and beyond the mission and ministry of the church. It must be clearly understood that the church's purpose is glorifying the Kingdom of God and this must be the starting point of the program.
• *Lack of results.* When members contribute to causes, even the church, they want to see the fruits of their labor. When funds are collected for a deemed purpose, those funds must
be delivered. Accountability is a necessary part of stewardship.
• *Lack of motivation.* Much time and attention may be given to launching the campaign but the excitement quickly feigns. Lack of continued motivation can quickly snuff out much

needed support to keep the campaign alive and well.

• *Competition.* When the stewardship campaign commences, all fundraisers should cease. Having both going on simultaneously taxes members' resources and confuses where loyalties should lie.

HOW TO MAKE IT WORK

Having addressed some of the reasons why stewardship campaigns fail, let's move our attention to some elements that will ensure success. First, keep in mind that the focus of the program must be God. God has provided all we need to further the Kingdom. It is our responsibility to correctly discern and utilize these resources. Corporate and individual prayer and fasting is one way to allow God to direct all efforts involved in the campaign. It will also direct contributors in their level of commitment. Success will be determined by the spiritual maturity, faith, commitment, models of leadership, and integrity of all those involved in the program.

Second, a preliminary planning committee comprised of the pastor, other clergy, officers, and heads of ministries and organizations may be gathered to discuss the stewardship campaign. It does not help to put a team of eleven soccer players into a game without positioning them. This will make them not play well because no one will know where he/she should be playing and what their responsibilities would be. Therefore the results will be disastrous. The same is for those who are going to work on the stewardship and tithing campaign. It is imperative that persons who are going to work the campaign be well informed to know what is expected of them. At the meeting, the following questions may be asked:

• What level of financial stewardship currently exists in the church?
• What is the potential level of financial stewardship in the church?
• What are the financial goals of this stewardship campaign?
• Are we sure we want to do this?

Using the information gathered at this preliminary meeting, the pastor will need to assemble his or her campaign team. These key members will have specific responsibilities in administrating the program. The leadership team will consist of:

• *Pastor*— The Pastor serves as the spiritual leader and instructor for stewardship; recruits personnel resources for leadership in the campaign; schedules program events and deadlines; and oversees the entire process and executive committee of chairpersons and other leaders of the church.

• *Campaign Chairperson*—The Campaign Chairperson assists in identifying and recruiting other personnel resources for leadership in the campaign and provides leadership in the entire process including planning, implementation, and member response.

• *Program Chairperson*— The program Chairperson provides leadership, coordinates initial and concluding events, gathers additional personnel resources to provide testimonials, and make solicitations during regularly scheduled services.

• *Response Chairperson*—The Response Chairperson tracks distribution and collection of commitment or covenant cards from members agreeing to sacrificially give and recruits personnel resources to canvas the congregation and make personal appeals to members.

• *Publicity Chairperson*—The Publicity Chairperson assists the pastor and campaign chairperson in developing the program's theme and logo; makes recommendations and implements methods of communicating the campaign to members via posters, banners, mailings, bulletin inserts, email distributions, website development, and telephone chains; and serves as liaison to the congregation.

The third element to ensure a successful stewardship campaign is timing. Once the pastor and campaign leadership are united on the overall program, specific planning begins. An official time period for the campaign's duration should be determined. This time frame can range from months to years. A realistic timetable for events, appeals, executive meetings, and progress checks should be developed and honored.

The date of commencement can be designated as the kick off or launch. The date of conclusion should also be identified. A celebration of some kind culminating the campaign success should be scheduled to share with the congregation what had been accomplished.

Once the campaign kickoff has occurred, the Response Committee goes to work. It is their task to make personal contacts with members and solicit a commitment to the campaign. Members may sign a Stewardship and Tithers Faith Covenant Card indicating their level of support. See Covenant Card for example. The Response Committee is responsible for collecting these instruments and following up with members to ensure their commitment is carried out. For those who may be hesitant about making a commitment, this is an excellent opportunity to share personal benefits and testimonies about such proportionate and sacrificial giving. The pastor may also want to invite stewardship specialists to the church to conduct seminars or preach on stewardship themes.

In order for the campaign to be successful, remember it must have integrity. That is to say, the program must be reasonable, reputable, and responsible. It must have quality. People want to see a well-defined and efficient system before deciding to get involved. Here then are some additional principles about implementing a stewardship program you may find beneficial.

TWENTY FUNDIMENTAL PRINCIPLES OF STEWARDSHIP

(These 20 principles are on a sheet of paper from my file. I do not know the origin, but they are worth sharing. If someone can help me, I will be very glad to give credit.)

1. Start planning early enough to provide ample time to accomplish.
2. People who have experienced for themselves the joy of being good stewards are more likely to be able to plan and conduct a financial enlistment that will help others

experience a similar joy (so we need to put good givers in charge).

3. People give more for what they understand better (so a year-round program of stewardship and mission education is needed).
4. People give more for what they have helped to determine (so they should be given opportunities to share in decisions about the work of the church).
5. People in any congregation are not all the same (so we need to formulate plans in ways that demonstrate concern for various members).
6. People benefit from making periodic reviews of their values, life styles, and contributions (so asking them to make a new decision about their giving is not an intrusion but a valuable service).
7. People do not respond as well if the same approach is used year after year (so we need to vary the methods we use).
8. People profit from the commitment and growth experienced by other Christians (so at least every two or three years we need to plan a financial enlistment that gives one person an opportunity to talk personally and privately with another person or family about giving money).
9. People give to people (so we need to maximize personal contact in all phases of seeking and receiving commitments, especially in years when no personal visits are planned).
10. About one-third of the people provide about three-fourths of the money (so we need to give priority attention to how we work with this one-third).
11. People do not graduate from the school of Christian giving (so we need to keep challenging our best givers to re-examine their giving).
12. People need to consider their total financial situation as they decide on their commitment (so we need to invite them to think about accumulated assets as well as current income).

13. All people do not face the same financial circumstances (so it is always wrong to suggest that a "fair share" is the church's budget divided by the number of members).
14. People do not usually take offense at being considered generous (so we can invite them to consider a significant increase in their giving without insulting them).
15. People give more dollars in response to a specific challenge (so we need to invite people to give a specific dollar amount or a specific percentage of what they possess).
16. Many people receive most of their income on a monthly basis (so we need to encourage these people to pay the bulk of their commitment on a monthly basis).
17. People need time, in privacy, to give serious considerations to their commitment (so we need to allow time between the occasion for the challenge and the occasion for the response).
18. People pay more attention to what is given special attention by the church (so we need to dedicate financial commitments in a special worship context, no matter what methods have been used to seek or receive such commitments).
19. People like to feel they are important to the church, that they matter (so we need to follow up when no financial commitment is received and we need to follow up when a financial commitment that has been received is not fulfilled).
20. People appreciate being appreciated (so we need to include ways of thanking people for their commitments and for their actual gifts).

TWENTY RECOMMENDATIONS FOR AN EFFECTIVE STEWARDSHIP PROGRAM

1. Make sure you are familiar with God's giving standard.
2. Study stewardship concepts.
3. Have well-planned meetings
4. Orientation for stewardship committee members and volunteers are a must.
5. Innovation is the key.

6. Strive for excellence.
7. Know why most stewardship campaigns fail.
8. Plan your work and work your plan.
9. Be selective when choosing the right people to serve on committees.
10. Develop the right stewardship climate in your church for giving.
11. Solicit support and counseling from stewardship specialists.
12. Don't try to manage more than you can handle.
13. Evaluate your strengths and weaknesses.
14. Learn as much as you can on stewardship.
15. If you fail in implementing a stewardship campaign, don't stop trying.
16. Maintain a clear focus that is consistent with the church's mission statement.
17. Keep fundraisers at a minimum.
18. Keep the congregation well informed.
19. Remain positive.
20. Stay prayed up.

A Definition of Stewardship
Stewardship is an acknowledgement of God's divine provisions and response to the Lord Jesus Christ redeeming grace, through a life of giving, and the proper management of God's resources.

Here are Ten Principles for Making Stewardship Work in the Local Church

1. A Biblical standard of giving must be the primary belief of your church.

2. Your church should have a Mission Statement.

3. Your church mission statement should have a strong stewardship position.

4. There must be ministerial participation in the stewardship of the church.

5. Officers and members should be challenged to examine their faith.

6. A well-planned stewardship program should be included in annual projections.

7. Seminars, workshops, retreats, and study groups should be implemented to broaden stewardship development and understanding among members.

8. An appeal for stewardship and tithing commitments should be given weekly.

9. A stewardship message should be included in the worship service bulletin.

10. Fund-raisers should be at a minimum.

FORMS AND CHARTS:

"THE YEAR OF TOTAL COMMITMENT"

A Commitment form

We believe that each of us is "CALLED TO MAKE A DIFFERENCE" in our home, community, and church. As an expression of your love and gratitude to God, members of (your church name) are being asked to examine their Christian stewardship. As an ongoing thrust toward becoming a total tithing church, we make a special appeal each week for you to consider becoming a tither.

This year, OUR GOAL IS TO HAVE _____ TITHING MEMBERS. As of today, (month/date/yr), _____ members have indicated they will be tithers.

STEWARDSHIP EMPHASIS
Nothing we do changes the past, but everything we do changes the future. By becoming a tither I can touch tomorrow, today, if I am willing to stretch out on faith. (An appeal like this should be done every week).

Return This Form:

Dear Rev._____

I (print your name_____
As an expression of my love and gratitude to God, I hereby make my decision to join you and others in being a tither.

PERCENTAGE GIVING CHART

INCOME

If your weekly/ annual income is:	$200 $10,400	$300 $15,600	$400 $20,800	$500 $26,000	$600 $31,200	$800 $41,600	$1,000 $52,000	$1,200 $62,400	$1,500 $78,000	$1,800 $92,600	$2,000 $104,00
And you are giving:				THIS IS THE WEEKLY DOLLAR AMOUNT OF YOUR GIVING							
1%	$2	$3	$4	$5	$6	$8	$10	$12	$15	$18	$20
2%	$4	$6	$8	$10	$12	$16	$20	$24	$30	$36	$40
3%	6	9	12	15	18	24	30	36	45	54	60
4%	8	12	16	20	24	32	40	48	60	72	80
5%	10	15	20	25	30	40	50	60	75	90	100
6%	12	18	24	30	36	48	60	72	90	108	120
7%	14	21	28	35	42	56	70	84	105	126	140
8%	16	24	32	40	48	64	80	96	120	144	160
9%	18	27	36	45	54	72	90	108	135	162	180
10%	20	30	40	50	60	80	100	120	150	180	200
12%	24	36	48	60	72	96	120	144	180	216	240
15%	30	45	60	75	90	120	150	180	255	270	300
20%	40	60	80	100	120	160	200	240	300	360	400

(Left margin spells vertically: P E R C E N T A G E)

Percentages are accurate only if the weekly giving is constant – even when the giver is absent from worship. Locate the present level of giving and drop down one box to calculate a one percentage point increase in giving.

WEEKLY PERCENTAGE GIVING GUIDE

ANNUAL INCOME $	WEEKLY INCOME $	WEEKLY GIVING ($) IF PERCENTAGE IS:					
		3%	5%	7%	9%	10%	15%
5,200	100	3.00	5.00	7.00	9.00	10.00	15.00
6,500	125	3.75	6.25	8.75	11.25	12.50	18.75
7,800	150	4.50	7.50	10.50	13.50	15.00	22.50
9,100	175	5.25	8.75	12.25	15.75	17.50	26.25
10,400	200	6.00	10.00	14.00	18.00	20.00	30.00
11,700	225	6.75	11.25	15.75	20.25	22.50	33.75
13,000	250	7.50	12.50	17.50	22.50	25.00	37.50
14,300	275	8.25	13.75	19.25	24.75	27.50	41.25
15,600	300	9.00	15.00	21.00	27.00	30.00	45.00
16,900	325	9.75	16.25	22.75	29.25	32.50	48.75
18,200	350	10.50	17.50	24.50	31.50	35.00	52.50
19,500	375	11.25	18.75	26.25	33.75	37.50	56.25
20,800	400	12.00	20.00	28.00	36.00	40.00	60.00
26,000	500	15.00	25.00	35.00	45.00	50.00	75.00
31,200	600	18.00	30.00	42.00	54.00	60.00	90.00
36,400	700	21.00	35.00	49.00	63.00	70.00	105.00
41,600	800	24.00	40.00	56.00	72.00	80.00	120.00
46,800	900	27.00	45.00	63.00	81.00	90.00	135.00
52,000	1,000	30.00	50.00	70.00	90.00	100.00	150.00
62,400	1,200	36.00	60.00	84.00	108.00	120.00	180.00
72,800	1,400	42.00	70.00	98.00	126.00	140.00	210.00
83,200	1,600	48.00	80.00	112.00	144.00	160.00	240.00
93,600	1,800	54.00	90.00	126.00	162.00	180.00	270.00
104,000	2,000	60.00	100.00	140.00	180.00	200.00	300.00

Prioritizing Worship Personally and Congregationally
William D. Watley

PRIORITIZING PERSONAL WORSHIP

Even though the incident occurred about a decade ago I remember it as if it were yesterday. Early one morning I was praying and asking guidance for the day. Those who have a regular prayer life know that there are times when we pray that we feel as if our words are hitting the ceiling and bouncing back into our faces. There are other times when life seems to either be put on hold, get worse or go backwards; when our prayers seem to be more routine than transformative. However, there are those times when we feel that we have made a connection and can feel the empowering and comforting presence of the Lord. The prayer session that I am reflecting upon was one of those special times when I felt that I was really communicating with my Lord and that his presence and the sweet savor of the Holy Spirit had come near. However, as I was praying and communing with my Lord through the Holy Spirit, I happened to glance down at my watch and remembered a business meeting that I was supposed to attend. I realized that if I was going to be on time I needed to cut my devotional time short and prepare to leave home, quick, fast and in a hurry. I felt a light tinge of guilt but I figured that the Lord would understand and that I would get back in touch with him later when I had settled down.

I went to my meeting as any conscientious person would and I was on time as any responsible person would be. However, soon after the meeting started I began to feel that I had made a mistake in interrupting my devotional time; leaving the presence of the Lord to attend the meeting where I was seen, made minimal contributions, and whose content I really cared little about.

I went to the meeting because I believed that as a community leader it was politically expedient to do so. However, I soon realized that this particular meeting, like so many others that I attend, was not really that important. I began to feel like an elder statesman in ministry that I have looked up to down through the years, after he had experienced a major heart attack. The doctor told him that he needed to take a nap every day. However, this minister could not see how he could accommodate the doctor's request considering his busy schedule and the many demands upon his time. During that time, while he was wrestling with the doctor's counsel and how and if he could obey it, another colleague who had suffered a heart attack called him on the phone and told him, "My friend, every day lay down and take a nap for an hour and a half and you will discover that nothing, absolutely nothing of significance would have happened while you were doing so."

I began to reflect over the truth that I had left the presence of the Lord to attend a meeting where "nothing, absolutely nothing of significance" was happening. I began to think about the fact that I could have gotten a breakthrough or an answer to a prayer or dilemma during that prayer session that I hurriedly left. I began to think about the fact that even if none of that happened and I just experienced the presence of the Lord, the sweetness of the Lord's presence was more than worth the sacrifice of missing this particular meeting where "nothing, absolutely nothing of significance" was happening. The God of the universe who looked from heaven's mercy window one day and called me, in spite of myself, to preach heaven's word to a dying and sin-sick world, had condescended to visit me in my humble abode, and I had the nerve to rush from that divine visitation to attend a meeting where "nothing, absolutely nothing of significance" was happening.

The Lord Jesus Christ, the incarnate presence of God wrapped up in human flesh, who loved me enough to die for my sins on an old rugged cross, and then had risen from the grave with all power in heaven and earth in his hands to assure my victory over every possible foe and force that can rise against me, had chosen to come to see about me. Yet I had the insensitivity to rush away from my Jesus to attend a meeting where "nothing, absolutely nothing of significance" was happening. The Holy Spirit, the abiding presence of God living among us had brightened my drab surroundings with power from on high and I had the mitigated gall to rush away from heavenly glory to attend a meeting where "nothing, absolutely nothing of significance" was happening. Can you imagine this infinitesimally insignificant piece of earth dust being presumptuous enough and callous enough to take the presence of the Almighty for granted to the point that he would put God on hold so that he could attend a meeting where "nothing, absolutely nothing of significance" was happening.

As I sat in that meeting and realized the stupid mistake I had made I asked God to forgive me and made a decision to leave that meeting where "nothing, absolutely nothing of significance" was happening, to return to my home, to something of significance by spending time with God. As I drove home, I prayed that God would be there to meet me and that I would be able to continue our time of worship, praise, and reflection as if I had never left. I am humbled and grateful to report that God heard me prayer and I was able to find God's presence right where I had left God's presence. I spent the time that morning where I should have spent it, in the presence of God. Later when I asked about the business meeting I had suddenly left without explanation, I found out that it had ended just as it was proceeding while I was there---"nothing, absolutely nothing of significance" happened.

The dilemma I faced that memorable morning and the poor choice I made regarding private worship time and other pressing matters on a schedule, is one that a number of committed, sincere, love-the-Lord, busy Christians face, both clergy and lay. I bring good news and bad news to persons who face the dilemma of prioritizing worship on a personal level while juggling the incessant demands that fall into the hands of busy believers and pastors. The good news is that one can actually have a lifestyle that includes a dynamic private worship life that grows deeper, richer, fuller, and sweeter as the years go by. The bad news is that the decision to maintain a private worship and devotional life does not get any easier over time. At this point in my life, I have been trying to preach the Gospel for about forty-six years and by this season one would think that prioritizing worship was second nature to me. There may be others for whom private worship is as natural as breathing and as easy as thinking. I sincerely wish that I were in that number. However, I must confess that even though I enjoy being in the presence of God and know that personal worship and devotional time is something I should do for my soul's health as well as the well-being of my ministry, prioritizing worship in my daily life is still something I must consciously make the time to do.

In a twenty-four hour day, a tithe of time is two hours and twenty-four minutes. I sincerely wish I could say that I give God a tithe of private worship every day. I sincerely try to give God at least an hour and a half of private devotional time that consists of one-half hour to forty-five minutes of Bible and other devotional reading, and an hour of prayer. However, there are some days when God gets an hour and there are other days when the words that the Lord spoke to his disciples in the Garden of Gethsemane also convict me, "So, could you not stay awake with me one hour? Stay awake and pray that you may not come into the time of trial; the spirit indeed is willing, but the flesh is weak."[1]

Why is prioritizing worship such a challenge among so many of us? I am not talking about crises worship because no matter how busy we are, when we have a problem or when we are facing a life or career threatening situation, or when the ministry or someone we love is in danger, we can find time to worship. Neither am I talking about sermon preparation time, even though that can also be a challenge for a number of persons who are so busy with other things during the week that the only time given to being in God's face and presence is either late Saturday night or early Sunday morning. Bodies that are fatigued, souls that are empty and minds that are distracted then desperately plead for some kind of word, any kind of word, to deliver to our congregation who gather with expectant hearts and curious and anxious ears.

My concept of private devotion or worship refers to time spent in the presence of God and reading the word of God simply because we love God. We are not trying to find inspiration for a sermon. We are not simply bringing our usual laundry list of needs. We are not in a particular panic or crisis mode. We have simply made time with God a priority in our lives regardless of what is swirling around us, our loved ones or the ministry or happening to us physically, emotionally and mentally. I must confess that for me the hardest time to find and keep is such quality time with the Lord. Why is such valuable time that I and so many other believer's love so difficult to find. Among the many reasons I could list are just three.

The first reason is the one that our Lord observed in his word of caution to the disciples in Gethsemane---"the spirit indeed is willing, but the flesh is weak." Sometimes we are simply so physically tired from all of our attention to lesser things that we are too physically drained to give time to things that matter.

Sometimes we become so wearied in running with "footmen" that we have neither the energy nor the inclination to spend time in the presence of the One who "gives power to the faint and strengthens the powerless." An example from my own life may help illustrate this point.

About thirty-eight years ago I was a pastor in a small rural town. Even though being a pastor in an urban context can be physically, mentally, emotionally, and spiritually draining, my personal experience has demonstrated that serving a small rural congregation where you not only live in a fish bowl, but are expected to be the point person for any number of issues that not only involve your flock but the community at large as, can also be very demanding. While serving in that place, I dealt with a young man in my congregation who had gotten into some difficulty with the local police department. After making an appeal on his behalf before the local magistrate, after one such incident, his mother said to me, "Reverend Watley, I really appreciate all that you do for me and my family. I wouldn't know what I would do without you." I thanked her for what she said. My only problem was that I took her words too seriously. Every time anyone needed me for anything I would try my best to be present whenever they called me. In time, I was promoted to another church. Soon after leaving that rural church I made a startling discovery. Those people survived very well without me. They survived after me, just like they survived before I came into their lives as pastor.

Many times, we wear ourselves down serving people as if they cannot live without us. The truth is that while they may truly appreciate all we do and while our ministries can have a definite impact upon their lives, the fact of the matter is that in our absence they manage to survive just as they did before we came into their lives. I raise this point because often in our efforts to minister to people we neglect ministry before and to the Lord. We become so worn down because we are serving and listening to people and meeting the never-ending demands of ministry, that we do not have any energy or time left to listen to or spend quality time with God. The reality is that our people, the church, the community, the denomination, and the ministry will survive, and do very well, if we take time to prioritize private and personal worship.

There have been times when I have been so physically drained from doing ministry and church that when I made the effort of doing personal worship I have fallen asleep. At such times, I have hoped that God understood the intent of my heart as I have sought God's forgiveness for my tiredness. I believe God does understand when we are so physically tired that we cannot focus on God. However, such times should be the exception rather than the rule, and when we find ourselves nodding and falling asleep during private worship on a regular basis, then perhaps we should take inventory of our activities. We may discover that the things that are preventing us from giving God attentive and alert personal worship are about "nothing, absolutely nothing of significance."

Another factor that works against consistent, quality devotional time is poor prioritizing. I began this article by describing an incident that demonstrated poor prioritizing on my part. The example of my choice of a meeting where "nothing, absolutely nothing of significance" was happening over time with God, demonstrates the reality that every day we must choose how we spend our time. Every day there are things and people that demand our time and attention. However, we can make decisions and choices about the legitimacy of a demand. Simply because something or someone demands our attention does not mean that the situation they consider to be life or death is really important or urgent.

Some people have a Chicken Little complex. They declare that they sky is falling every time they encounter any kind of problem or difficulty. Some people believe that every inconvenience, bump in the road, change in their plans, interruption in their schedule, or decision requiring serious thought or new direction is a major crisis. Some people's lives are like a soap opera. They move from one sequel of drama to another, all of which amounts to a sum total of "nothing, absolutely nothing of significance." Certain persons and situations have no problems intruding themselves into our lives and demanding we give them the time and attention they feel they deserve.

As responsible shepherds and care givers, we must have the maturity, the sense, the wisdom, and discernment to decide what is a legitimate demand and what is not, and prioritize our time and energy accordingly. I am not suggesting we become callous or insensitive regarding the mole hills some people call mountains or the ditches that some people consider to be seas. An uninterested and arrogant dismissing of problems that others consider to be crises can become a little fox that destroys the vine of a pastoral relationship. Neither am I suggesting that we become Pharisaical or obsessively neurotic about our time with the Lord. Our time with the Lord is not to be viewed as some good luck charm that will result in bad luck if we do not keep it.

Genuine emergencies and unexpected events occur that will sometimes interfere with time we have allotted to be with the Lord. Emergencies and unexpected and unavoidable interruptions occur with our immediate and extended families, our spouses, our members, the facilities, and us that require immediate attention. Sometimes our children become sick or run late for school. Our spouse has to deal with a crisis in her family that involves our time and attention. Sometimes we oversleep or we are mentally fatigued. We receive an early morning or late night call about a break in, a broken furnace or a broken pipe that is causing a flood at the church or some other problem related to the building. God understands emergencies and unexpected interruptions. We must attend to those matters and consequently we may not be able to keep our scheduled time with the Lord. If such is the case, so be it.

The Lord understands emergencies and unexpected interruptions we have no control over that cannot be dismissed or delegated to others, which require our attention and time. My point is that every call, demand and interruption is not an emergency or crisis. We must decide what constitutes a real emergency and

238

prioritize time and attention and worship accordingly. God will help us handle real emergencies and legitimate demands. However private worship time should not be held hostage to any and every demand and interruption that cries out for immediate attention. There are some things, and even people, we must *gently* press a mental call-waiting or hold button upon so that we can prioritize worship lest we leave the presence of God to attend to interruptions and self-perceived emergencies that amount to a sum total of "nothing, absolutely nothing of significance."

Prioritizing private worship can be a challenge because of physical weariness, because of poor prioritizing, and third, because of poor planning. Granted emergencies and unexpected interruptions can disrupt the good intentions of the most disciplined and thorough planner. However, emergencies and unexpected interruptions do not occur everyday. We handle emergencies and the unexpected as they arise, but our lives should not be governed by exceptional situations. Prioritizing private worship is a challenge not because of the emergence of the unexpected and intrusive emergency or the unforeseen accident. Prioritizing private worship is a challenge because of our poor planning. Personal worship will not occur unless we intentionally plan to do it. Personal worship will not occur unless we purposively set aside time to do it just like we set aside time to do anything else that is important to us. There is nothing wrong with making a daily date with God. There is nothing wrong with setting aside time to talk with God and be in the presence of God. There is nothing wrong in guarding that time, holding it sacred and not allowing anything other than emergencies and unexpected interruptions to interfere with that time.

Time set aside for God is not time that is available for business meetings. Time set aside for God is not time that is available for counseling or meeting demands of members who have an emergency that is in their minds but not one in reality. Time set aside for God is not time that is available for conversations with friends and colleagues. Time set aside for God is not free time

239

that is available for house chores or paying bills. Time set aside for God is not time that is available for opening mail and catching up on deskwork. Time set aside for God is not time that is available for reading emails or working on the Internet. Time set aside for God is not sermon preparation time. Sermon prep time is work time during which we are actively preparing to speak on behalf of God to God's people. Time set aside for God is the time when God can speak to us about us and about our relationship with God. Sermon preparation time should flow out of our private worship time. When we reach a point that sermon prep is burdensome and tedious and fresh sermon ideas are rare, the reason may very well be our lack of private time with God.

Mark 3: 13-15 tells us, "He [Jesus] went up the mountain and called to him those whom he wanted, and they came to him. And he appointed twelve, whom he also named apostles, to be with him, and to be sent out to proclaim the message, and to have authority to cast out demons." The Lord called the twelve apostles to first "*be with him,*" to be in special relationship with him. The first identifiable reason the scriptures give for the calling of the twelve was not to proclaim the message or to exercise authority over demons, but to simply be in relationship with the Lord. Message and ministry were the outgrowths of being with the Lord, of spending time with the Lord. Failure to prioritize personal worship during which we are simply with the Lord, neglects a fundamental purpose and core component of our calling. We are not first called to preach or baptize converts, or visit the sick, bury the dead or comfort the bereaved. We are first called to be with the Lord.

We are not first called to guide the young, or counsel the troubled, or engage in other forms of ministry to others. We are first called to be with the Lord. We are not first called to raise money, balance budgets, erect buildings, or wrestle power from saints and church leaders whose primary claim to fame is their standing in the community of faith. We are first called to be with the Lord. We are not first called to establish mega or major ministries, build a name for ourselves, or to help the saints prosper, or to become financially secure ourselves. We are first called to be with the Lord. We are not first called to be either political or ecclesiastical power brokers or celebrities in our own minds. We are first called to be with the Lord. Everything else we do should be an outgrowth of what the Lord first called us to do—"to be with him." In other words, *time set aside for God is time set aside for God.*

In the midst of very busy and demanding schedules, how do we set aside time to be with God? We set aside time to be with God by setting aside time to be with God. I recognize that everyone has obligations, commitments, and meetings that we must attend. However, we have more flexibility in scheduling a number of things than we sometimes are inclined to admit. Secretaries and administrative assistants cannot over book us without our consent and cooperation. Funerals cannot even be scheduled without our consent. Therefore, if we do not have time to be with God, *"it ain't nobody's fault but ours."*

We schedule time based upon our body clocks. Since I am a morning person, I am most comfortable setting aside the morning as devotional time. However, persons with different body clocks, those who are night persons, should feel free to prioritize worship at the times that fit them. Whether late at night or early in the morning, the issue is not the time of day but the commitment to set aside a certain period every day to be with God. There may be times when we may schedule afternoon time to be with the Lord. Sometimes I will take a prayer break in between appointments or have my administrative assistant leave a half an hour or so free in a day when I am going to be in the office so that I can go into the sanctuary and have quiet time with the Lord. I am convinced that most prioritizing worship can be done with consistency without neglecting any of our other responsibilities when we make it a real priority and plan to do it. Being too busy to pray is being too busy. Being too busy to worship privately is being too busy. Too busy to study the word of God for our own good, is being too busy. Being too busy to just be with God is being too busy.

Whenever I begin to feel as if I am too squeezed to spend daily quality time with God, I think about Dr. David Yonggi Cho. Dr. Cho, as many of us already know, is the pastor of the world's largest church. The Yoido Full Gospel Church in Seoul, Korea, which Dr. Cho heads, has a membership numbering around 830,000 souls. Dr. Cho started with five persons who were members of his own family. During that time, he developed the discipline of praying at least two hours every day. That discipline has continued to this day. The phenomenal size and growth of his ministry had not impeded his personal time with the Lord. Consequently, when I am feeling pressed and too busy to schedule time with the Lord, I think about Dr. Cho. If he can do it while pastoring and administering a ministry that numbers into the hundreds of thousands, why can't those of us whose ministries are far smaller find time to prioritize worship? I am inclined to believe that the issue is not simply our busy schedules, demanding members, or family pressures, but our commitment, discipline, and determination to prioritize worship.

I mention determination, because of something that Dr. Cho mentions when he speaks about his prayer life. According to Dr. Cho, even though he has been praying two hours every day for forty years, every single day during all that time as he prepared for prayer, he has heard the devil say, "Don't pray today; pray tomorrow." Prioritizing worship is such a challenge not only because of physical fatigue, poor prioritizing, and haphazard planning. Prioritizing personal worship is a challenge because it is also spiritual warfare. Every time Dr. Cho plans to pray, he hears the voice of the Biblical paradigmatic symbol and representative of evil and sin known as the devil, telling him not to do so. And so will we!

Satan wars against prioritizing personal worship because such time not only brings us closer to God and renews us for ministry, it also strengthens us in our daily battle against the principalities and powers that come against us in any number of ways and through any number of voices to distract, discourage, and break our spirits as we seek to "bring good news to the poor...[to] proclaim release to the captives and recovery of sight to the blind, to let the oppressed go free, to proclaim the year of the Lord's favor."[3] The conflicts and battles that we fight every day that undermine and make difficult our efforts to be faithful to the ministries entrusted unto our care are only the reflection of a deeper spiritual warfare and engagement that is taking place in another realm. Time with God sharpens, equips, and helps us keep perspective of the real struggle in which irritating and even hellish humans are only pawns. The cross was a weapon that Satan tried to use to defeat God's plan for salvation. However, the Lord's prayer time in Gethsemane and his surrender to the will of the Heavenly Father meant that no weapon formed against him, not even a heinous, painful, and disgraceful cross could get the victory over him.

PRIORITIZING CONGREGATIONAL WORSHIP
The Lord understood the importance of prioritizing worship and that is the reason he instructed the disciples not to leave Jerusalem until they received the promise of the Father, which was the baptism of the Holy Spirit. The Lord had already given them authority over demons and disease. In his resurrected state, the Lord had breathed the Holy Spirit upon them and had given them authority as instruments and vessels of the Holy Spirit to forgive and retain sins. Before his ascension, the Lord had given them the great commission and an international mandate. He told them, "All authority in heaven and on earth has been given to me. Go therefore and make disciples of all nations, baptizing them in the name of the Father and of the Son and of the Holy Spirit, and teaching them to obey everything that I have commanded you. And remember, I am with you always, to the end of the age."[4]

However, before the disciples were to go anywhere or do anything with all that had been poured into them and spoken over them, a lighted match needed to be thrown onto their kindling potential. The light switch had to be turned on to reveal the electricity that had been wired into the house. The faucet had to be turned on so that the water in the pipes could flow. The knob had to be turned on so that the gas that was already in the stove could burst into flame. Thus, in obedience to his command the disciples assembled in expectation of receiving something. They did not know what or whom they would receive. They did not know who or what the Comforter, the Paraclete or the promise of the Father was. How it or he/she would feel or what it or he/she would do. However, in obedience to the instructions of Jesus they assembled in an upper room in Jerusalem during the Jewish festival of Pentecost. And after a ten-day prayer meeting, when the Day of Pentecost was fully come, when they were not only in one place but also on one accord, they received more than they expected. Suddenly a sound came from heaven like the rush of a mighty wind that filled the whole house. Cloven tongues of fire appeared over each of their heads as each of them spoke in other languages as the Holy Spirit gave them utterance.

The worship and praise of the believing community was so passionate and powerful that a great international throng gathered in amazement and curiosity about the multi-linguistic approbations to Almighty God that was being expressed by those whose Galilean accents identified their ethnic heritage. There were some in the crowd who sarcastically questioned the sobriety of those who were giving forth anointed and Spirit filled praise. However, Simon Peter, under the anointing and speaking from the overflow of the Holy Spirit, stood up boldly. As he informed his listeners about the fulfillment of ancient prophecy that was taking place in their midst, he boldly proclaimed to them the Gospel of the Lord Jesus Christ. When Peter finished preaching, there was such a conviction among his hearers that three thousand souls were added to the church that day.

The mission, outreach, growth of the church, and the international spread of the Gospel began with passionate worship and praise. The Holy Spirit did not fall on the Day of Pentecost when the members or leadership of the church were balancing budgets, planning programs, visiting the sick, and serving the needy. The Holy Spirit first came to and fell upon the church when it was gathered in worship. After the outpouring of the Holy Spirit came upon the church as it was gathered in worship the word of God tells us,

Awe came upon everyone, because many wonders and signs were being done by the apostles. All who believed were together and had all things in common; they would sell their possessions and goods and distribute the proceeds to all, as any had need. Day by day, as they spent much time together in the temple, they broke bread at home and ate their food with glad and generous hearts, praising God and having the goodwill of all the people. And day by day the Lord added to their number those who were being saved. ⁵

Great worship and passionate praise on the Day of Pentecost set the tone and determined the character of the church's ministry and power to reach others. Great worship and praise also released an unusual unction of generosity and giving among the saints.

Great worship and passionate Spirit filled praise should serve as the foundation and seedbed of the church's life mission, outreach and programming. Great worship and passionate Spirit filled praise, as distinct from artificially-contrived-feel-good-jump-to-the-music-entertainment-and-emotional-catharsis that has no lasting impact or implications, provides the church with impetus and power to fulfill the Lord's kingdom vision. Great worship and passionate Spirit filled praise should be the center of the church's life and the fulcrum for the church's ministry. Great worship and passionate Spirit filled praise should have overflow and set the atmosphere for attitudes and actions that are present in the church staff who are involved in the day to day administration of church business.

Great worship and passionate Spirit filled praise should overflow and set the atmosphere for attitudes and actions that are present in the counting room where the tithes and offerings are tabulated and prepared for bank deposits; and in the elder, deacon, vestry, trustee, and steward board and other business meetings that take place during the week. Great worship and passionate Spirit filled praise should have overflow and set the atmosphere for attitudes and actions that are present in auxiliary, club, and other ministry meetings that often spend too much time fellowshipping, gossiping, griping, and eating, in between Sunday services.

Too often in many of our churches, there is a Grand Canyon size divide between what happens on Sunday morning and the attitudes and actions that are manifested among saints throughout the week. The early church grew because the outside community saw the fruit and evidence of worship and praise manifested in the spiritual power, generosity, love, caring and service of the saints among themselves first and then towards others. Perhaps one of the reasons that the aftermath is so anemic of what passes for worship and praise in the present is that we really do not know what worship and praise are.

The early church assembled to seek the presence and the non-material promise of God. The early church assembled to glorify and praise the name of Jesus. Worship then is the adoration, reverencing, and glorification of God. True praise is the outward manifestation of an inward adoration and reverence. Many of us give God praise without true worship. We can raise our hands in praise that recognizes the greatness of God without hearts that are in loving adoration and reverence of God. The church always has more "praisers" than worshippers. Everything and everyone can and should praise the Lord. When we consider the greatness of God's glory, everything and everyone should praise the Lord. However, everything and everyone that praises the Lord has not yielded his or her hearts in loving adoration and reverence or submission to God's word and God's will. Raised and clapping hands, uplifted voices, stomping and running feet, powerful and praising tongues, and inspiring music can be given without hearts that have been yielded to God and eyes that are single to the glory of God.

Those who were gathered in the upper room on the Day of Pentecost gave such powerful praise because their hearts were so totally yielded. When one has a yielded heart that truly adores, reverences, and glorifies God, there will be afterglow and overflow that abides long after the benediction is pronounced. This afterglow and overflow will produce the fruit of the Spirit in which the gifts of the Spirit can flourish and accomplish their purpose in the body of Christ. In the process, God is glorified, the saint is edified, the devil is horrified, backsliders are reclaimed, and sinners are brought to the foot of the cross. Perhaps the reason that the saints were assembled ten days in the upper room was that it took that long for hearts to be grounded, yielded, and prepared for the sudden outpouring of the Holy Spirit.

True worship and praise then are about God not us. Worship is not a narcissistic focus on our needs, wants, and feelings. Worship is not about our getting "something" from the service. Too many of us believe that the purpose of praise going up is to get "blessings to come down." Praise is not a political manipulation of God's ego to get blessings to come down. God is not some self-serving despot with a weak ego that must be stroked before we can get our needs supplied and our wants and wishes granted. Praise exalts and focuses on the *Blesser* ("from whom all blessings flow"), not those who want to be blessed. God inhabits the praises of God's people not God's pawns, who are fawning and groveling for goodies and divine favor. God's people are not those who simply say "Lord, Lord," but those who do the will of God, the Heavenly Father of Our Lord and Savior Jesus Christ.[6]

God's people are those who have been called by God's name who have humbled themselves, who are prayerful, who seek the face of God and have turned from their wicked ways.[7] God's people are those who are in covenant and loving relationship with God. God's people are those who have confessed the Lord Jesus Christ as Savior and Lord and who are living out the process of being "saved, sanctified, Holy Ghost filled and fire baptized." God's people are those with adoring and reverencing hearts that yield lives that cause them to worship God in spirit and truth. When such people offer praise, God inhabits the physical and outward expressions of their adoration and tabernacles among them. When God tabernacles among us, God brings everything we need. When God tabernacles among us, miracles are available, healing is available, breakthroughs are available, and answers to prayers are available. When God tabernacles among us, grace that is sufficient and strength that is made perfect in weakness are also available to bless us even when God says "No" to some of our specific prayers.

Worship and praise have powerfully lasting impact and significance when we truly understand and practice them. Worship and praise have powerfully lasting impact and significance when we prioritize them. We really do not prioritize worship. We schedule worship but we do not prioritize it. Many times our worship services consist of running through a checklist of items on the bulletin, rather than an effort to please, adore and glorify God. Sometimes we are so busy making sure that everyone's ego is satisfied so they can perform the part they have planned and practiced or we are so focused on making sure that every "i" is dotted and every "t" crossed in terms of the tradition so no one will be offended or uncomfortable, that we do not have time to worship. Sometimes we are so busy taking care of church business that should be addressed at a later business meeting or calling names or recognizing and thanking everyone who made a contribution or thought about making one, that we do not have the time or inclination to worship God. Sometimes we are so busy looking for mistakes and things that went or were said wrong that we do not have the time or inclination to really worship. Sometimes we, as church leaders, are so busy or distracted by our personal agendas, or hitting at our foes, that we do not lead the congregation in worship of Almighty God who alone is worthy.

While we say and pray for the coming of the Holy Spirit, when the Spirit comes, we panic and do not know what to do or how to welcome, receive, or abide in the presence of the Holy Spirit. While we say we want the Holy Spirit to have the Spirit's way, our real desire is that the Holy Spirit make a brief non-intrusive guest appearance and fit into our liturgy without disrupting it too much or staying too long. We know approximately when worship should be over. We have our after church plans based upon "church should be letting out" or adjourning at a certain time. Therefore, if or when the Holy Spirit comes we expect the

Holy Spirit to have whatever "it's" way (we sometimes forget that the Holy Spirit is not an "it" but a personality), in a manner that does not interfere with our plans or the way we do things "around here."

One of my favorite illustrations of this tendency, that I have used on any number of occasions, occurred many years ago at a couple of churches when I was relatively new and young as a pastor. There was a service when the presence and move of the Holy Spirit were so powerfully manifest that I knew that the time had come to deliver the message. I got up midway through the service and announced that it was preaching time and called for the hymn of preparation. I was surprised at the number of notes that came to the pulpit that said, "You forget to call to recognize the visitors," or "You forgot to call for the announcement about the bus ride," or "You forgot the offering". I explained to the congregation that we were following the lead and the flow of the Holy Spirit and would get to these items at a later point in the service. The next Sunday I put a sentence before the first item of worship, that remains in the bulletin and says, "The order of service is under the direction of the Holy Spirit and is subject to change without notice".

Since that time the congregation knows that the move of God and the presence of the Holy Spirit is the Order of the Day in worship. I believe in planned worship and in things being done decently and in order. I do not believe in giving God sloppy and haphazard worship. However God the Holy Spirit is not the author of confusion.[8] Therefore, when the Holy Spirit moves among us, we lay aside our plans and order because the Holy Spirit does all things well. The purpose of an order of worship then is not to bind, constrict, or restrict worship, praise, and the movement of the Holy Spirit, but to help set the atmosphere and plan a welcoming context for the manifest presence of the Holy Spirit. Whenever or however the Holy Spirit manifests divine presence, our worship plans become secondary and we give thanks that our planning and preparation were inviting and welcoming enough, and the atmosphere was conducive enough for God to be glorified and the Holy Spirit to bless those who have a heart for worship as well as the passion for true praise.

Planning and preparation then are not antithetical to the move of God or the manifest presence of the Holy Spirit. The presence of the Holy Spirit in worship completes the plan. The presence of the Holy Spirit in worship is affirmation, confirmation, and validation of a worship plan that has come together. Powerful worship is planned worship. Many times, our latter day worship is anemic because of a faulty understanding and practice of the meaning of worship and praise, because we tend to prioritize our orders of worship rather than true worship, and because we do not plan appropriately for worship with the consistency that ushers in the consistent presence of God. The Day of Pentecost was planned worship on the part of heaven. After ten days of the disciples fumbling and stumbling, holding elections, working through their unresolved issues, they were gathered in one place and on one accord in mind, spirit and heart. Then, suddenly the heavens opened and the church was baptized with power and fire from on high.

When the gift of tongues became disruptive, Paul told the church at Corinth, "What should be done then, my friends? When you come together, each one has a hymn, a lesson, a revelation, a tongue, or an interpretation. Let all things be done for building up."[8] Paul was not trying to curb or limit the move of the Holy Spirit but to provide a context for the flow of the Holy Spirit. Many times, we approach worship with a kind of casual, uncoordinated, and lackadaisical approach that limps along from month to month, week to week, and sometimes year to year without much thought about improvement and enhancement. Our trustees, stewards, deacons, elders, ushers, choirs, and other auxiliaries meet regularly. These groups would not think of not meeting regularly, even if they had no real business to discuss. While we will meet to regularly discuss business and controversy, real and imagined, many times we do not meet regularly to discuss how worship can be enhanced to glorify God and bless God's people. There are some churches that have not looked at their order of worship for decades even though everything else and everyone else has changed, including the worship leaders and participants.

Often we prepare separately---the preacher prepares a message; the choirs practice old songs and occasionally come up with a new one; the ushers get together to plan their next fundraiser, work out their internal issues, and go over their marches and procedures when anniversary time draws near, the nurses make sure their supplies and uniforms are in order and the technicians check the mikes. And on Sunday morning we all do our part with the hopes that everything falls together. However, sometimes our efforts fall apart because we have not done any planning and reflection on how we all fit together and if the way we fit together is the best way for worship to happen in this day and age and for a congregation that may have changed since the order of worship was set or fell into place years ago.

All of the separate planning from the constituent components of worship is well and good. Some practice, planning, and preparation is better than none at all. However, at what point do the various constituents look at what we do and say, and the tradition behind them and ask ourselves, "Why do we do this? Do we still need to be doing this? Is there a better way to do this? What is this procedure or custom or tradition adding to the total experience of worship? How does it flow or fit in with the other components, parts and aspects of worship? How does this thing we love to do so much, and in which our ego is invested in so much, fit in with the present church, the present congregation, the present worship style of the congregation, and the present leadership and vision of the present pastor? And most important---Is God glorified in what we are doing or are we just comfortable in doing this because we have always done it this way?

Many times our approach to planning worship is that of fixing squeaking hinges or repairing what is wrong. If the mikes are squealing or too loud or too weak, then we fix those. If there is a problem with the choir or dance ministry or praise team, we fix those or try to. If there is a problem with the ushers or with the bulletin we try to straighten those things out. And if the sermon is too long, too loud, irrelevant or irreverent, we either complain and grumble or suffer it to be so, go somewhere else or try to get another preacher.

We are accustomed to looking at worship in terms of its parts. However, we need to plan worship holistically and not simply try to patch up and repair the weak elements we have isolated and made the scapegoat for whatever goes wrong with worship. Ask some of us what is wrong with our worship and we will complain about the choir and/or its director or the music, the attitude of the ushers, the length, loudness or quietness of the service or the preaching. Very few people think about looking at the worship experience as a whole. Perhaps the whole worship experience needs restructuring. Sometimes the various elements of worship forget that they make up a whole and that what Paul said about the body of the church also applies to its various elements of the worship experience. Paul wrote to the church at Corinth:

Indeed, the body does not consist of one member but of many. If the foot would say, "Because I am not a hand, I do not belong to the body," that would not make it any less a part of the body. And if the ear would say, "Because I am not an eye, I do not belong to the body," that would not make it any less a part of the body. If the whole body were an eye, where would the hearing be? If the whole body were hearing, where would the sense of smell be? But as it is, God arranged the members in the body, each one of them, as he chose. If all were a single member, where would the body be? As it is, there are many members, yet one body. The eye cannot say to the hand, "I have not need of you," nor again the head to the feet, "I have no need of you."...If one member suffers, all suffer together with it; if one member is honored, all rejoice together with it.[9]

The preaching, the music, the sound system, the hospitality of the ushers, the alertness of the security, the attitude and mood of the leadership (clergy and lay), the mood of the congregation, the lighting, comfort and cleanliness of the sanctuary, together

252

contribute to worship experience. If any of them is off kilter or not functioning well, then the whole worship experience can suffer. People receive the message and enjoy the music, and worship in the context of the total experience. Visitors from whom new members come look at the whole worship and church experience before making a decision to receive Christ and join a particular church. Visitors attend our worship experience after having viewed television worship services that have had the opportunity to edit out the normal flubs and flaws of live real time worship. Visitors attend our worship services after having watched secular television programs that have a seamless flow of movement. While none of our worship is perfect, we should always strive for an excellence, not simply for the sake of appealing to media shaped congregants and visitors who attend our churches. We should always strive for excellence in worship because Almighty God is too great and has been too good to us for us to be content with giving God mediocre, ill prepared, half-baked, half-hearted, half-thought out, fragmented, and patched-together worship and praise.

As I grew to recognize the importance of the total worship experience in terms of my own context, I organized a Worship Council that meets with regularity. At first we met monthly, but we now meet bi-monthly. Since I believe that the pastor is chief liturgist and that worship should be a pastoral priority, and since I have learned that people pay attention and consider important what the pastor focuses upon, I chair and attend the Worship Council. In addition to myself, top executive staff, the key musicians, the president of our leading choir, representatives of the steward and trustee boards (our two key policy making boards), my administrative assistant, as well as representatives from the dance or worship arts ministry, security ministry, media and sound ministry, and usher and hospitality ministries are all expected to sit on the Worship Council.

We discuss any special worship services that may be coming up, as well as how our ongoing worship services can be improved. We discuss what we went wrong over the past several weeks and what went very well. Each area has the opportunity to talk about any challenges they may be facing and we together we try to offer suggestions to help any aspect of worship that is encountering difficulties. Since I am the presiding officer, I set the tone for the meeting, part of which is to make sure that everyone stays on point, that all egos are checked at the door, and that we do not digress into other areas of the church's life that do not come within the purview of the Worship Council.

Since I pick out the hymns, I give them the hymns for the upcoming eight weeks, which they are invited to comment upon. The music ministry usually has much to say about my selection of hymns. We try to keep the meetings to an hour and no more than 90 minutes at the maximum. I believe this small investment of time has helped the worship experience to be enhanced and to have better flow. Does this mean that we get it right or that our worship experiences move without human and technical errors? Absolutely not! That is the reason we must have regular meetings. We meet and make plans and things still go wrong. However, we earnestly and sincerely work at framing a solid, viable, prepared, welcoming, and flexible context for the presence of the Holy Spirit in the congregational worship. I believe that God honors our efforts in spite of our errors. While every church is different, I believe every church can still plan to frame a rich worship experience that honors God and in turn blesses the people of God who assemble to exalt the name of the Lord Jesus Christ.

A WORD OF WARNING AND A WORD OF WINNING
Before ending this discussion on prioritizing worship in our personal lives and congregationally, I must give this word of warning. Worship can be one of the most controversial, contentious, and church dividing areas of congregational life. The story is told of a sincere older gentleman who said, "I'd do anything to have my children and grandchildren in church again. They've lost touch with the faith. The church means everything to me, and it breaks my heart that my own family members don't attend anywhere". His eyes watered with emotion as he spoke the sentiments of his heart. A friend responded, "You'd do anything?" Would you change your taste in music? The older

254

gentleman responded without hesitation, "I can't do that."[10] This man's words and attitudes reflect the sentiments of many sincere believers when it comes to "tampering" with the worship service. For many people, worship traditions and music they have become comfortable with represents a sacred cow they are not prepared to easily part with without a fight or without much "weeping and wailing and gnashing of teeth."

Someone has observed that in church life, "There are no wars like music wars." More than one person has commented that the choir seems to be the seedbed for the devil's activity in the church and that the devil seems to break loose in the choir quicker than anywhere else in the church (with the possible exception of the finance room). Why is worship such a volatile issue in the life of the church and why do church choirs tend to be such potentially explosive tinderboxes? I am no scholar but I am inclined to believe that music and worship tend to become so divisive because they focus on giving God glory. Even though they may become involved in other things, choirs are organized for the primary and sole purpose of giving glory to God. The worship life of a church is focused on giving glory to God. Anything that is designed to give glory to God and anyone whose ministry is focused on giving God glory will become targets of the wiles of Satan. Satan will seek to disrupt and destroy anything that seeks to give glory to God. Satan will seek to corrupt and seduce anyone who seeks to give glory to God. This is the reason that choirs, singers, ministers of music, psalmists, musicians, praise leaders, in addition to clergy, need to be constantly lifted in prayer. They become especially vulnerable to the wiles of the enemy.

Sometimes, Satan will use saints who have good hearts and intentions but who have become so attached to their own conceptions or misperceptions that they fear and fight any change that threatens their sense of comfort and home in a world where they are often made to feel homeless and alien. The older gentlemen who felt that giving up the old familiar music he liked was too much of a sacrifice to make, even for the possibility of his children and grandchildren coming back to church, falls into this category.

Sometimes, Satan will use the blessings of our giftedness to seduce us. Attention, pride of accomplishment, comfort, perceived power, popularity, success, and a taste of the riches and glory of the world can make persons susceptible to the wiles of the enemy. Those who are in leadership and those whose ministry puts them in the spotlight or in position to receive attention, pride of accomplishment, comfort, perceived power, popularity, success, and a taste of the riches and glory of the world, such as clergy and leaders of worship and music, are especially vulnerable to the wiles of the enemy. Whether the attention, pride of accomplishment, comfort, perceived power, popularity, success, and a taste of the riches and glory of the world is bestowed by adoring worldly fans or by sincere believers who are grateful because they have been blessed by our gifts that have been magnified by the presence of the Holy Spirit, the pull of the flesh, pride, and the aphrodisiac of power can be very seductive and alluring.

If we are not prayed up and grounded in the word and will of God, Christ's vision for his kingdom and his church, and if we are not attentive to the guidance and the anointing of the Holy Spirit, our priorities and perception can become easily skewed and misdirected. We can begin to think that ministry really is all about us, rather than God's glory. When we forget the God and goal of ministry, we can become involved in the turf wars that sometimes take place between pastors and leaders in the music ministry. Perhaps one of the reasons for so much confusion between those in pastoral leadership and those in music leadership is that we are fraternal twins in the same womb, in the same tight and confining environment and under the same pressure and are fighting for survival and breakthrough into another dimension. Like Esau and Jacob we come forth seeking dominance, resenting and coveting gifts, and attempting to supplant each other. Rather than responding to our "twin-ness" we fight over our differences, without paying any attention to the real enemy who is attempting to defeat the best possible combination of leadership, gifts and vision for the glory of God and the edification of God's people.

When we prioritize worship, expect the enemy to war against us. Sometimes the war takes the form of seduction of sincere saints, the seduction of self, and the seduction of saved leadership. Whatever forms or means worship and praise wars take, and no matter what human personalities are involved in the battles, we must remember, "we wrestle not against flesh and blood, but against principalities, against powers, against the rulers of the darkness of this age, against spiritual hosts of wickedness in heavenly places."[11]Sometimes the face of the opponent is that of an overbearing and cheap pastor, an egotistical minister of music, a star struck palmist or soloist, a money hungry musician, a fussing choir member with a turned up nose and a downcast spirit, a faithful church sister who cannot handle all of that loud music, a kind old gentlemen who loves the church and loves the Lord but holds on to certain music as if they were the embodiment of Christ himself, or a recalcitrant member who looks for any reason to fight and raise hell.

However, the real enemy behind the human faces we see and the human voices we hear is always a spirit that seeks to defeat empowering worship and praise that glorifies God and uses worship revisions and enhancements as another means to further divide the people of God and distract them from their mandate to "make disciples of all nations." There are times when the best course of action for those engaged in worship wars is to take a breath, stop the threats, find their way back to their praying ground, and rephrase the prayer of David in Psalm 139: 19, "Search [us], O God, and know [our] heart[s]; test [us] and know [our] thoughts. See if there be any wicked way in [us], and lead [us] in the way everlasting."

Satan seeks to defeat worship because worship, and the adoration and reverencing of God and praise, the recognition of God's greatness, authority, and goodness defy whatever claims the enemy makes regarding whatever dominion he thinks he has. Since worship and praise defy and challenge the rule of Satan, worship and praise are potent weapons for God's people. Thus worship and warfare go together. I find it interesting that the Book of Revelation, which contains more scenes of warfare than any other book in the New Testament, also contains more worship and praise than any other book in the New Testament. Those who seek to enhance the worship and praise of God's people cannot escape warfare and the wiles of the devil to defeat them. However, the assurance of the word of God is that those who have a heart for the Lord, who seek the face of God above all and through it all, no matter what sacrifices are involved; those who persevere in God glorifying worship and praise, that make all things and people new, no matter what the opposition or circumstances, will triumph at last.

According to the vision of John the Revelator given to him on Patmos, those who prioritize worship privately and congregationally, those who persist in giving glory to God no matter what the context or immediate consequences, are victorious in the end. God will be glorified and God's people edified in the process. John declared:

> *After this I looked, and there was a great multitude that no one could count, from every nation, from all tribes and peoples and languages, standing before the throne and before the Lamb, robed in white, with palm branches in their hands. They cried out in a loud voice saying, "Salvation belongs to our God who is seated on the throne, and to the Lamb!"*
> *And all the angels stood around the throne and around the elders and the four living creatures, and they fell on their faces before the throne and worshiped God, singing, "Amen! Blessing and glory and wisdom and thanksgiving and honor and might be to our God forever and ever! Amen!"*
> *Then one of the elders addressed me, saying, "Who are these, robed in white, and where have they come from?" I said to him, 'Sir, you are the one that knows." Then he said to me, "These are they who have come out of the great ordeal; they have washed their robes and made them white in the blood of the Lamb.*

For this reason they are before the throne of God, and worship him day and night within his temple, and the one who is seated on the throne will shelter them.

They will hunger no more, and thirst no more; the sun will not strike them, nor any scorching heat;

For the Lamb at the center of the throne will be their shepherd, and he will guide them to springs of the water of life, and God will wipe away every tear from their eyes."[12]

---

[1] Matthew 26: 40b-41
[2] Luke 4: 18
[3] Matthew 28: 16-20
[4] Acts 2: 43-47
[5] Matthew 7: 21
[6] II Chronicles 7: 14
[7] I Corinthians 14: 33
[8] I Corinthians 14: 26
[9] I Corinthians 12: 14-21; 26
[10] Robert Schnase, Five Practices of Fruitful Congregations, Nashville: Abington Press, 2007, pp. 45-46.
[11] Ephesians 6: 12 (KJV)
[12] Revelation 7: 9-17

Opening Pandora's Box: Reflections on Sexuality for the Bible-Based Church
Teresa Fry Brown,

Greek mythology contains several different variations of the story of Pandora whose name means source of troubles. Some versions conclude Zeus, the head Greek god, created Pandora out of earth as a punishment for humanity after Prometheus embezzled fire from heaven and gave it to mortals. Without her knowledge, the gods gave a beautiful jar or box to her as a wedding present, filled with all the world's misery and evils. Although warned never to open the box, Pandora's curiosity consumed her. A world full of evil, misery and sorrow immediately was released. She quickly replaced the lid, horrified at what she had done. Some versions, however, contend that under the lid, hope for the world remained.[1] In contemporary language one is said to "open Pandora's box" when the conversation turns to issues that others avoid discussing or the topic is so complex that there is not enough time to fully discuss it. Such is the case with discussions of sexuality and the church.

James B. Nelson, in his classic text *Embodiment*, defines sex as the biologically based character of being male or female and anything connected with sexual gratification or reproduction. Conversely, sexuality is defined as the symbolic meanings, psychological and cultural orientations that involve the entirety of one's personhood, self-understanding and way of being masculine or feminine the world.[2] Ethicist, Traci West, defines sexuality as key to our sensory perceptions, emotional life and our affect or presence with others. Sexuality includes our minds and our bodies. Sexuality reflects our presence with and as God created beings. Sexuality is both individual and communal.[3] In the same text, Christian social ethicist Alton Pollard defines sexuality as our erotic orientation, our attraction to the other sex, same sex or both. Sexuality, in Pollard's view, includes our self-understanding and ways of being in the world with our sexual roles, affection, genital activity, physiological arousal, or our capacity for sensuousness.[4] Sexuality refers to more than sexual organs (genitalia) and to much more than sexual intercourse. It is a way of living in a body as a person with sexual drives that bear on each person's way of thinking, feeling, and acting. The two terms may be intertwined in Bible-based churches or faith based discussions leading to pronouncements about one's actions apart from one's personhood or defining one's level of faith development by one's adherence to or suspension of cultural standards.

On any given Sunday one may hear liberating, life affirming sacred rhetoric, preaching moments, choir selections, Bible studies, or Sunday School lessons that recognize the promise of God that all are welcomed into the kingdom. One may also hear sermons, proclamations, testimonies, prayers or other forms of religious discourse that intentionally marginalize, ignore, oppress, or denigrate particular members of God's human family due to their gender, sexuality or sexual orientation. Judgmental language about "loving the sinner and hating the sin", jokes about one gender's weakness and another's strength, innuendos about "Adam and Eve not Adam and Steve", creation of ecclesiastical "Don't act/don't' tell policies or euphemisms about sex and sexuality may abound in the pulpit and pews.

Pandora's faith talk box overflows with conversations pertaining to homosexuality but comparatively little is said about sexuality. The church reflects on why one sin demands rigorous public scrutiny and punishment and another sin is glossed over as personal, private and accepted as "everyone is dong it" behavior. If one believes the biblical text" all have sinned and come short of the glory of God" who sets the standards of acceptable sexual behavior? What is said about clergy responsibility for personal sexual behavior or complicity in sexual harassment or abuse? Where is the congregational discussion of sexual surrogacy as men and women view the pastor as their "husband" or "wife"? How long will we endure the *"wink wink"* or *"hint hint"* about the length of so-called Holy hugs and kisses as the membership passes the peace?

Is anyone responsible for ending the discussions on who is dating whom? How did we reach the point where all the "real" men have access to the "Master's Meat" (selected young women's sexual favors) due to the stress, needs, and ownership of men of faith, senior male pastors or visiting ministers? If "God is no respecter of persons" why are all the "real" women weak "receptacles" for men, out of order if they enter ministry, castrating men if they head households or are victims of sexual shaming as "bad women" if they become pregnant or tell someone about an unwanted or unwarranted proposition? What is the origin of the spoken and unspoken mythology that all the "gay" men are in the choir, are all child predators, or are all in need of deprogramming-pray it away sessions, or lessons on hyper masculinity by "real" men? Should churches remain selective by focusing on one category of sexual misconduct? Who is willing to not only open Pandora's Box but also to engage in honest, sans uncomfortable, smatterings of whispers, pointing and laughter discussion of not only homosexuality but also each believer's personhood as sexual beings?

The following essay will briefly delve into a few considerations of sexuality in Bible-based churches. The essay serves as a resource for ongoing discussion rather than the definitive answer to the following questions. What is at the source of either the seeming preoccupation or pubic silence on issues of sexuality? How do leaders of Bible-based churches speak of God's love and care in one breath, and castigate God's children in another? Why is the subject of sexuality both inflammatory and ignored? What are some biblical imperatives, commandments, laws that speak to sexual behavior? Why are some texts routinely used to describe the sexual behavior of particular groups while other texts are routinely omitted that describe the sexual behavior of others? Is there even residual hope of honest and ethical church based conversations on sexuality?

Lord, How Come We Here?
Church history scholar, Gayraud Wilmore, writes that the nineteenth century religious revivalism known as the "Great Awakening" and the subsequent development formative of nineteenth century religious institutions taught, "Cleanliness was next to Godliness". In order to be fully accepted as humans in society one was required to exhibit middle class manners and morals. Sex of any type was deemed "dirty" according to various interpretations of biblical ordinances and laws. This led to a form of conservatism in mainline denominations that allowed "communal values to at times override biblical legalism", making tolerant exceptions to the rule for sons and daughters of congregants and clergy.[5] There were instances of men and women being separated even in worship to shield men from "seductress" women who might lead them to "sins of the flesh". The First Great Awakening was closely followed by two intertwining movements that solidified rules, standards, and expectations of men and women in *genderized* roles in home, church, and society.

The so-called "Cult of True Womanhood" that developed in the 19th century (1820-1860) defined womanhood through cardinal virtues. This emanated from Victorian standards and delineated the proper place of primarily white women in society. Piety meant that women were naturally religious, moral, virtuous, and more open to the call of conversion and consolations of religion than men. It was a woman's duty to teach the children about God and insure that her spouse was religious. This strengthened the family and protected the republic. Women were to be pure and asexual. Men, on the other hand, were sexually rampant and could not help themselves. They had to depend on women to assist them in denying their urges. Women were to be submissive and accept subordination to their husbands who ruled by divine ordination. "Female influence" was to be exercised gently, subtly or one was deemed unfeminine. Finally, a woman was to be domestic. Her sphere was home, household tasks, nurturing and bearing children.[6] The church was a desirable setting for men and women; however, men were rulers of public and private castles.

Conversely, the second Great Awakening (Protestant revivalism) took place from 1795 to 1830. The movement prompted American women to actively evangelize families and neighbors. The primary outcome of the revivals was holiness as directly tied into charisma. This meant a new authoritative power in position and religion with one's personal access to the divine. The coupling of a women's call to proclaim and the Holy Spirit enabled women leaders to achieve self-empowerment and priest personal autonomy. They were empowered to minister to the people by bringing meaning and healing to their lives. Charisma enabled women to found religious institutes and inspire movements outside patriarchal mainstream religions. There was a social expectation of leadership due to the move of the Holy Spirit in the life of men and women.

Women who responded to their calls to leadership, ministry, and teaching were charged with being part of the "feminization of the church," in which the lack of male participation in churches or religious communities was attributed to –and often blamed upon-

- women's presence and personalities, women such as them. In a 1921 article in the *AME Review*, the editor describes the crisis created by "Silly Women Masquerading in the Name of Religion". He castigates them as generally ignorant, public nuisances, grotesque caricatures, which "carry, ostentatiously, a Bible, and adorn themselves with crosses, crucifixes, rosettes, or badges..." He charges women with being too loud, too conspicuous, and too visible, reminding his readers that women's work was to be with the poor or with children in the role of stewardess or deaconesses.

> ...*the horde of irresponsible "evangelists" and women in religious garb, bearing different names, are attaining such proportions that pastors should refuse to recognize them. ...as a rule, they can sing and are glib with a slangy harangue which may create a temporary attraction for the crowd.*[7]

Apparently in an attempt to placate or perhaps silence these very women, the editor ends his comments by saying women have always had a place in the church as prophets, evangelists, and ministering saints. The implication is that women who work quietly in the background will be elevated for their good works while those who seek a more visible—and particularly preaching--role are an embarrassment to the church. The editor was apparently entrenched in the larger culture's ideology of true womanhood, which understood the domain of women as being the home –to be kept immaculately...for men, whose domain therefore was any area outside the home, including the church.

Women instead were to be pure, chaste, and virginal, eternally available for the needs and pleasures of men. So although women were responsible for teaching men and children about faith,[1] for reading the Bible, leading prayers, and teaching religion in the home, they were castigated for doing so in public. Little has changed as ordination wars and patent statements by some men about women's roles abound at least until their daughters, mothers, sisters, or wives express a call to a previously "male" leadership role. Others swim against the tide when the women in their lives tire of writing papers, editing sermons, suffering silently working in the church or supporting the husband's ministry while suppressing their own God given gifts and talents and a new vision, revelation, "Rhema word" or new take on a text leads them to believe women can in fact do ministry.

Unlike sex, which is a biological concept, gender is a social construct specifying the socially and culturally prescribed roles that men and women are to follow. Gender identity may be affected by a variety of social structures, including the person's ethnic group, employment status, religion or irreligion, and family. Socialy acceptable gender roles originate in community and persons are accountable to the power structures in that chosen community for either living into those roles or rejecting them. In a number of faith systems, denominations and local churches gender roles are ascribed using the leadership's interpretation of specific biblical texts and assessment of social cultural needs. Abilities, responsibilities, religiosity, and piety along gender lines are entrenched. There are special conferences, programs, and ministries to "attract" men to the church—women purportedly having driven them away. These restoration programs are established to give men a sense of strength, power and purpose; reclaim their godly" masculinity, "headship", and role as women's "covering". Men are said to be made in the image of God but women are weaker vessels, made from men, who need to be submissive, controlled, nurtured, protected, and subservient.[7]

Women are being denied ordination or their ministerial orders are being rescinded. In some denominations women are removed from lay leadership positions to make room for more men—a phenomenon I talk about as senior pastors "birthing baby boys and killing all the baby girls". Women are said to be "out of order" if they head households regardless of the reason for absent or even limited male leadership. Male responsibility for abandoning women and children, absenteeism due to imprisonment, loss of employment, incapacitation due to illness, or basic demographic or census information indicating women out number men in every age, racial, and ethnic group is not indicative of all women willfully "trying to become men". The root of the matter is deeper. The argument is not new. The numerous social constructs of gender roles, sex and sexuality, just as in the nineteenth century, are based on traditional, inerrant, literal, liberal, figurative, denominational, individual or collective, interpretation of the biblical text.

For the Bible tells me so...
Many Christians believe that scripture is a source of revelation that bears witness to the Word of God. There is attention to how the text reveals God's pattern for our lives and disclosure of how we are to engage and love God, others and ourselves. The individual understanding a particular text is dependent on the perception, comprehension, integration, use and relationship with the words either on paper or heard. Other considerations of textual meaning include knowledge of the language of the text, the translation of the text, authority given the text or the one presenting the text, context in which the text is read or used, effective learning channels for receiving the text and communal or individual interpretation and/or acceptance of the text. There are, however, instances of a form of bibliolatry that elevates Christian scripture above God's revelation in Jesus Christ. Bibliolatry refers to the worship of the bible - taking it so seriously and so literally that it becomes the entire focus of religious devotion, even to the exclusion of everything else. It is the excessive adherence to a literal interpretation of the Bible or extreme devotion to or concern with books.[8] There is a difference between rigid love of the words in the printed book and understanding of the revelation of the living Word of God. What are some of the textual descriptors of sex, sexuality and gender roles? How does the biblical text inform us about marriage, intercourse, rape, sexual immorality, prostitution, fornication, and homosexuality? There are approximately three hundred fourteen texts regarding sexuality in the biblical text depending on translation.

Regardless of which Creation story one reads God formed humankind as male and female (Genesis1:26-28). Said to be made in the image of God, humanity ranks above and has dominion rather than dominance over animals due to our God given thought processes, emotions, and needs. The man (*adam*) in Genesis 1:26-28 ("him") represents the human species ("them") made up of male and female. Each reflects the image of God.[8] Each is responsible, as fully God-made and breathed into humans, to work together to increase the human population, to share in God's benefits and to obey God. The Creation story in Genesis 2:18, 20-22, depending on one's interpretation of the text, is used to substantiate women are less than, the complement, the helpmate, the corresponding opposite, the equal, the essence of men due to her creation after man from his rib. In the Hebrew Bible and the New Testament of the 3000-3100 named persons only 137-170 are women, often associated with the place of their birth.[10] The dearth of women's stories in the biblcial text is cited as evidence of their minimal importance in the grand scheme of God's world. One rebuttal to the evidence may be that the social context and gender of the historian is a determanent of whose story is told rather than one's influence or importance.

The Old Testament is filled with stories and rules about sex. The Bible virtually lacks terms for the sexual organs, being content with such euphemisms as "foot" or "thigh" for the genitals, and other euphemisms to describe coitus, such as "he knew her" (Genesis 4:1;) or "to know" to mean sexual intercourse or the sexual act union of desiring and knowing (Genesis 30:14-15.) Use of terms for penis or vagina usually are met with gasps, blushing, or frowns as if no one ever uses the terms. This is one of the points when adults pretend that everyone arrived by "Immaculate conception" or that one only talkes about genitilia behind closed doors. The biblical text with figurative language or the languae of the day at least speaks to sexual intercourse. One might wonder how healthy congregations would be if there was honest and mature dialogue about physical sex, why God created distinctive body parts for men and women, and the benefits of using the real names of our sexual organs rather than infantile, street, or cultural media names.

In ancient Israel the primary purpose for sexual desire was to create life or procreation (Genesis 3:16) as a mirror of the creative nature of God. Although they were viewed as the man's property, women were "co-producers of children with Yahweh. The more male children women produced the greater their social status.[11] This measuring stick carried over into periods of American enslavement where women were given birth prizes for the more marketable children she birthed. In biblical times, sex was to be used with care due to the risks of death from childbirth. Casual sex without marital or family bonding was against societal norms. The perpetuation of one's name through the birth of male children (See Numbers 27, 36 the Daughters of Zelophehad exception to the rule) and assurance of property rights meant sexual relations were essential to the survival of society and entire households. In the three versions of the wife/sister stories, Abraham and Isaac try to pass their wives off as their sisters and almost endanger peace in the land (Gen 12, 26 and 20). Sex was about continuity not some salacious "dirty" act. Sex was created on purpose and for a purpose. A human critique of a God given act is responsible for the current idea that moral people do not have sex. Sexual immorality is about causal sex absent love, respect or commitment. Biblical love is creative.

There were inflexible laws about sexual hygiene in the biblical text. Any emissions from the body (semen and menstrual blood) were considered unclean. A menstruating woman was unclean (not to be touched) for seven days, and anything she touched or sat on was also defiled (Leviticus 15:19-24). Many women today speak of menses as a "curse" and something dirty rather than evidence of the potential for child bearing. Emission of semen after intercourse is also cause for ritual impurity for men and women. Both had to bathe in water to be purified (Leviticus 15:16-18). "Nasty" people are those with questionable hygiene and those whose sexual practices are public knowledge. Communicable or sexually transmitted diseases are rarely discussed in churches other than the occasional health fair or a World AIDS Day wear a red ribbon for "those" people Sunday.

One of the reasons for excluding women from ministry is that they may be menstruating. No thought is given to the possibility that a woman may have had a hysterectomy and would not emit blood or the man who may have an ejaculatory moment while serving in the church. Finally, the Song of Solomon is one of the most sexually explicit books in the Bible yet is rarely preached or taught. It holds beautiful language that would be instructive on how to language love, sex or relationships. In spite of all the resources available in the biblical text the topic of sex is avoided as if the very discussion would cause listeners to perform rampant sexual acts in the midst of worship or a nod is given to puritanical standards that such things are not discussed in "mixed company."

Marriage was an expression of a social unit signifying kinship and family patterns. Women often were married soon after menarch. Women had to be virgins at marriage but the Bible never mentions male virginity. If it was determined that the bride was not a virgin she was stoned to death (Deuteronomy 22:12-21). Women's life expectancy was shorter than men usually due to childbirth.[13] Men married later in life generally after he was able to support a household. Marriage defined the extent of a man's ownership, control of people and property. Women were considered the property of her father, male head of household, brother or husband. Women had minimal rights and, as was the case in the Cult of True Womanhood, women's domain was the home. Because she had little or no source of income the woman depended on the man in her life for support.

Part of the argument about "uppity" women today is that women often have a source of income and are able to live alone, work to help support the family, or may be the higher or only financial source for the family due to illness, unemployment or under employment or absence of men in th family. The charge is that women are trying to be men. Perhaps the reason is that the Biblical economic, cultural and family structure allowed women to remain at home not working but the current structures demand that women contribute to the household in order for families to survive. One's social location of privilege allows for men to be the principle "breadwinner" while other locations demand everyone in the family to work just to make ends meet. This is an economic reality not a challenge to the man as head of household or women trying to destroy masculinity.

Sexual intercourse for any reason other than to protect the integrity of the family unit (Exodus 20:14) is called fornication.[14] This includes various acts of sexual immorality, behavior against the norms and standards of society, especially being a harlot or whore. Men were privileged to have sexual relations with married women within the bounds of law. If he could afford it, a man's household could include a number of women, termed polygamy. Polygamy (many wives) and concubinage (a marital sexual arrangement often following a woman's voluntary consent or involuntary enslavement due to debt, war, etc) were regularly practiced in the Old Testament. Concubines, such as Hagar or Zilpah, were in a recognized martial or extramarital relationship but were legally inferior to the legitimate, often barren, wife. A concubine's status varied with the number of her male children. The double standard of the sexual activities of men and women is not new.

In the Old Testament there were numerous social regulations regarding adultery, incest, rape and prostitution are determinants in the males' property rights over women. Men were carrying out acts to protect themselves but women were cast as doing something "unnatural". Prostitution was considered natural and necessary as a safeguard of the virginity of the unmarried and the property rights of husbands (Joshua 2:1-7). A man did not sin if he visited a prostitute (Proverbs 6:26) but the prostitute sinned. A woman whose father was not in ministry (priesthood) was allowed to be a prostitute (Leviticus 21:9).

Contemporarily, rape is the defined, as unlawful sexual intercourse with a woman against her will. The biblical text describes several instances of rape (Genesis 34:1-4), a gang rape (Genesis 19:4-8), and incest (Genesis 19:31-39), and prostitution (Gen 38:15-17). If a man raped a woman who was unmarried or was engaged he had to marry her without any option for divorce

271

(Deuteronomy 22:28-29). A man desecrated the property rights of another man if he raped an engaged woman. There is no mention of the emotional or physical damage done to the violated woman. In one well-known biblical story, her brother Amnon rapes Tamar. Her father, David, is angered but does nothing. Tamar goes to live with her brother, Absalom. He eventually avenges the rape by having his brother killed. Tamar's voice of protest is heard prior to and immediately after the rape, and then her voice is never heard again. She had no rights, not even to her body. Little has changed over the centuries. Women are blamed for causing the rape due to her attire, inferred provocative mannerisms, belief that women enjoy rape, men own women anyway so it is not a big deal, or women's failure to say "no" loud and long enough for the perpetrator to understand she means that she wants to preserve the sanctity of her own body[15]. In reality, this felony offense happens to men, women and children with more than 60% of rapes perpetrated by a person the victim knows.

The Biblical text clearly condemns adultery as a sexual sin and a violation of property rights. Adultery is defined as having sex with another man's wife or concubine without his permission, not as having sex outside of one's marriage. It was consensual intercourse by a married woman with a man other than her husband's right. The rationale was that adultery might establish paternity issues and economic loss[16] There was a belief that an adulterous man was not violating his own marriage but someone else's. Adultery was a capital offense (Leviticus 20:10), with a punishment of death by stoning for both the man and the woman if the woman was married (Deuteronomy 22:22). In the twenty first century, adultery is generally described as any sexual relationship, outside of marriage by a man or a woman.

The New Testament world indicates some modification in rules of gender engagement. Although there are a large number of single persons mentioned in the New Testament stories it is difficult to know if they never married, were separated from or living apart from families or widowed.[17] Although public conversations between single men and women were forbidden,

Jesus routinely held faith dialogues with lone women. Women are blessed (Mary), priests (Anna), homeowners (Martha), business owners (Tabitha), queens (the Candace), teachers (Pricilla), head of households (Lydia), single mothers (Canaanite woman), deacons (Phoebe), disciples (certain women in Luke 8), teachers, greedy (Sapphira) and sinful (woman anointing Jesus" feet). The depiction of the status of women is quite different from the Old Testament. Women had voices and actual dialogue. Women and men seemed to be in some cases equals in spite of some of Paul's writings. Regulations in some Bible-based churches pertaining to the length of women's hair, head and lap coverings, type of attire, makeup and jewelry are composed from the interpretation of the Pauline letters on submission and sexual immorality.

There are seemingly more rigorous rules concerning sexual conduct in the New Testament as compared to the Old Testament. There are approximately seventeen topics on sex and sexual behavior included in First Corinthians alone. Paul addresses moral values, gender roles, sexuality, sexual desire, physical anatomy, family structures, marriage, child rearing, love, decision-making, communication, assertiveness, shared sexual behavior, and religion. The sacredness of the body, mutual sexual pleasure and responsibility of intimacy are included in the text attributed to Paul. In the New Testament, the word, *porneia*, is used to mean any act of sexual immorality such as voluntary sexual intercourse with an unmarried person (1 Corinthians 7:2); adultery (Matthew 5:32); lust (Mathew 5:28); divorce based on infidelity (Matthew 19:3-9) and prostitution (Revelation 2:14).

Harlots and prostitutes are lifted up as the ultimate "bad women" in the biblical text, although redeemed like Rahab after some great act that saved men. To call a woman a prostitute was also a routine interpretation when a reader was unable to figure out how the "good" woman became an integral part of a Biblical story line. One has only to study, for example, the case of Mary of Magdela to understand the veracity of this claim. Mary is a victim of mistaken identity. Although there is no Biblical evidence that she was ever a prostitute; the fifth century Pope Gregory identified Mary as a *peccatrix*, a sinful woman, using her as a model for the repentant sinner. He mistranslated the word *meretrix*, a prostitute. Many decided that the reason she was with Jesus was that she was so repentant she had no choice but to follow. Some even confused her with Mary the sinner, and Mary of Bethany from the gospel as one in the same. It took 14 centuries (1969) before the slanderous characterization began to change.[18] There was an established practice that good women or named women were the exception to the rule or exemplified proverbial "virtuous" woman who knew her place, loved God and although working, was doing so to make her husband's life better. Mary of Magdela was too independent, and therefore must have been redeemed from the most heinous profession a woman could have in order to dedicate her life to following Jesus. There are numerous specialized threshing floor conferences, books, sermons, and songs about a woman's need to "be slain in the spirit", "come clean about her past," tell it all," and "be delivered."

The most contentious subject in Pandora's Box is homosexuality. The term, while having no equivalent in Hebrew or Greek, was coined in the nineteen century in reference to same gender sexual relations. This was not the inception of such relationships just the naming of the particular type of relationship. There are a number of allusions to same gender loving and same gender relationships throughout human history. One has only to read classical literature, peruse various forms of media, recount family histories, or observe life to become aware of same gender relationships. A quick web search reveals that persons have even questioned the relationships of Jonathan and David, Ruth and Naomi, Paul and Barnabas, Jesus and the disciples, as possible same gender loving paradigms. Even in church culture, if some members are unable to discern if a man is in a heterosexual relationship, an anecdotal assessment of his mannerisms, voice, attire, martial status, carriage, and absence of a family results in a default determination that he is gay. Because women are more likely to be single, divorced, or widowed the determination of her sexuality is not a priority. This seems to be a nod to the church idea that family structures need a male figurehead and the gay man is endangering that structural necessity. The preoccupation with the subject matter is at times mind-boggling.

The Biblical text contains only four to six verses about sexual activity between members of the same sex depending on the translation and interpretation of the texts. Genesis 19:1-13 (infers sex male-male gang rape); Leviticus 18:22, 20:30 is about men lying with men, punishable by death); Romans 1:18-32 (violation of purity laws, unclean and dishonorable.[19] 1 Corinthians 6:9-10 (sense of licentious, loose, or lacking in self-control); Timothy 1:8-11; and Jude 7 (sex with angels). The New Testament words imply one is "soft" or is a male or female prostitute. The sense that men participating in these sexual activities are *demasculinized* may add to the fervent critique of persons who name themselves homosexual rather than the socially acceptable "strong" man. Critiques of the mannerisms of males as to effeminate, posturing or walking as "like a woman", attire as being "girly", or fear of hugging or even handshakes with men deemed "funny" abound in churches. Tentative acceptance of gay men as long as they are contributing to the worship experience yet condemning them when their services are no longer needed is a curious program. The reality is that there are same gender loving people who fear public "outing". Some are encouraged by supervisors or leaders to "hide" in pulpit and pew closets in order to continue in ministry or worship in peace. Others remain in loveless marriages in order not to embarrass the family and to have children not confiding in spouses until divorce, death or disease. Some fear emotional, physical, and verbal attacks by the same people who speak about God's love or "all have sinned and come short of the glory of God" creates a counterintuitive rationale to worshiping God in spirit and in truth.

The Leviticus texts, in particular, blatantly condemn same gender sexual behaviors regardless of the translation cited.[22] According to the biblical text, persons violating these laws are to be put to death. It is interesting that the same people of faith who immediately charge that homosexuality and any disease associated with homosexual or lesbian persons are to die but fail to review the biblical text for other death penalty cases. There are many other behaviors, in the biblical text, that result in the death penalty. They include murder (Genesis 9:5-6), perjury (Zechariah 5:4), striking or cursing father or mother (Exodus 21:15,17), disobedience to parents (Deuteronomy 21:18-21), theft (Zechariah 5:3-4), Sabbath desecration (Numbers 15:32-36), treason (1Kings 2:25), sedition (Act 5:36-37), adultery (Deuteronomy 22:24), incest (Leviticus 20:11-12,14), promiscuity (Deuteronomy 22:21-24), bestiality (Exodus22:19), sodomy (Leviticus 18:22; 20:13), and rape of an engaged virgin (Deuteronomy 22:25). Selective use of texts to determine one groups' residence in heaven or hell while overlooking everyone's responsibility to live by all God's commandments, rules, laws or regulations must be reevaluated. Every person has the moral obligation to live responsibly not just same gender loving persons.

Regardless of why one selects a text, interprets a text or uses a text homiletics scholar, Ronald Allen, states that one must consider its appropriateness to the gospel and ask oneself "Does this text affirm that God loves each person (and all parts of nature) with unconditional love? Does this text call for justice (that is, relationships of love in community) for each person and all constituents of the natural world?"[23] Old Testament scholar, Renita Weems, states that the result of faithful and just use of the biblical text is "the oppressed are liberated, the last became first, the humbled are exalted, the despised are preferred, those rejected are welcomed, the long-suffering are rewarded, the dispossessed are repossessed, and the arrogant are prostrated."
[23]Any use of the biblical text that purposely demeans, denigrates or disenfranchises another child of God on the basis of gender, sex or sexuality is a misappropriation of the text. The repercussion of proof texting, using texts out of context or selectively using texts to identify or castigate one to the exclusion of another has serious repercussions. The power of our words even use of the Word of God can lead to psychic damage to persons seemingly devalued even by God, acceptance

of domestic violence as deserved by women, sexual harassment of men and women, and community brokenness even as persons preach and teach the love of God.

Is There Still Hope in Pandora's Box? Reflections of Possibilities

Remembering that some versions of the Pandora's box myth state that *hope* was left inside the box one might wonder if in spite varied interpretations, misinterpretations, disagreements, challenges, charges, jokes, innuendos and euphemisms if there is any hope for honest and full conversations on sexuality and the church. The Biblical text speaks of being transformed by the renewing of our minds. Justice is a process of deprogramming our thoughts about self and others, engaging institutions, social structures and persons who seek to enslave us and imagining new and different ways of living as God created people in God's created world. This requires an assessment of why and how we use texts about sex and sexuality in the church. Why are we citing texts? Is the purpose of teaching, preaching or discussing sex and sexuality punitive for one type of love over another, one gender over another, or one age group over another? Is the purpose preventative and protective in a concerted effort to expose congregants to God's rules for living and loving God, others and self, to protect and maintain family units, or to stave off disease? Is it a nod to be politically correct, to follow a particular line of thought about sex, or avoidance of candid discussion of what we do not know about the subject matter? Do Bible-based churches develop a theology of the body and sexuality based on a consideration of the Image of God? What are the standards of moral accountability for sex and sexuality in the church? How do we teach members to be responsible for their own lives and how they use or care for the body God gave them?

Content or issues of sex and sexuality are more than homosexuality but how we each live as beings created by God. Topics on what the Biblical text and our lived experiences say sex and sexuality might include: issues of infertility, pregnancy, rape (stranger and acquaintance), prostitution and those who use the services, abortion, genetics, marriage, blessings of sexual relationships, inter-racial marriage, domestic violence, harassment, incest, child abuse, divorce, responsible sexual behavior, blended families, still births, celibacy (chosen, vocational), singleness (chosen, vocational, through death of a partner), AIDS and STDS, "living together", sexuality and those physically challenged, pornography, marriage of the mentally challenged, teen-age sexuality and pregnancy, day care/parenting, sexual surrogacy, touching, abuse, infidelity, and disease. These topics must be supported through Bible study, confidential discussion groups, intergenerational presentations, and professional presentations rather than isolated sermons.

The residual hope in this Pandora's box is that thinking people of faith understand there are no exceptions to the rules. All persons must reassess what our sexual behaviors are. We must under gird the sermons, songs, testimonies, and prayers with messages of how God wants life to be and reconstruct community so that all persons are able to move to where God wants it to be. One must challenge the listeners and self to a thorough examination and fuller personal engagement of the Biblical text. The leadership must relay hope for change from present realities to future possibilities. Finally, there must be critiques of the inequities in interpersonal relationships, families, communities, and churches and in the world. The result will be *emancipatory* knowledge through care filled and careful re-reading of the biblical texts. It means the hopeful, personal and communal empowerment to talk about and understand sex and sexuality without laughter, euphemism or innuendos. At the end of the day, perhaps the healthy thing for Bible-based churches to do is to open Pandora's box and begin the Godly rather than worldly journey of healthy and hope filled sexual lives that value all persons.

[1] http://www.merriamwebster.com/dictionary/pandora's;http://www.answers.com/topic/pandora;
[2] http://www.newworldencyclopedia.org/entry/Pandora's_Box.
[3] James Nelson, *Embodiment*, Minneapolis, Augsburg, 1978, 14-13; 17-18, 112-129
[4] Traci West, "Ethical Black Ministerial Practices" in *Loving the Body: Black Religious Studies and the Erotic*, Anthony Pinn and Dwight Hopkins, editors, (New York: Palgrave/McMillan) 2004, 38.

[5]Ibid. Alton Pollard, "Teaching the Body", 318.

[6] Gayraud Wilmore, "What we can learn about he texture of Christian ethics by observing how African American congregations have historically dealt with issues related to sexuality", San Francisco: The Covenant Network of Presbyterians; 2006, 3.

[7]Susan Hill Lindley, *"You have Stept out of your Place": a History of Women and Religion in America*, (Louisville: Westminster John Knox Press, 1996) 52-54.

[8] *A.M.E. Review,* Vol. 38, No. 2, October 1921. 89.

[9]Hill Lindley, 52-54.

[10] Jonathan Walton*, Watch This! The Ethics and Aesthetics of Black Televangelism,*(New York: New York University Press, 2009)*,* 119-121, 129-130, 141, 143.

[11]http://education.yahoo.com/reference/dictionary/entry/bibliolatry

[12] http://www.biblestudytools.com/dictionaries/bakers-evangelical-dictionary/sexuality-human.html

[13]Carol Meyers, general editor, *Women in Scripture*, (Grand Rapids: Eerdmans, 2001), 33.

[14] Lyn M. Betchel, "sex" in *Eerdmans Dictionary of the Bible,* 1192-1193.

[15] Jon L. Berquist, in "marriage" in *Eerdmans Dictionary of the Bible,* David N. Freedman, editor. (Grand Rapids: Wm B. Eerdmans, 2000), 861-862.

[16] Allison A. Trites, fornication" in *Eerdmans Dictionary of the Bible*, 469.

[17] http://www.ncjrs.gov/App/publications/Abstract.aspx?id=151023

[18]Heindrik L. Bosman, "adultery", in. *Eerdmans Dictionary of the Bible*, 23-24.

[19]Berquist, 862.

[20] Carol Meyers, 120-122. See also http://www.pbs.org/wnet/religionandethics/week712/feature.html

[21]L. Wm Countryman, 'homosexuality" in *Eerdmans Dictionary of the Bible,* 602-603.

[22]Walter Wink, "Biblical Perspectives On Homosexuality" in *The Christian Century*; 7 November 1979.

[23] Ronald A. Allen, *Preaching: An Essential Guide* (Nashville: Abingdon Press, 2002) 52.

[24] *Renita Weems, Reading Her Way through the Struggle: African American Women and the Bible", Stony the Road We Trod, Cain Hope Felder, editor, (Minneapolis: Fortress, 1991) 57-77.*

YOUTH MINISTRY

Din Tolbert

When I was a child, I talked like a child, I thought like a child, I reasoned like a child. When I became a man, I put childish ways behind me. Now we see but a poor reflection as in a mirror; then we shall see face to face. Now I know in part; then I shall know fully, even as I am fully known. And now these three remain: faith, hope and love, but the greatest of these is love.

1 Corinthians 13:11-13 (NIV)

In thinking about "how to do youth ministry," we might do ourselves a great service by reading and reflecting on the entirety of 1 Corinthians 13. Love is, after all, the message that saves us. You can be the most eloquent speaker with the largest vocabulary and an impressive storehouse of knowledge, but if the youth you serve can't perceive your love for them and your investment in their lives and well-being, your ministry may get people's attention, but it will not be transformative. You can have great programming that impacts a community and a brand recognized for setting the standard in youth initiatives, but if there isn't the time taken to connect with your young people, you'll have a revolving door ministry.

Ultimately, Christian ministry is not about persuasive preaching or even good church – no more than any construction process is about the tools used to accomplish it. This calling is about inviting people into relationship with the divine and walking with them to understand our responsibilities, expectations and potencies as imperfect people loved by a perfect God. As difficult as this walk is, people need to know that they are loved through it. And, whether it's fair or not, Christian leaders are the representatives of both human and divine love. By our action, God can seem present and involved – dwelling among his children – or absent and disinterested – too busy doing stuff to stop by and see about His people. I'm simply saying our quest toward more perfect love needs to be central if we are going to do ministry, youth ministry in particular.

Though all of 1 Corinthians 13 ought, therefore, be the reminder that guides our doing, I believe verses 11-13 speak volumes to us about the mind and the method of the youth minister. As I look through the text, I am struck by an incredible series of questions that practically beg us to ask ourselves what it really means to be a child. What does it mean to talk like a child? To think like a child or reason like one? How much can we use our own childhood as a frame of reference for understanding the answers to these questions today? Some of us may be quite a few years separated from the congregations we deal with and, though some things are constant throughout the years, we may drastically miss the mark if our method for understanding the actions of our youth is simply to imagine what we were thinking at their age.

Within the framework of this major conversation, I want to pose a bunch of questions and offer some wisdom for you to hold up against your life and your experiences in youth ministry thus far.

Whatever fits; feel free to use. Whatever doesn't, shelve it for now but keep track of it. I do believe you'll find it handy at some point. Whatever raises your eyebrow, use it to facilitate discussion and build relationship with people you've identified as key contributors to your development in ministry, whether they are senior leadership, nephews and nieces, or the people you've felt led to minister to.

Being a Child

Over the past year, I've seen some remarkable things happen in the lives of young people around the world. Via the internet, I watched a 6 year old pianist and composer switch effortlessly between classical and jazz but on that same website I saw news footage of a teenager being beaten to death by his peers. Closer to home, I saw a 12 year old actor, filmmaker and educational advocate inspire his generation to envision new possibilities and realms of success but I've also counseled young men and women who knew the weighty harshness of this life all too well. Our young people are capable of immense good and unthinkable wrong. They live in a world of so much privilege, access to information and connectedness to diverse cultures and opportunities, and yet they are not distant from dangers, concerns and obligations that can make us wonder, "How old are you again?"

How does a child approach the concept of genius or paradigm shifting? How does a teenager understand death caused by his or her own hands or deal with their recovery from great loss? Is their cognitive processing dictated singularly by their age, or do these mature experiences and concepts signify mature thoughts about them? Can we so easily assume that there is a general way of childlike thinking and that it is, by definition, less advanced than the adult way of thinking? What are the implications for how we hear and value these "underdeveloped" thoughts, particularly when they challenge our firmly established ways of understanding? Do we treat young people like they are thinking in meaningful ways about things that matter or do we treat them like they are only capable of imagining juvenile, inconsequential things? I believe that the young people we minister to are thinking very powerfully about their agency in this world, and about what structures of power seem responsible for shaping their environment. Their thoughts are not meager and they need to be affirmed. For me, this means there are three things Shekinah Youth Church has got to give voice and credence to in our ministry to youth: the individual, the thought, and the language or culture that the thought is breathed through. All three are valuable and worth hearing, as well as discussing.

Affirming the Individual
One of the biggest, most damaging misconceptions about youth ministry is that it's just a stepping-stone to a "more significant" position. Now this myth is so tricky to deconstruct fully because, as most effective lies are, it's based in truth and reinforced by practice. I do think that the individual who maintains effectiveness and relevance for a youth population, despite a widening cultural gap, is the exception rather than the rule. There is some logical basis for saying that you shouldn't be in youth ministry (in a conventional sense) all of your life but an opposite, and equally non-beneficial, extreme is to treat youth ministry like a transitional period where you do just enough to get noticed by the powers that be. Frighteningly, many churches do very little to dissuade this latter kind of thinking. Whether it's inadequate funding or strained resources for youth initiatives, it can seem like church culture treats youth ministry as something "not yet relevant." But God forbid that we, as youth ministers, ever adopt this attitude. We've got to see, even when nobody else sees, that youth ministry is the most important ministry to the continued existence of the church. Youth have to be told and shown that we value the privilege and the awesome responsibility of being present for them because there is no church of tomorrow without pouring into and empowering the youth of today. These young people are up against a lot and they need committed and caring people to help bend their outlook toward hope and direct their devotion toward God.

That being said, I have never understood "affirming the individual" to mean saying "yes you can" to every request or pumping a person up with encouragement for things that he or she is not good at, but rather helping them find their vein or niche and then putting my time, effort, and resources into developing them along that line. So, I think a primary goal in affirming individuals is learning what type of individuals you're dealing with. It might not be realistic to organize a ministry wide behavioral style assessment like the DiSC® or a personality type indicator like the Myers-Briggs, but getting to know the different personalities in your church can be done in any number of ways.

A starting ground that I've found helpful, and less overwhelming than doing in-depth, one-on-one character studies of every member of Shekinah, has been to pay close attention to the dominant and emerging personalities in the ministry. There are about 7 or 8 who have come out of their shell and really found comfort and/or benefit in talking to me as pastor "+ friend." Each one has their own type of crowd that they attract/are attracted to and each one requires a different type of affirmation or encouragement. By treating them as representatives or spokespersons of those larger groups (assuming in-group commonalities of motivation and make up), I can employ fairly accurate perspectives and practices that affirm the group by just using raw information about the general needs of the individual. Here are a few generalized examples based on real life accounts I've witnessed (I've left all instances gender neutral to leave space for you to match youth from your own ministry context where appropriate):

M – "M" is the individual that, selfishly, I want to be the poster child for the success of the ministry. I want before and after pictures of "M" on the brochures we put out on ministry fair tables because this is my proof that God dwells with us and can work on ANY heart. "M" comes from a difficult background and visibly wears the scars, while attempting to keep everything else below the surface. Over time "M" began to open up, get more involved in ministry and, just as I was ready to feel accomplished, "M" messed up in a MAJOR way. This is not a single occurrence either. It follows a pattern (perhaps when triggered by significant changes in environment or comfort). How do I deal? Well, as opposed to letting the wind get knocked out of me and doubting the work (which was my very real, very human reaction for a season) I learned to find the disconnect (find the last virtue that was solidly placed and then find the one "M" didn't fully get) and repair it by using the major offense as a teachable moment to secure that "floater" in place. This method has, more often than not, yielded positive results in ministering to "M"'s in-group, characterized largely as:

- Strong and silent
- Having an absentee father
- Having an incapacitated (sick, disabled, drug addicted) or well-intentioned, but ill-equipped mother

O – "O" is an older teenager, a transplant to the ministry and the somewhat reluctantly used poster child. I cannot deny the obvious attributes: self-starter, high capacity, committed to tasks, and fiercely intelligent. But neither can I ignore the presence of "O"'s slightly divergent concept of morality and responsibility that has served him or her well for the years prior to becoming a part of the ministry. Though behavior is mostly exemplary, every once in a while there is a minor offense that reminds me of the complex nature of the person I'm dealing with. Affirming "O" is tricky because he or she is so self-reliant and suspicious of being steered towards indoctrination with my value system. The success I've had has come from acknowledging the value of "O"'s strengths while challenging areas of weakness harder than I would most. I find that the pre-existent values are not flawed so much in what they espouse as they are dangerous in the things they leave unattended to. "O"'s in-group is characterized largely as:

- Talented and bright, but existing as outcast
- Having a sense of identity and pride (cultural, organizational, ideological) that is bolstered by the dynamic personality in the group
- Non-conforming to social expectations or roles

E – "E" is another transplant like "O", but he or she is the poster child I feel guilty about claiming. "E" seemed to have had things pretty well figured out before he or she even knew who I was. There's a supportive family background and the sense of a legacy to live up to. I can't really take credit for shaping "E" to this point. On my worst days, I can really just hope to maintain his or her pre-existent good. On my best days, I hope to build upon a very good foundation. Affirmation has been accomplished by being sensitive to the moment and available when I was needed. Though it did not appear to be that often, when those moments came around, they were some of the most rewarding experiences in my ministry. "E"'s character is attractive to a wide range of groups, so he or she doesn't belong exclusively to one. Even a close look at the people "E" hangs out with the most reveals both individuals with shared traits and those attracted to, or desirous of, those traits. If I had to come up with some shared characteristics I would say they:

- Possess significant, yet well-hidden esteem issues that belie their confident air
- Are considered "friends" by more people than they would give that same term to
- stand out everywhere they go, but still believe they can blend into crowds

N – "N" is the one that I would have missed, had it not been for the grace of God. "N" had been under the radar, sitting in or near the back, talking during service and leaving immediately after it was over. It was, therefore, extremely surprising when I realized how much "N" had ingested the core values and concepts I'd been espousing. What's more, "N" had been authentically finding and living the hope in the gospel and the proclamation of it. In his or her in-group (which is more mixed than "E"s but is constant, insofar as it is almost always the same group of diverse people) "N" had even begun to mini-teach the gospel, indeed emerging as one who had been made a "disciple from a distance."" "N's in-group can be characterized as:

- A hodgepodge of dynamic personalities, though not necessarily all invested in the ministry to the same extent

- Having extensive social networks, the majority of whom they stay in close contact with
- Appearing to be activated all of a sudden when they are given a sense of ownership of a task or activity

Do these types sound like any of your young people? Take a minute to think about the makeup of your ministry. Who are your dynamic personalities? How have you been successful in encouraging them or affirming them? What kind of people makes up their in-groups? After determining types, it's important to give them assignments or get them involved in activities that challenge them according to their strengths and build them up in their areas of weakness. *"N"*, for instance, was given the opportunity to speak to the church from the pulpit about a topic that we had a shared concern about. When *"N"* addressed the congregation, we were able to highlight some areas for strengthening, like pacing and stage presence, but we also boosted *"N"'*s confidence regarding a natural knack for language, impressive exegetical talents and a capacity for community organizing. When word of mouth got around that *"N"* would be speaking, we had a boost in church attendance (that has only moderately tapered off), as friends poured in to hear "one of their own."

There are some clear risks involved – maybe the young person will get cold feet, maybe more weaknesses than strengths will be highlighted and you'll have to repair fragile egos, etc. – but the greater danger is not showing young people that the church is a place for their empowerment. I've realized that youth want structure and responsibility and they recognize the necessity and benefit of it, but much of the apprehension we see comes from them feeling like they have no ownership of the process – like they have no voice. This can be overcome by showing them that the tasks we give them have been constructed with them in mind and not just randomly assigned.

To this end, it helps to pay attention to other supporting information that you may have noticed, e.g. that some people thrive when given a particular type of assignment or that certain cross-groups of people work really well together. When you begin to incorporate an understanding of personality and/or behavioral types into this type of ministry analysis, you can leverage the dynamic personalities to mentor and develop some of the less invested people in their spheres of influence. What you impart to them in your one-on-one interactions can be duplicated and you also reinforce the affirmation of your core group by letting them know that you trust them with the responsibility of interpreting, managing and expanding the work of the ministry. Good affirmation is bolstered by expectation. If a young person knows that you anticipate a return on your investment, they realize the value you place on what you're putting in (sacrifice of time, energy and giving of resources) and, in turn, recognize the value you must see in them to make the investment in the first place.

Affirming the Thoughts
But of course affirmation isn't just about finding healthy challenges that urge them to *do* something, but it's also about saying: "I trust you with this challenge to think or imagine something. I trust that you are mature and capable enough to wrestle with some difficult questions about this matter that I am telling you is critical and important." Doing youth ministry well means simultaneously helping young people recognize their duty and power in Christ and facilitating their healthy process from children to adults. Putting away childish things and becoming an adult in Christ is not something one just does intuitively. It is a rite of passage facilitated by ministers who empower youth to step up from an introductory-level faith in God and commitment to Him. Doing youth ministry well, therefore, has got to mean putting ownership in the lap of the young person, giving them time and a safe environment to grapple with their faith and seek answers to the difficult questions.

The most incredible part of the Pastoral vision of the Reverends Floyd and Elaine Flake in creating Shekinah Youth Church in 1992 was that it designated a space where youth could cringe from the harshness of God's discipline, cry when His sovereignty didn't match up with our expectations, balk at how His objective standards didn't seem fair – in general, be disappointed by God and the church – and fall right back in love with Him, time and time again, in our own language. Because at the end of the day, the overwhelming results of this type of ministry are young adults with a strong faith that allows us to manage ourselves relationally to the situations and people that we meet in life.

It is not the case that every successful youth ministry must have its own building, but it must be founded upon the intention that having a building represents. That is the desire of leadership to give young people the resources to engage the whole of scripture – not just the pre-approved parts – and walk it out in their everyday living. We have to get a little bit dangerous, be willing to sacrifice mindlessness and listlessness in favor of thinking and action, in order to affirm the thoughts of these youth. We have to respect the fact that they have the ability to think very deeply about their relation to God and God's relation to everyday life.

Your young people are probably not quoting Karl Barth's Doctrine of Creation (thank God mine aren't), but you've got to see "Why don't I fit in?" as more than their emotional longing. That question is a deep, theological pondering about what is right and can reasonably be expected in the course of human life. Because significant questions like this exist in their minds, we can't afford to avoid them, whether they seem like priorities or not. For when we make God the invisible authority, seeing all and knowing all, but curiously silent on matters that are not our moral concern, we create double minded youth who ideate an uninterested God. So what it seems like they're asking is the same question? Who cares that they're attention seekers? Somebody in the room doesn't get it and will benefit from your re-explanation. Maybe you've not explained it sufficiently enough. Perhaps they think they're asking a different question and you're just hearing it the same. Which is the greater harm: repeating or rebuking?

And when we do tackle these questions, we can't skate around the difficult truths with answers that sound good but don't mean anything. There is real concern in their minds about us saying (and then never expounding upon) stuff like: "God is good and holy, can't stand the sight of unholy things, and that there is no wrong or imperfection in Him" because when they take a snapshot of our world, there IS so much wrong, so much ugliness, so much sin and degradation. What is going on? How do we explain this? How can the Earth be the Lord's and everything in it as Psalm 24:1 suggests? How can it be and what does it mean, "by Him all things consist" as Colossians 1:17 tells us? What do you really think young people do cognitively with the appearance that humanity has more direct interaction from a devil (and the "haters" he employs) who wants to steal from us, kill us and destroy us than from God who wants to love us and gift us with more abundant life? Daily experience, to the uninformed mind, suggests this very thing and if our preaching, teaching and ministry don't deal with it (note, not dismiss it or ignore it) then we are implicit in the corrosion of faith and the perpetuation of ignorance.

It may be difficult, unpleasant or scary to talk to your young people about God as the only uncreated, sovereign being, and whether His omnipotence and supremacy mean that ALL other things, including the devil and "bad times," are subject to Him (not equally powered opposition to His authority) but they're having this conversation with or without you. Every ghetto-glamorization that streams in through the headphones of their mp3 players, every hyper-sexualized billboard or television show is another inquisition into the location and power of God in relation to human activity.

Let's make it practical: If you were to ask your youth why bad things happen to good people, what would they say? If none of your Biblical understanding comes through in their answer, pump the brakes, cancel the concert and have that conversation. Talk about the tension of re-imagining God in a way that tries to make sense of His fundamental characteristics against the backdrop of the brokenness of this world He created. Dive deeply into the definition of redemption that restores the hope that God has not once taken His eye off of His people, and there is a plan that incorporates every good thing and every bad thing that has ever happened into this process of reclaiming humanity to its first love. Let your calling to this ministry challenge *your* understanding and stretch *your* faith because God is bigger than you envisioned when you first said yes. And give your young people snapshots and postcards of your journey along the way. They don't have to be there at every depth you plumb or every height you scrape, but they really can handle the introduction and the guided conversation of the challenging thoughts that bring you there.

And furthermore, when the concert does happen, it ought to feature an artist that will echo lyrically what God has given your ministry spiritually. An artist with a following, who's got good production and exciting talent is great, but they're better – and dare I say ONLY purposeful — when they give your young people another way to hear and remember what God has already been saying about His omnipresence, omnipotence, omniscience, and grace (which encompasses His lavish love and His ridiculous mercy) through the other facets of your ministry. All this talk of music brings us right to our conversation about affirming the culture of your congregation.

Affirming the Culture
In your wise age, I invite you to look back on your own faith formation. Think of *how* you learned the lessons that drew you closer to God. Think of the sermons that have added to your understanding of the Gospel message and your Christian responsibility. Think about what types of people helped put things in better perspective for you. Think also of the alone time, the moments when nobody else was around and it was just you and Jesus. You were shaped by that silence. By synthesizing what you remembered from all you'd been taught and what you were feeling, you found the constancy of God and the true intentions of your heart. It wasn't easy to learn how to prefer God's will over yours or to subject all of you to all of Him, but you had the understated privilege of language. The Bibles and

accompanying literature you read were all written in familiar translations. Those preachers, teachers and friends that really reached you all spoke your language when they encouraged you to give yourself up and reach toward something more significant. Affirming the culture of your young people simply means not putting them at the disadvantage of trying to hear a God who speaks in a language they don't understand.

I believe that greater degrees of maturity, compassion and faith are necessary in order to see this affirmation of culture as an exercise in showing youth a God who is sensitive to their need to be understood and to understand. Without these points of growth, these enablers of objectivity, our traditions become our default and we say: "I cannot allow this culture to invade the church" or "I don't see how Christ can exist in this culture." Perhaps the biggest culprit in the crime of dismissing an entire culture is the subjective value we place on the words "traditional" and "contemporary." Neither of these two words is synonymous with "holy" or "right," which means that when we disallow the expression of culture in church, we may be passing off what is preferential as what is necessary. Again, to translate, we may be aligning a holy, untamable God with our way of thinking (instead of vice versa) in a manner that makes God inaccessible to the younger generations that would otherwise seek Him. Without knowing your specific context, it's difficult to forecast what, specifically, "affirming the culture" will mean for you, but I'll use a familiar issue to illustrate the general process of steering the conversation toward values, integrity, and godliness and away from preference.

There's a familiar debate that has yet to be fully resolved regarding whether or not hip-hop is an acceptable form of music to be used in liturgy. In this debate, hip hop is most often set in contrast to hymns and spirituals, the latter being assigned greater weight or authenticity. Thinking specifically of the African-American church tradition (since it is the one with which I am most familiar), hymns and spirituals have undoubtedly had a great historical significance, so there is value in them as vehicles of expressing Biblical truths that are relevant to Black culture, struggle and spirituality. There is nothing about them that is intrinsically holy though, just as there is nothing about hip hop that is intrinsically wicked. Both genres use lyric, melody, and rhythm to tell a story. The only divergent point relevant to the question of hip-hop's suitability as a liturgical art form is the intent. If we say that spirituals are expressions of a religious faith and songs of protest against inhumane activity that challenges such faith and if we say that hymns are songs of adoration or prayer directed toward God, and this is what makes them acceptable for liturgical worship, then we must ask whether hip hop can accomplish similar aims. The only suggestion that it can't, is the perception that, throughout its history, it has not popularly done so.

This is a different conversation. Instead of saying traditional forms are worthy while contemporary forms are not, we're now articulating why the tradition has been so important and seeing if contemporanetcy can carry that torch if given a fair chance. We are saying that our relationship with Christ is the best tool we have to affect the change we're trying to see so the music must be representative of that. We sing these songs because they brought us through so much and they were anchors of our faith, which is not to say that a differently constructed song can't be an anchor as well, but we want to impress upon youth the importance of having, that be their aim. We don't want youth to use the same ear for sacred, Christian music as they do for music in the world. We don't want them to evaluate its worth on the same level. They should want it ultimately because it moves them, not simply because it makes them move. This is a point that we can raise with our young people to encourage the critical thinking they're already doing while also adding a new, usable dimension to it.

We can affirm hip-hop while challenging our young people to evaluate the culture behind it according to a relevant standard (e.g. holiness, its contributions to their process of maturation). In so doing, we can bridge all three affirmations, individual, thought and culture, by:

1. Acknowledging how the individual has been shaped by "culture as potential formative agent" and letting that knowledge mold the space, instruction and opportunity provided
2. Trust individuals to consult the instruction they've received and use the tools made available in order to process a response to the portions of the culture that do not move them towards understanding duty and responsibility in Christ
3. Not dismissing the culture entirely because we don't prefer it or fully understand it, because dismissing it means ignoring a powerful vehicle for instilling time-tested values in a generation that requires ownership before investment.

The solution isn't to let the culture run rampant and form the dominant impression of your ministry. On the contrary, by teaching the Biblical and historical values that inform the tradition you're comfortable with AND listening for a response from their contemporary perspective, you provide a meeting place. It is here that these essential statements can be made: "To speak your language through your cultural filter in this church, it must maintain the truths of the Christian reality. Even as we affirm the validity and suitability of your culture we maintain that Christ must be over it – Christ has got to dictate what you practice and what you say in culture." Giving them voice and agency in determining this is the bedrock of producing enduring Christians. For when this generation has to confront the dominant world culture of their day, the opportunities you've given them to actively choose Christ over something will prove its own worth.

Conclusion
We've covered one conceptual starting point of ministry that may be helpful as we envision, pray and work for success as ministers to youth. Why this particular point? I think that, for one reason or another, we tend to stop really thinking about

children when we become adults, as if the admonition to become men and women and put childish thoughts, speech and reasoning away gives us license to disregard the inner workings and outward expressions of children, even as we serve them in a ministerial capacity. How can we have conversations about efficacy, endurance and excellence with such a flawed foundation? So I hope that I've given you some food for thinking about what it means to be a child.

I know, however, that a great deal more goes into being successful at ministry than the ideology behind your praxis inside of the church. What about the self care that is so important for making sure that we don't become the hurt people that, in turn, hurt other people? What about tapping into resources to learn from? They're all questions that could probably take their own individual chapters to answer but I want to provide some brief insights into them, again leaving space for you to employ your analytical and creative skills to see how the advice might be put to use in your life. The keyword that I want you to keep in mind as we go through these points is "balance." We all need balance and if we deny that need, it will make demands in unexpected ways, at unexpected times and in unexpected places. "I would never do that" turns into "I can't believe I did that" when appropriate attention is not paid to your needs as an intellectual, emotional, physical and, of course, spiritual being. These insights come from much trial and error and I've found them to offer me a reprieve from the madness that is youth ministry:

Stay <u>Connected</u> to the Youth
- Be intentional about doing "out of church" activities with them
- It will help you see their humanity & keep them from being "objects that confirm your ministerial worth when they're present and deny it when they're absent."
- Don't just dwell among them
  - > Actively listen, critique and offer support for their vision
  - > Learn from them

You will learn how to do your job more efficiently, which will translate into less time being spent brainstorming about what kind of programming to develop or what hermeneutic lens to employ in order to craft relevant sermons. Less time in preparation means more time for other things.

Get an Accountability Group
Select a group of people that you feel comfortable talking through difficulties with
- They should be peers (as much responsibility as I give my young people, I cannot advocate making them my confidants) that you don't always need to qualify your statements around
- It helps if they have known you over one or more significant transitions in your life so that there's a shared understanding of the background information that informs the stance you take on a particular issue.
- "Who is ministering/can minister to me?" becomes a very urgent question the deeper you get into ministry. Getting this group together early on can eliminate the resentment that can come from feeling like the people you spend the most time with are incapable of ministering to you.

Sounding boards are invaluable at this stage in your life, because you have a great and weighty responsibility upon your shoulders that you can do immeasurable good or seemingly irreparable harm with. The danger exists not only in dropping this responsibility and shaking up lives in the process, but also in carrying it erroneously.

Know That People are Watching – Be a Healthy Public Figure
Take ownership of what it means to "act accordingly."

- Allow scripture and wise counsel (Pastor Flake and Co-Pastor Elaine have been invaluable to me in this regard) to confirm for you what your action should be. Don't feel hard pressed to conform to standards imposed by people that wouldn't even attempt to measure up on their own scales.

Expand your concept of what ministry is
- If ministering to you always looks like Sunday morning, then it will always be more performance than organic. Ministry is what we do with the life that we live, so live your life and when you find opportunity to tune into the needs of others, do it in the context of the current moment
  - ➢ For instance, if you're on the basketball court, and a youngster who was picked last is exhibiting body language consistent with low self-esteem, it's okay to forego the altar call in favor of just passing him the ball for an open shot.

Make no mistake. There is an external expectation – on the part of those that have made your title your primary identification – that, since you're a minister, you will follow a script of what they think you can say, how they think you should act, where they think you should go, etc. But you made your profession of faith to God. His is more than enough of a standard to try to live up to. Be diligent about it, but also be healthy about it.

Build Relationships – Save a Life
- Get to know the other people that are doing what you're doing as well as those who have done it before you.
  - ➢ Start in your area – there is so much capacity within a 1 mile radius of your church (after school & youth mentoring

programs, gyms, jobs that are hiring, etc.)
> Get a community calendar going to cut down on multiple ministries/ organizations doing similar events at the same time
- Break out of the "ministry as competition" model.
  > There are so many youth who need Jesus, and each one is wired differently, with different languages through which they process and communicate back at their optimal level.

Networking and sharing resources with other ministries allows you to learn what other types of differently-wired ministries there are that might serve similarly wired young people better and keep them from falling through the cracks of a ministry that cannot connect to them

After all of this, I want to reiterate that my intent was to provide you with a framework and some measuring points for your own success in youth ministry. Rather than giving you a step-by-step model that has worked for me, because you are not me, I wanted to inspire your passion for doing your own potent, personal ministry. Please allow me to put the capstone on that work by giving you another perspective on the awesome significance of what you do. In 1 Corinthians 13, verse 11 is a very peculiar interjection to an otherwise seamless train of thought. If you read verses 10-13 without verse 11, "now" is seen as a period of lack – during the "now" we know and prophesy in part, and we see only a poor reflection. "Then," on the other hand, is the time when perfection comes and imperfection disappears, when we see face to face and know fully, even as we are known fully. I can't speak for you, but I would certainly much rather be in the "then" than the "now."

But in verse 11, the values of "then" and "now" seem to switch. Then = childhood/past. Now = manhood/present, where the ways of the past are discarded. Can "then" ever really become disposable? Life says probably not - as one grows, the ways (or outward expressions) change but ingrained thought patterns and basic motivations never seem to vary too greatly. Scripture seems to say preferably not: "I tell you the truth, unless you change and become like little children, you will never enter the kingdom of heaven." (Matthew 18:3) Seeing Jesus say this, we see Him examining the human life, not according to all that we've accomplished in the "now," but to our ability to recall and reclaim our "then." In our adulthood, responsibilities, jadedness and the illusion of self-sufficiency cloud our vision and relegate us to partial knowledge. But in our childlikeness, Christ finds something worth granting entrance into the Kingdom of God. What "then" will your young people reclaim? When they are called to go back to basics, what foundational messages will they have to stand on? My brother, my sister, you a visionary charged with pouring into these young people something real and true and potent. You have been entrusted with training up children in good ways that they will not depart from so as they get closer to glory, the condition of their hearts will be right before God. That is significant work.

299

BIOGRAPHIES
(alphabetical order)

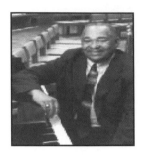 **DR. JAMES ABBINGTON** is associate professor of church music and worship at Candler School of Theology at Emory University in Atlanta, GA. Prior to coming to Candler he was a professor of music in the Department of Fine Arts at Morgan State University in Baltimore, MD. From 1998-2003, he was associate professor of music at Shaw University in Raleigh, North Carolina, chairman of the Department of Visual and Performing Arts and director of the Shaw University Concert Choir. He received the B.A. in music from Morehouse College in Atlanta, the M.Mus. and D.M.A. in church music and organ from The University of Michigan in Ann Arbor. At Michigan, he was a student of Marilyn Mason.

He was minister of music and church organist of the Hartford Memorial Baptist Church in Detroit, MI from 1983-1996 and National Music Director of the Progressive National Baptist Convention, Inc. from 1990-1994. He has been conference organist, assistant director of accompanying, lecturer, and clinician for the Hampton University Ministers' and Musicians' Conference for twenty years and was appointed Co-Director of Music in 2000.

Dr. Abbington is an associate editor of the *African American Heritage Hymnal* (GIA) and is the Executive Editor of the African American Church Music Series for GIA Publications. He is the author of *Let Mt. Zion Rejoice: Music in the African American Church* (Judson Press), *Readings in African American Church Music and Worship* (GIA), co-author of *Waiting to Go! African American Church Worship Resources from Advent through Pentecost* and *Going to Wait! African American Church Worship Resources Between Pentecost to Advent* (GIA).

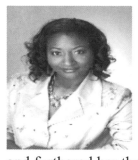

REV. DR. CECELIA E. GREENE BARR is an honors graduate of North Carolina Agricultural and Technical State University with a BS in Industrial Technology in Manufacturing. She studied Early Childhood Education at the University of the District of Columbia and furthered her theological education at Princeton Theological Seminary and Ashland Theological Seminary earning a Master of Divinity degree and a Doctor of Ministry degree respectively. She currently serves as the pastor of Trinity A. M. E. Church in Detroit.

Dr. Greene Barr's methodology and philosophy of ministry were molded by the effective tutelage of the late Rev. Dr. Samuel D. Proctor.

Dr. Greene Barr is a life member of Delta Sigma Theta Sorority, Inc., and has served four years as Midwest Regional Chaplain. As such, she has conducted workshops during Regional Conferences created specifically for chapter chaplains and has often preached the gospel message at Delta prayer breakfasts, Founder's Days and Regional Revivals. In previous years she also served as a volunteer for Big Sisters of the Washington Metropolitan Area.

Dr. Greene Barr is the author of Guide My Feet: Ministry Transformed through Mentoring, and a contributing author in, *This is My Story: Testimonies and Sermons of Black Women in Ministry, The African American Pulpit* (Summer 2005).

In 1999, Rev. Dr. Greene Barr founded *Sharing Faith Ministries, Inc.*, a Kingdom-based ministry promoting spiritual maturity. A key component of *Sharing Faith* is the weekly Internet newsletter she writes and publishes, "The E-Word". For more information about her ministry, see www.ceceliagreenebarr.com.

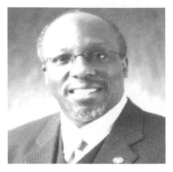

REV. DR. CHARLES E. BOOTH received his Bachelor of Arts Degree from Howard University, Washington, DC, earned his Master of Divinity Degree from Eastern Theological Seminary, Philadelphia, PA, and received his Doctor of Ministry Degree (Proctor Fellow) from United Theological Seminary, Dayton, Ohio.

In 1978, he was called to be Senior Pastor of the Mt. Olivet Baptist Church, Columbus, Ohio, where he has faithfully served for over thirty-one years. Under the leadership of Dr. Booth, the Mt. Olivet Baptist Church completed a 2.1 million dollar building program consisting of a 100 seat Martin Luther King, Jr. Memorial Chapel, an administrative wing, twelve classrooms, expanded fellowship center, a heating and cooling system, new kitchen facility, and property acquisition.

In addition to providing pastoral leadership to the Mt. Olivet Baptist Church, Dr. Booth currently serves as Professor of Preaching, Trinity Lutheran Seminary - Columbus, Ohio, and has also published his first book titled, **Bridging the Breach: Evangelical Thought and Liberation in the African-American Preaching Tradition** (Urban Ministries 2000).

Dr. Booth has traveled the world preaching and teaching the Gospel and received many significant invitations including guest lecturer and preacher at the Hampton Ministers Conference; guest preacher to enlisted service persons and their families - Kaiserlauten, Germany; North American Preacher, Baptist World Youth Conference - Buenos Aires, Argentina; Baccalaureate Preacher at Lincoln University, Morehouse College, Howard University School of Law; and Guest Revivalist at many churches throughout the US, Europe, South America, Central America, and Africa.

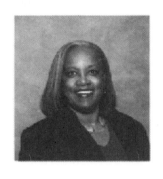

REV. DR. TERESA L. FRYE BROWN is an Associate Professor of Homiletics at the Candler School of Theology and Director of Black Church Studies at Emory University in Atlanta, Georgia. She obtained a Doctorate of Philosophy in Religious and Theological Studies from the Iliff School of Theology and the University of Denver, with an emphasis in Religion and Social Transformation (1996). Additionally, she earned a Master of Divinity from Iliff School of Theology (1988), a Master of Science degree (1975) and a Bachelor of Science degree (1973) in Speech Pathology and Audiology from the University of Central Missouri (formerly Central Missouri State University) in Warrensburg, Missouri.

Dr. Fry Brown has over thirty-five years teaching experience in academic and ecumenical settings across the United States and internationally. She has presented numerous workshops and seminars including those in homiletics, church administration, African American health and family issues, ministerial relationships, voice and diction and worship. Additionally, she has served as guest preacher and lecturer at a variety of religious and secular seminars, educational conferences, revivals, special events and ecumenical worship services.

Dr. Fry Brown is a prolific author whose latest books include *Delivering the Sermon: Voice, Body and Animation in Proclamation,* Fortress Press (2008) and *Can A Sister Get a Little Help?: Advice and Encouragement for Black Women in Ministry,* Pilgrim Press (2008) Dr. Fry Brown is the Assistant Pastor and Minister for Worship and Arts at New Bethel A.M.E. Church, Lithonia, GA.

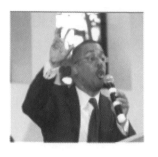

REV. DR. PATRICK CLAYBORN was born and raised in Memphis, TN by two loving parents – John and Lois Clayborn. After completing his primary and secondary education in the Memphis City Public Schools, he attended Morehouse College and Georgia Institute of Technology in Atlanta, GA. There he earned undergraduate degrees in Mathematics and Electrical Engineering respectively.

After completing his undergraduate work, Dr. Clayborn answered the call of God on his life and enrolled in seminary. While there, he met and married his wife Rev. Sheri Smith Clayborn. He then earned the Master of Divinity and Master of Theology degrees from Candler School of Theology at Emory University in Atlanta, GA. Dr. Clayborn also served as an adjunct instructor in the Philosophy and Religion Department of Spelman College.

Alongside his educational pursuits, Rev. Clayborn pursued ordination in the African Methodist Episcopal Church and served on the ministerial staff of Big Bethel AME Church in Atlanta, GA. He is an ordained itinerant elder in the Atlanta North Georgia Annual Conference. After ordination, Rev. Clayborn was accepted into Drew University in Madison, NJ, and earned the Master of Philosophy and the Doctor of Philosophy in Liturgical Studies with a focus on Homiletics. While at Drew, he served as an adjunct Homiletics Instructor at New Brunswick Theological Seminary in New Brunswick, NJ, a Religion Instructor at St. James Preparatory School in Newark, NJ, and also served on the ministerial staff of St. James AME Church in Newark, NJ.

Dr. Clayborn currently serves as the Assistant Professor of Homiletics at Methodist Theological School in Ohio.

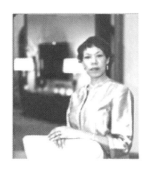

REV. DEBRA HAGGINS O'BRYANT, M. Div. is a licensed and ordained minister of the Gospel of Jesus Christ. Most recently, she has served as the Interim Pastor of the Historic Queen Street Baptist Church in the City of Norfolk, Virginia. President, Dr. William R. Harvey, recently appointed Reverend Haggins O'Bryant, University Chaplain at Hampton University. *She becomes the first woman to hold that position in the 140-year history of the University!* She is the pastor of the Memorial Church on the beautiful campus of Hampton University.

As chaplain, Rev. Haggins O'Bryant serves as Director of the Religious Studies Program and handles all religious affairs for the university. She currently serves as the Executive Secretary and Treasurer for the 10,000 member Hampton University Ministers' Conference and Choir Directors' and Organists' Guild. *She is the first woman to hold this position in the 95-year history of the conference!* The Hampton University Ministers' Conference is the largest interdenominational gathering of African American clergy of its kind in the world.

She has earned these academic letters: Bachelor of Science *(B.S.)* degree in Early Childhood Education from Paine College, Augusta, Georgia and the Master of Divinity *(M.Div.)* degree from the Samuel DeWitt Proctor School of Theology, Virginia Union University, Richmond Virginia. She has also earned advanced degrees from Old Dominion University: a Master of Science in Education *(M.S.Ed.)* in Secondary School Administration and a Certificate of Advanced Studies *(C.A.S.)* in Higher Education Administration.

Reverend Haggins O'Bryant counts among her greatest accomplishments and blessings, the birth of three wonderful sons: Charles O'Brian, Steven Marcus, and Bradley Alexander Haggins. She is also the ecstatic grandmother of four beautiful grandchildren Isaiah Jamal, Kyle Elijah, Kayla Elizabeth, and Jaden Marcus Haggins. She has one beautiful daughter-in-law, Neketa Haggins.

307

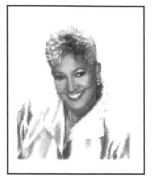

REV. CYNTHIA L. HALE, D.MIN is the founding and Senior Pastor of the Ray of Hope Christian Church in Decatur, Georgia. Ray of Hope has an active membership of 5,000 and an average of 1,500 in worship each Sunday morning. The church has been recognized in the book, *Excellent Protestant Congregations: The Guide to Best Places and Practice*, as one of 300 excellent Protestant congregations in the United States.

Dr. Hale received her Bachelor of Arts degree from Hollins University in Virginia, holds a Master of Divinity degree from Duke University and a Doctor of Ministry degree from United Theological Seminary. Dr. Hale holds five Honorary Doctor of Divinity degrees, with the most recent conferred by the Interdenominational Theological Center, Atlanta, Georgia.

Dr. Hale has established a mentorship program known as Elah Pastoral Ministries, Inc. to assist in the spiritual as well as practical development of pastors and para-church leaders. In September 2005, she convened her first Women In Ministry Conference that hosted women from various stages in ministry. In 2006, she was elected to the office of Necrologist for the Hampton Ministers' Conference. She is also a contributor to the book, "*Power in the Pulpit II: How America's Most Effective Black Preachers Prepare Their Sermons.*"

Selected by Sen. Barack Obama and the Democratic Party, she gave the opening invocation at the 2008 Democratic National Convention and was privileged to participate at the National Prayer Service for the inauguration of President Barack Obama.

Dr. Hale has received numerous honors and recognitions, and has preached the Gospel of Jesus Christ in Africa, Australia, Europe, the Caribbean, and South America

308

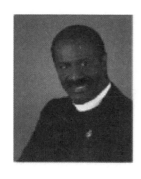

BISHOP GREGORY INGRAM, D. MIN. was elected and consecrated the 118th Bishop of the African Methodist Episcopal Church in the year 2000. His first appointment as a Bishop was to the Fifteenth Episcopal District, which comprises Angola, Namibia and most of South Africa. Bishop Ingram has served as President of the Council of Bishops and is now the proud Episcopal leader of the Tenth Episcopal District, which encompasses the entire State of Texas. Under his anointed leadership Bishop Ingram introduced the 10 Point Partnership Plan, a strategy for improving every aspect of life for the people of the Tenth Episcopal District through (1) Church growth and evangelism, (2) Economic development, (3) Education, (4) Health and Human services, (5) Management, marketing and administration, (6) Missions, (7) Political Empowerment, (8) Creation of a Resource Inventory Bank (R.I.B.), (9) Spiritual Entrepreneurship, and (10) Stewardship.

Prior to his election to the Episcopacy, Bishop Ingram served 13 years as the Senior Minister of Oak Grove African Methodist Episcopal Church in Detroit, Michigan. Under his leadership, 2,600 members joined and more than 1,420 became tithers. Bishop Ingram has distinguished himself throughout African Methodism for his expertise on Stewardship and Tithing. He has authored a number of publications that are heralded throughout African Methodism. Included among them are Equipping the Saints for Service, The Spiritual Aptitude Test (S.A.T.) Manual for African Methodism: A Textbook for Teaching New Members and Nurturing Others in the Church, The African Methodist Episcopal Church Pastor's Journal and Quarterly Conference Record Book and The Joy of Giving 'More than Enough".

Bishop Ingram holds a Bachelor of Arts degree from Wilberforce University, a Master of Arts degree in Teaching from Antioch College, a Master of Divinity degree from Garrett Evangelical Theological Seminary and a Doctor of Ministry degree from United Theological Seminary.

309

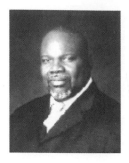

BISHOP T.D. JAKES is a quintessential leader known for his service to the church and the global community.

Bishop Jakes has global reach through missions around the world, record-breaking events, and weekly, with his diverse congregation at The Potter's House, where he shares his message of hope, inspiration and God's love with over 30 thousand members in Dallas, Texas. The Dallas-Fort Worth community is also home to Clay Academy, the college preparatory school for leaders of the next generation; the Metroplex Economic Development Corporation, a resource for aspiring entrepreneurs; and Capella Park, a charming single-family housing development.

Having written over 30 books, Bishop Jakes is a New York Times best-selling author several times over! One of his most recent runaway successes, *REPOSITION YOURSELF: Living Life Without Limits*, has over a half-million copies in print in less than a year's time! His message is also communicated in print and broadcast media through interviews and features in Time, Forbes, and Essence magazines, the Washington Post, USA TODAY, CNN, Fox News and more. His life-enriching wisdom is highly sought after, from the pulpit to TV screens across the country—as seen on his many appearances on the Dr. Phil show.

His worldwide outreach is strengthened by his weekly television broadcast, The Potter's Touch, which reaches millions of households globally. From the small screen to the silver screen, Bishop Jakes has added the title of filmmaker to his list of pursuits, transmuting his message of empowerment and encouragement into *WOMAN THOU ART LOOSED: THE MOVIE*—his first motion picture. This moving story of a woman plagued by the ills of domestic abuse highlights Bishop Jakes' emphasis on social issues. His latest film, *NOT EASILY BROKEN*, is the tale of what happens when calamity meets an already-troubled marriage. The movie—the first of a multi-picture deal with SONY—is directed by Bill Duke and stars Morris Chestnut, Taraji P. Henson, and Jenifer Lewis and hit theaters in early 2009.

From Dallas to Washington DC to Nairobi, prison inmates, Hurricane Katrina evacuees and Kenyan natives alike have been touched by the message of faith and God's love through the ministry of this servant and pioneer.

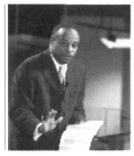

PASTOR JOHN K. JENKINS serves as the Senior Pastor of First Baptist Church of Glenarden, located in Landover and Upper Marlboro, Maryland. Coupled with the support of his wife, Trina, Pastor Jenkins has been the Senior Pastor of this thriving metropolitan church since 1989. In February 1987, Pastor Jenkins was called to serve as the Senior Pastor of the Union Bethel Baptist Church in King George, Virginia. He faithfully served there until December 1989, when he returned to FBCG to become its seventh pastor.

Since his installation, the church membership has grown from 500 to more than 9,500 active members. Under his leadership, the church has over 100 ministries that meet the diverse needs of the congregation and community.

Pastor Jenkins' ministry extends beyond the walls of the First Baptist Church of Glenarden into the metropolitan area. Pastor Jenkins serves as chairman and board member to several community organizations, where he is Chairman to Project Bridges (a coalition of churches devoted to improving the quality of family life), and Trustee for Bethel University and Chairman Emeritus to SHABACH! Ministries, Inc. (a non-profit entity of the First Baptist Church of Glenarden). He also serves on the Board of Directors for Great Dads, Greater Prince George's Business Roundtable, National Association of Evangelicals, Skinner Leadership Institute, Teen Challenge, Vision 360 and a local bank.

Pastor Jenkins travels extensively around the United States and throughout the world preaching and teaching the Gospel of Jesus Christ.

Since 1973, Pastor Jenkins has devoted his life to winning lost souls for the Kingdom. Countless testimonies attest to his passion for "Develop Dynamic Disciples."

In 2001, Pastor Jenkins received an honorary Doctorate of Divinity from Southern California School of Ministry in Inglewood, California.

311

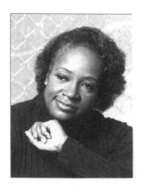

DR. CAROLYN A. KNIGHT received her Bachelor of Arts degree from Bishop College in Dallas, Texas and was awarded Master of Divinity and Master of Sacred Theology degrees from Union Theological Seminary in New York City where she studied under her mentor, Dr. Cornel West. She also holds a Doctor of Ministry degree from the United Theological Seminary in Dayton, Ohio.

Under the influence of her godfathers the late Rev. M. C. Williams of Los Angeles, California, the late Dr. Frederick G. Sampson of Detroit, Michigan and her spiritual father, the late Dr. Samuel D. Proctor of New York City, Dr. Knight developed a love for preaching and the pulpit. She has served in the pastoral ministry in pulpits in Denver, Colorado; Dallas, Texas; Rochester, and Harlem, New York. For many years she also served as Assistant to the Pastor of the Canaan Baptist Church of Christ in Harlem where she was mentored in pastoral leadership, organizational strategy and finance by The Reverend Dr. Wyatt Tee Walker, former chief of staff to Martin Luther King Jr.

Dr. Knight is the founder and president of "CAN DO!" Ministries; a progressive, preventive youth advocacy ministry dedicated to the cultural, social, intellectual, and spiritual well being of youth and young adults.

For ten years, Dr. Knight served as Assistant Professor of Homiletics at The Interdenominational Theological Center in Atlanta, Georgia where she had the primary responsibility for teaching and training students in the art and craft of sermonic design, development and delivery. Dr. Knight has served as adjunct professor at LaGuardia Community College and New York Theological Seminary and as the permanent part-time professor of preaching at her alma mater, Union Theological Seminary.

She serves on numerous boards and committees; among them are Harlem Congregations for Community Improvement and the advisory board of the *African American Pulpit* of Judson Press.

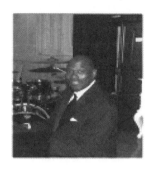

MIN. TOMMIE J. ("TJ") MARTIN, began his music career at the tender age of 7 as a child prodigy, and playing more than five instruments by the time he was 9 years old, including bass guitar, French horn, viola and cello. Immediately recognized for his unusual and extraordinary talent, he began playing bass guitar for his apostolic home church in Newark, NJ at 7 years old.

Later in life, he served in the Air Force for 6years and lived in Italy, Spain, and Germany. While in the Air Force, he was chosen to be a part of Tops in Blue, a select group of the best musicians in the military who tour across the globe. While traveling with this group, he learned to speak four new languages and performed in front of audiences in various locales throughout Europe that at times numbered in the thousands.

Once home from the Air Force, he joined the Church Of God In Christ, and was later ordained an Itinerant Elder at the Mount Zion COGIC Church in Sacramento, CA. He was active in their Music and Performing Arts Ministry and Evangelism Department until he came to join the music staff of St. James AME Church in Newark, NJ nearly 21 years ago. Under the leadership of Dr. William D. Watley, Ph.D., Min. Martin has nurtured and faithfully served several musical groups, including The Inspirational Mass Choir, Youth Choir, Select Ensemble and the Praise Team.

Min. Martin's musical influences include Oscar Peterson, Art Tatum, and Richard Smallwood among others. His gifts have made room for him and given him the opportunity to work with several well-known gospel artists, such as Dorothy Norwood, Cissy Houston, Edwin Hawkins and others.

313

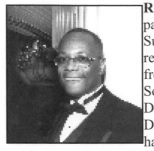

REV. J. MICHAEL SANDERS has pastored Fountain Baptist Church in Summit, New Jersey since 1983. He received his Bachelor of Arts Degree from Benedict College in Columbia, South Carolina, and a Master of Divinity Degree from Duke University School of Divinity in Durham, North Carolina. He has also been awarded an honorary Doctor of Divinity degree from Benedict College and an honorary Doctor of Humane Letters degree from Florida Memorial University.

Rev. Sanders is a Life Member of the NAACP and Alpha Phi Omega National Service Fraternity. He is also a member of American Baptist Churches, the National Baptist Convention, U.S.A., Inc., and the Lott Carey Baptist Foreign Mission Convention.

Rev. Sanders has led Fountain Baptist to be a strong supporter of mission, giving $400,000 to the United Negro College Fund and $30,000 to aid churches in Haiti. Additionally, for the last five years, Fountain has given a minimum of $100,000 annually to the Lott Carey Baptist Foreign Mission Convention to assist overseas missions.

Under Sanders' leadership, Fountain purchased a $300,000 office building in Johannesburg, South Africa and donated it to the Baptist Convention of South Africa to serve as the National Headquarters for the Convention. In 2006, the church made a two-year commitment for a $1 million donation to help with relief efforts in the Gulf Coast. This donation was realized in 2007.

Rev. Sanders is a member of the Summit Interfaith Clergy Association, former Moderator for the Middlesex Central Baptist Association, and former President of the Lott Carey Baptist Foreign Mission Convention.

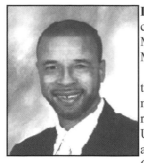 **DR. FRANK ANTHONY THOMAS** currently serves as the Senior Pastor of Mississippi Boulevard Christian Church in Memphis, Tennessee. Having fulfilled the requirements for the degree of Doctor of Philosophy with a major in Communications, Dr. Thomas received his third doctoral degree from the University of Memphis in May 2008. He has also earned a Doctor of Ministry degree from Chicago Theological Seminary in Chicago, Illinois, a Doctor of Ministry degree in Preaching from United Theological Seminary in Dayton, Ohio, and an honorary Doctor of Divinity degree from Christian Theological Seminary in Indianapolis, Indiana. He received a Master of Divinity degree from Chicago Theological Seminary, a Master of Arts degree in African-Caribbean Studies from Northeastern Illinois University in Chicago, Illinois, and a Bachelor of Arts degree from the University of Illinois at Champaign-Urbana.

Dr. Thomas has taken his pastoral experience, his love of African American preaching and his abilities as a scholar to McCormick Theological Seminary in Chicago, Illinois where he has taught Preaching in an adjunct capacity for many years at the doctoral level in the Doctor of Ministry in Preaching Program and in the Master of Divinity Program

Dr. Thomas wrote his first preaching method book, *They Like to Never Quit Praisin' God: The Role of Celebration In Preaching,* in 1997 (Pilgrim Press). In 2001, Judson Press published, *What's Love Got To Do With It? Love, Power, Sex and God,* a collection of essays on the intricate connections between love, power, sex, and God. The book has been so successful that a special workbook, *What's Love Got To Do With It? Love, Power, Sex and God: The Workbook* was released by Judson Press in January, 2002. Chalice Press released his most recent book, *The Lord's Prayer In Times Such as These,* with September 11, 2001 as its central focus. Dr. Thomas and Rev. Martha Simmons co-edited, *9.11.01 African American Leaders Respond to An American Tragedy (*Judson Press, December 2001). The book sold out of the first print run of 10,000 copies in two months.

Dr. Thomas has been the keynote speaker and lecturer at seminaries, universities, and Bible colleges. In April 2003, he was inducted into the Martin Luther King, Jr. Board of Preachers of Morehouse College.

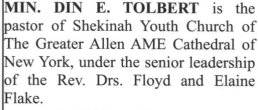**MIN. DIN E. TOLBERT** is the pastor of Shekinah Youth Church of The Greater Allen AME Cathedral of New York, under the senior leadership of the Rev. Drs. Floyd and Elaine Flake.

A 2004 graduate of Cornell University (B.S., Communication), and a 2010 M. Div. candidate at Union Theological Seminary (concentration in Preaching and Worship), Min. Tolbert is also an alumnus of several scholarship and skill building organizations, including The Jackie Robinson Foundation and the DeVos Urban Leadership Initiative.

As a product of the church he now pastors, Minister Tolbert knows first-hand Shekinah's proficiency as a training place for grounded, intelligent and capable leaders. He is committed to teaching the Word of God with integrity, and instilling the standard of excellence in the young people he pastors.

DR. LEE P. WASHINGTON is Senior Pastor of Reid Temple African Methodist Episcopal Church, located in Glenn Dale, Maryland. Dr. Washington's extraordinary vision, unconventional leadership and prophetic calling led the Reid Temple membership in relocation from Washington, D. C. to a Lanham, Maryland property on five acres in 1989. Membership at the time of relocation was 300. Faced with overwhelming odds, Dr. Washington and Reid Temple faithfully endured the struggle. He received by revelation the theme, "HAVE FAITH IN GOD," and within three years the membership grew to over 1,500 worshipers. Reid Temple's membership now well exceeds 8000 persons and has over 80 innovative ministries to combat and confront personal issues in the lives of God's people.

Reid Temple's current facility-The Worship Complex, offers state of the art audio/visual technology with a seating capacity over 3000. It also houses a bookstore, credit union, commercial kitchen, 1000 seat multi-purpose fellowship hall, two story office administrative wing, separate choir dressing rooms, outdoor amphitheatre, recording studio, nursery, ministry rooms, and 1000 spaces for parking. The Reid Temple Academy is also connected to the Worship complex with grades Pre K through 8, combined to assist in fulfilling kingdom purposes.

Dr. Washington is a spiritual activist, sought after for his pragmatic approach to ministry and as a gifted preacher and teacher. He has been featured in the Washington Post, Washington Times, Bowie Gazette, PG Post, Sentinel, Washington Informer and numerous news related articles.

Dr. Washington's educational achievements include: Doctor of Ministry from Howard University, Washington, D. C., Masters of Divinity from Howard University Washington, D. C., Bachelor of Science in Behavioral & Social Science from the University of Maryland, College Park, Maryland, and Associate's degree from Community College of Baltimore, Maryland, General Business degree, Cortez Peters Business College.

317

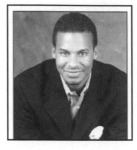

REV. MATTHEW L. WATLEY is the Executive Minister to the more than 8,000 members of the Reid Temple African Methodist Episcopal Church, *one church in two locations*, where the Reverend Dr. Lee P. Washington is the Senior Pastor. Reverend Watley has oversight of the churches' 7 corporations, 50-person staff, and 80 ministries. He also led in the design and development of a $32 million facility, which was completed in December 2004 housing a worship center, elementary school, credit union, bookstore, music and video studios, and banquet facility. Each Sunday, Rev. Watley preaches at the Reid Temple North Location's morning service and the evening service at the Glenn Dale location. These services are attended by hundreds of students from Howard University, the University of Maryland, and Bowie State University.

He was selected to serve on a special commission sponsored by the Ford Foundation to assess Non-Governmental Organizations in the Republic of South Africa. While serving as Graduate Assistant at the Andrew Rankin Memorial Chapel, Reverend Watley also served on the Board of Trustees of Howard University. On September 10, 2001, Reverend Watley founded **Power Lunch,** a non-denominational noontime worship service. Today hundreds of workers from the public and private sector gather at the historic Union Station in Washington DC to listen to his messages. In 2005 Power Lunch began its expansion to other cities. There are now Power Lunches in Suitland, MD, Baltimore, MD, Columbia, SC, Columbus, OH and Atlanta, GA.

Rev. Watley received a Bachelor of Arts in Political Science and Master of Divinity from Howard University, and holds an Executive Masters degree in Leadership from the Georgetown University McDonough School of Business.

REV. WILLIAM D. WATLEY, Ph. D. has served as Senior Pastor of the historic St. James African Methodist Episcopal Church in Newark, NJ for over 25 years. Under his leadership the membership has more than tripled and the annual church income has increased by 700%.

He established the St. James Social Services Corporation which oversees a feeding program and food pantry that dispenses over 89,000 meals annually, a clothes closet that distributes over 20,000 articles per year, an Intergenerational After School Care Program and Safe Haven Summer Peace Camp for children, as well as various emergency service, mentoring, literacy and employment training programs for adults. In addition, Rev. Watley is the chairperson of the Board of Directors for the 220 unit St. James Towers.

Most recently, Dr. Watley has launched a contemporary, multicultural Sunday worship service which is held in the suburban Essex County area and a Dot.com ministry that makes the weekly worship services, sermons, bible studies, and prayer ministry easily accessible to the masses via the Internet where viewers from over 45 countries regularly log on.

Dr. Watley has preached on the continents of Africa, Asia, Australia, Europe, and South America in addition to the island nations of Cuba, Barbados, Bahamas, Bermuda, and Trinidad.

A mentor and educator, Dr. Watley served as President and Distinguished Professor of Religion of Paul Quinn College in Waco, Texas. He has served as a visiting professor at the New Brunswick Theological Seminary, New York Theological Seminary, and Princeton Theological Seminary as well as a guest lecturer at Harvard University, Andrew Rankin Memorial Chapel at Howard University, and Payne and Turner Theological Seminaries.

A prolific author, Dr. Watley has written nineteen books and has authored several booklets and articles. He is the founder and C.E.O. of New Seasons Press, the publishing division of William Watley Ministries.

He has served on the Board of Directors for Beth Israel and Horizon/Mercy Hospitals, the United Negro College Fund and the Fund for Theological Education. In addition, he has been a member of the Advisory Boards for First Union Bank, the African American Pulpit, and the Interpreter's Bible Commentaries.

Dr. Watley received his Bachelor of Arts in Theology from St. Louis University and a Master of Divinity from the Interdenominational Theological Center. He received a Master of Philosophy and his Doctor of Philosophy-Ethics from Columbia University. In addition, he completed post-doctoral work at the Ecumenical Institute in Celigny, Switzerland and Harvard's Institute for Educational Management.

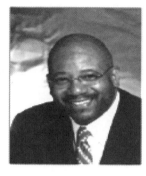

REV. DR. RALPH DOUGLAS WEST is the Pastor and Founder of Brookhollow Baptist Church, Houston, TX. From its initial membership of 32, Brookhollow has grown into a thriving congregation of over 15,000 families meeting in three locations. Along the way, because of the broad reach of its ministries in the Houston metropolitan area and around the world, Brookhollow Baptist Church affectionately became known as "The Church Without Walls."

Pastor West holds a Doctor of Ministry degree from Samford University's Beeson Divinity School, Birmingham, AL; a Master of Divinity degree with Biblical Languages from Southwestern Baptist Theological Seminary, Ft. Worth, TX; and a Bachelor's Degree in Religion and Philosophy from Bishop College, Dallas, TX. Pastor West has also completed advanced studies at Cambridge and Oxford Universities and received an honorary D.Div. Degree from the Interdenominational Theological Center at Morehouse School of Religion, Atlanta, Georgia and Paul Quinn College, Dallas, Texas.

Pastor West's philosophy of ministry includes a belief that the church and the academy are mutually dependent upon one another. For the academy, the church provides the impetus for its work and directs its course. For the church, the academy illuminates its sacred text, informs its worship, and articulates its faith. Pastor West's ability to connect the esoteric with the practical makes him a sought after speaker who has lectured at institutions such as Princeton Theological Seminary, Morehouse College, and Samford's Beeson Divinity School. Pastor West also serves as adjunct professor of preaching at Truett Seminary in Waco, TX.

Pastor West is the author of *Finding Fullness Again: What the Book of Ruth Teaches Us About Starting Over*, (B&H Publishing, May 2006). In 2008, Pastor West released *Left Alone,* a powerful book on finding strength for life's mysteries, impossibilities, and uncertainties.

321

USING RESEARCH TO IMPROVE
NURSING PRACTICE:
A GUIDE

Using Research to Improve Nursing Practice

Other books in this series:

CURN PROJECT STAFF

PRINCIPAL INVESTIGATOR: **Jo Anne Horsley, R.N., Ph.D.**
School of Nursing, The University of Michigan

CO-PRINCIPAL INVESTIGATOR: **Donald C. Pelz, Ph.D.**
Institute for Social Research, The University of Michigan

MNA LIAISON: **Joan S. Guy, R.N., B.S.**
Michigan Nurses Association

RESEARCH UTILIZATION PROGRAM:

Director: Joyce Crane, R.N., M.S.N.
School of Nursing, and Institute for Social Research
The University of Michigan

Research Utilization Training Staff: **D. Jean Wood, R.N., Ph.D.,** Faculty Associate
School of Nursing, The University of Michigan
Katherine Crabtree, R.N., M.S., Faculty Associate
School of Nursing, Michigan State University
Suzanne Brouse, R.N., M.S., Faculty Associate
School of Nursing, Michigan State University

Protocol Development: **Margaret A. Reynolds, R.N., M.S.,** Research Associate
School of Nursing, The University of Michigan
Karen B. Haller, R.N., M.S., Research Associate
School of Nursing, The University of Michigan
Janet D. Bingle, R.N., M.S., Faculty Associate
School of Nursing, The University of Michigan

Consultant: **Ronald G. Havelock, Ph.D.**
Institute for Social Research, The University of Michigan

COLLABORATIVE RESEARCH PROGRAM:

Director: Maxine E. Loomis, R.N., Ph.D.
School of Nursing, The University of Michigan

Staff: **Kathleen P. Krone, R.N., M.S.,** Faculty Associate
School of Nursing, The University of Michigan

DATA COLLECTION AND MANAGEMENT:

Data Management: **Laura Klem, A.B.,** Senior Research Associate
Institute for Social Research, The University of Michigan
Lynn Levin, M.P.H., Research Associate
Institute for Social Research, The University of Michigan
Linda Shepard, B.A., Research Associate
Institute for Social Research, The University of Michigan
Patricia Tomlin, M.A., Research Associate
Institute for Social Research, The University of Michigan

Research Assistants: **Jane Anderson, R.N., M.S.,** Data Analysis
School of Nursing, The University of Michigan
Mary Best, R.N., M.S., Data Editor
School of Nursing, The University of Michigan
Judith Fry, R.N., M.S., Data Collection
School of Nursing, The University of Michigan
Cheryl White, R.N., M.S., Data Collection
School of Nursing, The University of Michigan

SUPPORT STAFF:

Editor: **Vivian Collier, M.Ed.**
School of Nursing, The University of Michigan

Principal Secretary: **Margaret Horn**
Institute for Social Research, The University of Michigan

Administrative Assistants: **Kathryn Horne, A.B.**
School of Nursing, The University of Michigan
Barbara Welmers
Michigan Nurses Association

USING RESEARCH TO IMPROVE NURSING PRACTICE: A GUIDE

CURN Project

Conduct and Utilization of Research in Nursing Project
Michigan Nurses Association

Principal Investigator:
Jo Anne Horsley, R.N., Ph.D.

This book is a product of the Research Utilization Program,
CURN Project.
Director:
Joyce Crane, R.N., M.S.N.

The manuscript for this book was prepared by:
Jo Anne Horsley, R.N., Ph.D.
Joyce Crane, R.N., M.S.N.
M. Katherine Crabtree, R.N., M.S.
D. Jean Wood, R.N., Ph.D.

This project was supported by the Division of Nursing, DHEW, Grant RO2 NU00542, and conducted under the auspices of the Michigan Nurses Association. The scientific work of the Project was conducted at The University of Michigan School of Nursing and Institute for Social Research, and at Michigan State University School of Nursing.

W.B. SAUNDERS COMPANY

A Division of Harcourt Brace & Company

Philadelphia   London   Toronto   Montreal   Sydney   Tokyo

Library of Congress Cataloging in Publication Data

Main entry under title:
Using research to improve nursing practice, a guide.

  (Using research to improve nursing practice)
  "This book is a product of the Research Utilization
Program, CURN Project."
  Bibliography
  Includes index.
  1. Nursing—Philosophy.   2. Nursing—Research.
I. Horsley, Jo Anne.   II. Curn Project. Research
Utilization Program.   III. Series.   [DNLM: 1. Nursing.
2. Research. WY 20.5 U85]
RT84.5.U74   1983   610.73   82-15661
ISBN 0-8089-1510-X

W.B. SAUNDERS COMPANY
A Division of
Harcourt Brace & Company

The Curtis Center
Independence Square West
Philadelphia, Pennsylvania 19106

Library of Congress Catalog Number 82-15661
International Standard Book Number 0-8089-1510-X
Printed in the United States of America

9 8 7 6

CONTENTS

ACKNOWLEDGMENTS

The work of the CURN Project could not have been completed without the participation of nursing departments in hospitals throughout the State of Michigan. In all, thirty-four nursing departments worked with the CURN Project staff in the following capacities: Research Utilization Program intervention (experimental) sites, Research Utilization Program comparison sites, and Collaborative Research Program sites.

Research Utilization Program: Intervention (Experimental) Sites

Detroit Memorial Hospital (Detroit–Macomb Hospitals Association), Detroit
Genesee Memorial Hospital, Flint
Grace Hospital Division (Harper–Grace Hospitals), Detroit
Harper Hospital Division (Harper–Grace Hospitals), Detroit
Henry Ford Hospital, Detroit
Hurley Medical Center, Flint
Lapeer County General Hospital, Lapeer
McLaren General Hospital, Flint
Metropolitan Hospital (Metropolitan Hospital and Health Center), Detroit
Midland Hospital Center, Midland
Mount Carmel Mercy Hospital, Detroit
Providence Hospital, Southfield

Rehabilitation Institute, Detroit
Saginaw Community Hospital, Saginaw
St. Joseph Mercy Hospital (Samaritan Health Center), Detroit
Sinai Hospital of Detroit, Detroit
South Macomb Hospital (Detroit–Macomb Hospitals Association), Detroit

Research Utilization Program: Comparison Sites

Emma L. Bixby Hospital, Adrian
Bon Secours Hospital, Grosse Pointe
Chelsea Community Hospital, Chelsea
Community Health Center of Branch County, Coldwater
Cottage Hospital of Grosse Pointe, Grosse Pointe Farms
W. A. Foote Memorial Hospital, Jackson
Holy Cross Hospital, Detroit
McPherson Community Health Center, Howell
Mercy–Memorial Hospital, Monroe
North Detroit General Hospital, Detroit
St. John Hospital, Detroit
St. Joseph Mercy Hospital (Catherine McAuley Health Center), Ann Arbor
Southwest Detroit Hospital, Detroit
Veterans Administration Medical Center, Allen Park
Veterans Administration Medical Center, Ann Arbor

Collaborative Research Program Sites

Bon Secours Hospital, Grosse Pointe
Children's Hospital of Michigan, Detroit
Henry Ford Hospital, Detroit
Little Traverse Hospital (Northern Michigan Hospitals), Petoskey
McLaren General Hospital, Flint
Rehabilitation Institute, Detroit

PREFACE

The body of scientific knowledge on which the practice of nursing rests is ever increasing. As a natural consequence, there is a growing urgency within the profession to have that knowledge become the basis for delivery of nursing care. This book represents one of the outcomes of a research project designed to develop and test a model to facilitate the use of scientific nursing knowledge in clinical practice settings. In this book scientific nursing knowledge is defined as knowledge that has been generated by research studies that used various methods of modern science to investigate nursing problems. The outcomes of these investigations include not only the research results, but also the scientific methods and technology used by investigators while conducting their studies.

One of the major barriers to the clinical utilization of scientific nursing knowledge arises from the varied contexts in which nurse

clinicians and nurse scientists work. Differences in the goals and methods employed by each are of primary importance. For example, nursing care is generally conceived of as individualized care; that is, patients receive care based on their unique needs (and the nurse's unique knowledge and skills). The focus is on individual differences of both patients and nurses. The nurse scientist, while cognizant of individual differences, seeks to identify and control phenomena, e.g., nursing interventions and patient outcomes, that are applicable to identifiable groups of patients and nurses. The nurse scientist tries to minimize the impact of individual differences. In order to produce a science of nursing practice, nurse clinicians and nurse scientists must recognize and appreciate this type of variance in each other's goals and methods.

This book attempts to move research and practice closer together by describing the processes involved in assisting nurses employed in inpatient settings to incorporate new research-based knowledge in their practice. An organizational rather than individual view of the processes involved in practice change has been adopted in the book. In so doing, the activities involved in making research-based practice changes are treated as the responsibility of the department of nursing, *not* of individual nurses. This is not meant to negate the valuable contributions that individual nurses can and do make. It simply recognizes that modifying practice involves such things as resource acquisition, staff development, and procedure and policy changes, all of which are generally beyond the control of individuals per se. This organizational approach to research utilization is put into operation by a group or committee that represents the nursing department. This group assumes the responsibility for carrying out the activities necessary to bring about desired research-based practice changes and assures that the knowledge of interest is not misused.

The research utilization process integrates the specific processes involved in transforming knowledge into practice activities, creating a climate for practice change, planning for and implementing the change, and evaluating the effects of a practice change. Each chapter is directed toward a specific aspect of the total research utilization process. Chapter 1 offers an overview of the research utilization process and introduces key concepts inherent in this process. Chapter 2 describes the factors that must be considered when initiating a research utilization program. Chapter 3 covers the identification of patient care problems, including how suspected problems can be validated, why such identification is necessary, and how the information can be used to promote change. Chapter 4

examines how to select research-based nursing practice solutions for the identified patient care problems, while Chapter 5 addresses how to adapt a given solution to meet the needs of a specific department of nursing. Chapter 6 focuses on how to plan for and conduct a trial of the nursing practice innovation; it provides a detailed step-by-step description of the planning process. Chapter 7 discusses how the evaluation data gathered during the trial should be used to determine whether to adopt, modify, or reject the practice innovation. Chapter 8 then discusses how to extend or diffuse the innovation to other relevant nursing units if a decision to adopt or modify the innovation has been made. One of the most difficult tasks facing change agents is how to maintain the quality of an innovation once the initial change activities are completed, and Chapter 9 discusses strategies for innovation maintenance.

The research utilization process described in this book was tested in sixteen departments of nursing as part of the Conduct and Utilization of Research in Nursing Project. On the basis of these "trials" we are confident that the process, when adequately implemented, will produce effective research-based practice changes.

Many people have contributed to the project that spawned this book. Special mention is indicated for some without whose vision and active support the project might never have happened:

The Council for Nursing Research of the Michigan Nurses Association (MNA) laid the groundwork for the project when it adopted "closing the gap between research and practice" as one of its primary goals. The project was carried out under the auspices of the MNA, and we thank the MNA Board of Directors, the Council for Nursing Research, and especially Joan S. Guy for their courage in taking up the challenge to close the research—practice gap.

Thirty-two nursing departments participated in the Research Utilization Program of the CURN Project. The directors of these departments and their respective staff members actively shaped the protocols and utilization process in the hope that they would be useful for themselves, their clinical colleagues, and the nursing profession.

The Regional Program for Nursing Research and Development Project, carried out by staff members from the Western Interstate Commission for Higher Education (WICHE), preceded our work in research utilization. Three members of the staff of that project deserve mention because of their tireless efforts to share the outcomes of their work in hopes that it would further our work. Janelle Krueger and Carol Lindeman, Principal Investigators of the

Project, and Jo Eleanor Elliott, Director of WICHE, demonstrated the true spirit of sharing knowledge and offering colleague support.

For the past five years, ten nurses have served as members of the CURN Project Advisory Committee: Amy Barbus, Mary Castles, Joan S. Guy, Barbara Horn, Ada Jacox, Corinne Bachle Kordyson, Carol Lindeman, Sally Lechlitner Lusk, Dorothea Milbrandt, and Carolyn Williams. They served us well over the years—questioning, offering advice, giving support, always encouraging, and expecting the best of what we had to offer, but never the impossible.

Doris Bloch, Chief of the Research Grants Section, Nursing Research Branch of the Division of Nursing, DHEW, has served as our project officer. Her vision of the intimate and interdependent relationship between research and practice was apparent from the earliest conception of the project, and over the years, she has served as a positive stimulus for our work. Further, her faith in a young, naive research staff never appeared to waiver; it sustained us when our faith sometimes failed.

We also want to acknowledge the work of the many staff members who learned, worked, created, enjoyed, and at times despaired as the project moved forward. Of special note are M. Katherine Crabtree and D. Jean Wood, who worked with us in writing this manuscript, and Ronald Havelock, who provided the basic model on which the work was based.

Donald Pelz was the Co-Principal Investigator for the project. Throughout the five years we worked together, he was a steady influence, bringing his knowledge and experience in the field of knowledge utilization to bear on the field of nursing. While never claiming to be an expert on nursing, he respected and sought to understand the aspects of our field that influence the process of research utilization. We thank him for his willingness to share of himself and to be open to others.

Jo Anne Horsley
Principal Investigator
CURN Project

Joyce Crane
Program Director
Research Utilization Program

School of Nursing
The Oregon Health Sciences University
Portland, Oregon
December, 1982

Chapter 1
INTRODUCTION

The purpose of this book is to help nurses use *research** as a basis for their practice. Transforming research into practice is a demanding task requiring intellectual rigor and discipline as well as creativity, clinical judgment and skill, organizational savvy, and endurance. *Research-based practice* reflects the characteristics of the research from which it is derived; it is precise and replicable, and produces predictable patient outcomes. Research makes known the links between the parts of the nursing process—assessment, planning and intervention, and patient outcomes and evaluation. Research-based practice involves the deliberate use of these known links between the parts of the nursing process; for instance, an assessment procedure identifies a need for a specific practice. Research is often viewed as mysterious and unfathomable, and sometimes it is. However, is also offers a very substantial and practical basis for nursing practice activity. This book focuses on the practical application of research findings, tools, and methods, and is intended to help nurses appreciate and feel confident about using research in their practice.

Research and *research utilization* are interdependent processes that help further nursing science. Together, they can be viewed as research activity. Societies support research activity because it furthers the attainment of societal goals by solving problems. The purpose of research is to identify and refine solutions to problems through the generation of new knowledge, while the purpose of research utilization is to get the new solutions used for the good of society. Neither process taken alone is sufficient to meet the needs

---

*See Appendix A: Glossary of Terms. The first reference to a term defined in the Glossary will be italicized and boldface in the text.

of society. Nursing, as a health care profession that exists to serve societal needs, must find ways to fulfill both purposes.

Research utilization is a systematic series of activities that can culminate in the change of a specific nursing practice. It can also recycle by raising more questions for researchers to answer, which leads to more solutions and so on. It involves the use of both the process and the product of research. The activities that comprise research utilization include (1) the identification and synthesis of multiple research studies in a common conceptual area *(research base)*; (2) the transformation of the knowledge derived from a research base into a solution or *clinical protocol*; (3) the transformation of the clinical protocol into specific nursing actions *(innovations)* that are administered to patients; and (4) a clinical *evaluation* of the new practice to ascertain whether it produced the predicted result.

This book addresses the issues involved with and provides guidelines for the last two activities. It is assumed that the reader has access to research-based clinical protocols.[1] The availability of research-based protocols is an essential aspect of the research utilization process. A protocol is a written document that transforms the individual studies in a research base into a synthesized whole, translates research jargon into clinical jargon, and addresses issues surrounding the use of the new knowledge in practice. A determination of the scientific merit of the research studies is completed prior to the development of the protocol, thus relieving the user from the responsibility for scientific merit review. This does not, however, relieve the user of the responsibility for reading, understanding, and using the original research to guide the development of practice innovations.

It is commonly understood that the professional nurse has an inherent responsibility for knowing about research in the field and for using it as a basis for practice. Unfortunately, it is a well-known fact that most nurses do not read research journals and have little opportunity to attend conferences at which nursing research is reported. For this reason, in this book research utilization is viewed as an organizational process to be carried out by and for the total nursing staff in a department of nursing. In order to bring about research-based practice change, nursing departments must establish mechanisms, such as committees or administrative units, to

---

[1]*This book is a guide to the implementation of 10 such protocols, each of which has been published as a separate book. The 11 books together comprise a series entitled* Using Research to Improve Nursing Practice.

conduct or direct research utilization activities.

Research utilization involves the use of both the processes and outcomes of research. This means that research findings are used to define new practices, and research methods are used to assist in implementing new practices with accuracy and in evaluating their impact on patients and staff. *Planned change* processes are viewed as an essential component of the overall research utilization process, since the resulting practice changes require alterations in values, behaviors, roles, and policies that affect both the staff members involved and the department as a whole.

PLANNED CHANGE PROCESS

"Planned change" is a conscious, rational, and deliberate process for bringing about change and innovation, which tends to make these changes more acceptable and beneficial to those involved. Inherent in the planned change process are a number of *change components* that interact over time. These components are as follows:

- The change: characteristics and requirements of the innovation itself (roles, procedures, technologies, etc.)
- The change agents: abilities and resources of those carrying out the change (the persons who plan and guide the change)
- The change targets: needs and capacities of those who will use or implement the change (the recipients of the change)
- The change setting: characteristics and resources of the setting in which the change will be implemented
- The rationale for the change: issues of need, cost/benefit, and predicted value that affect the change process
- The change strategies: approaches or means used to bring about the change (including facilitative, re-educative, persuasive, and power strategies)
- The timing of the change: placement of change events within the context of a time frame that considers other activities occurring within the organization and phasing likely to facilitate or impede the change

The process of planned change can be structured as a form of problem-solving, as a rational step-by-step process by which individuals, groups, or organizations meet their needs. Figure 1 is a typical model consistent with the planned change approach.

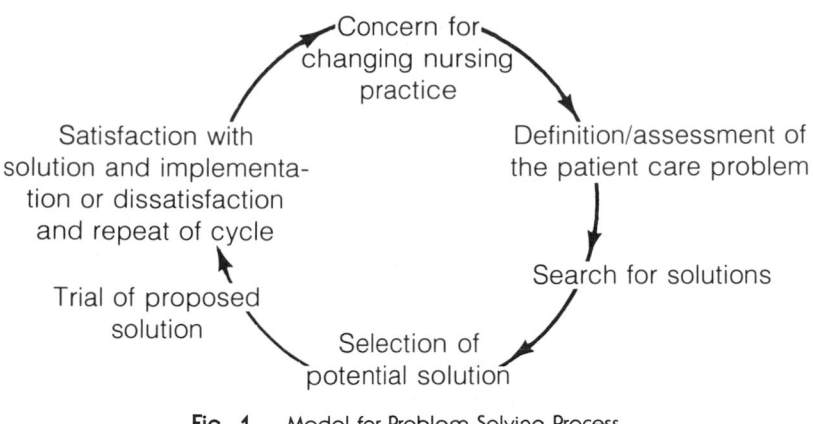

Fig. 1. Model for Problem-Solving Process.

This handbook presents such a rational, step-by-step approach to research-based innovation in nursing practice. A problem-solving model for planned change was selected because most nurses are very familiar with problem solving as a model for identifying and meeting patient care needs. Aspects of a problem-solving model that deserve particular attention include (1) creating a climate for change, (2) resistance to change, and (3) general planning activities.

Creating a Climate for Change

A basic requirement of planned change is providing effective communication about new ideas to all who are concerned with the intended change. This communication should be carried out in such a way that those involved are likely to become receptive to the innovation and willing to support the change and participate in carrying it out. Both administrative and practicing nurses must perceive some need for the change if it is to succeed; therefore, early efforts to foster awareness of the need for change are essential to establishing a receptive climate. Early identification of those who will need to be contacted for sanctioning or supporting the effort lays the groundwork for facilitating the change. Planning for the participation of all relevant persons within the system increases the likelihood that they will be supportive of the change and communicate that support to others as the change effort proceeds.

Even when change agents have been initially successful in creating a receptive climate for change, interest and motivation to carry out and maintain the change can waiver and thereby decrease

the long-range success of the change effort. Several factors influence people's ability to maintain interest and motivation for change across time: perceived need for the change, length of time required for bringing about the change, awareness of progress of the change effort over time, feedback about their participation, and reinforcement or reward for their ongoing participation.

Resistance to Change

No amount of careful planning eliminates *resistance to change,* which is a natural and inevitable human response to attempted alterations in the way things usually are done. Resistance to change can be a useful safeguard that limits the rate and scope of change and protects individuals from excessive disruption and disorganization. Resistance shows up as behavioral responses that serve to maintain the status quo in the face of efforts to change it. The reasons why people resist change are many and complex. Any or all of the following factors may be involved in resistance responses:

- *Personal or psychological factors* such as personality traits or need for self-esteem
- *Social factors* such as role or group identification, or social status
- *Cultural factors* such as traditions or belief systems
- *Organizational factors* such as authority, hierarchy, division of labor

It is important to note that while these factors may be sources of resistance, they can also function as sources of support for change.

When resistance arises during the change process, it is most useful to view it as a signal calling for careful assessment of the source and significance of the resistance, and the options for dealing with it constructively. Those who plan for change can often use their knowledge of the people and the setting to anticipate major sources of resistance in advance of their occurrence. Careful attention to anticipated or actual sources of resistance can help shape the change plan in ways that increase the probability of its success.

General Planning Activities

Implementing a research-based innovation is a complex system change worthy of deliberate and careful planning. Planning allows those individuals responsible for the change to anticipate needs as

well as possible obstacles or sources of resistance, and to take the necessary actions to ensure that the innovation will be well supported, well received, and likely to be successfully adopted. Planning for complex change in nursing departments requires the change agents to conceptualize numerous events and relationships in a time-and-system dimension and in a continuously changing progression toward the goal.

A master plan is needed in order to organize the tasks involved in the change according to a projected timetable. Such a plan helps the change agents to anticipate periods of greatest activity, clarify responsibilities, coordinate tasks, and gauge progress. A typical master plan for carrying out a trial and implementation of a research-based innovation involves 12 major planning activities.

1. Design the form the innovation will take in the particular hospital setting.
2. Design an approach to evaluating the effects of the innovation and the process for carrying it out.
3. Identify and delegate the tasks to be accomplished in implementing and evaluating the innovation.
4. Set up a feasible time line and sequence the tasks accordingly.
5. Obtain formal and informal organizational sanctions.
6. Plan for a trial of the innovation on a small scale (usually on one nursing unit).
7. Acquire necessary internal and external resources, such as personnel, materials, budget and support, and consultation.
8. Anticipate sources of resistance and plan strategies for dealing constructively with them.
9. Prepare for implementation of the innovation: organize and train staff involved, prepare materials, etc.
10. Plan for evaluation of the innovation: organize and train staff who will be involved, establish *interrater reliability,* prepare data collection tools and procedures, prepare for data analyses, etc.
11. Ensure that all who are involved in the trial are informed and prepared to carry out and support the change.
12. "Walk through" the plan to identify gaps prior to its implementation.

These planning activities attempt to account for the interaction over time of the change components. The planning activities are neither discrete, nor must they necessarily occur sequentially. More

specific information about planning for a research-based change in nursing practice will be discussed in detail in a later chapter.

RESEARCH UTILIZATION PROCESS

Producing research-based practice change involves the use of research outcomes, research methods, and planned change processes. The research utilization processes described in this book develop these three separate components into an interrelated whole. Each step in the process depends on two or three of the components to aid in the definition of a set of practice actitives and materials, or in the definition, collection, and utilization of data that support movement toward the desired practice change. Seven steps have been identified and developed and are listed below to provide the reader with an overview of the total process (Horsley, Crane, & Bingle, 1978; see Appendix B).

Systematically Identifying Patient Care Problems

This step involves the use of research methods and planned change processes and is directed toward setting a climate for change and identifying specific *patient care problems* for which solutions are desired. Inherent in this step are such activities as encouraging staff participation in the change process, quantifying patient care problems for which research-based solutions are available, and making data-based decisions regarding selection of the innovation to be considered for implementation. The emphasis on data-based decision making leads to consideration of such issues as techniques and ethics of data collection, response rate, summarizing and analyzing data, organization of data for decision-making purposes, and reporting strategies.

Identifying and Assessing Research-Based Knowledge to Solve Identified Patient Care Problems

This step involves the use of planned change concepts in combination with the previously obtained patient care data to assess and select research-based protocols. This step addresses ways to minimize the risk of clinical misutilization of research. Two potential sources of misutilization are of major concern: that which occurs if invalid knowledge is used as a basis for the innovation, and

that which occurs if valid knowledge is misunderstood and an innovation does not accurately reflect what is known. Several aspects of identifying and assessing research-based knowledge are emphasized here: the quality of the original research and the resulting clinical protocol, as well as the need to develop an understanding of what a specific protocol offers and how it fits the identified patient care problems (that is, is it a solution to the identified problem or to a different problem). A beginning assessment is made of whether the organization has, or can acquire, the resources needed to implement the innovation.

Adapting and Designing the Nursing Practice Innovation

This step involves a careful, detailed assessment of the protocol and original research in order to develop an understanding of the requirements and limits of the research base for an innovation, followed by a detailed examination of whether or not the requirements can be met in the specific nursing department. When research-based knowledge serves as a basis for viable nursing practice innovations in a particular setting, it is essential to understand the requirements and limits of the research base, the characteristics and resources of the service setting, and how these two factors interact. This step addresses how research-based knowledge is translated into specific practice activities that (1) are adapted to meet unique organizational requirements and (2) maintain the integrity of the research base.

Conducting a Clinical Trial and Evaluation of the Innovation

In this step, planned change processes and research methodologies are used to implement the innovation on a small (pilot) scale and evaluate its effectiveness in solving a patient care problem. A clinical trial and evaluation serve to limit the opportunity for misutilization by identifying problems with the innovation prior to large-scale implementation. A clinical trial also tends to decrease resistance to the innovation by making the pilot change less permanent and more dependent on data that support wide-scale implementation. Activities involved in this step include developing materials to support the innovation, carrying out staff development, collecting evaluation data, and implementing the innovation on one unit.

Deciding Whether to Adopt, Alter, or Reject the Innovation

This step involves analyzing the evaluation data in combination with understanding the research base and planned change concepts, in order to come to a decision regarding adoption, modification, or rejection of the innovation. This step entails organizing, summarizing, and displaying data in preparation for decision making about adoption or rejection of the innovation. Simple descriptive statistics are used for purposes of analyzing the evaluation data. Patient outcome data, both baseline and postintervention, are reviewed for predicted results and are compared with outcome data from the research base. Process data are similarly reviewed; apparent relationships between process data and outcome data are noted and interpreted. The evaluation outcomes are reviewed in light of cost–benefit considerations. When the analysis is completed, reports are prepared to be used in the decision-making process.

It is important to consider to whom the data might be presented (director of nursing, nursing staff, physicians, hospital board, others), and how to display the data to serve the intended purpose. This step culminates in an organizational decision to adopt the innovation as orginally designed, to adopt it with modifications based on the trial experience and made within the limits of the research base, or to reject it. It is important that all of these options be considered as viable and acceptable potential outcomes of a successful trial.

Developing the Means to Extend (or Diffuse) the New Practice Beyond the Trial Unit

In this step, planned change concepts and a clear understanding of the research-base requirements are combined in planning for large-scale implementation of the innovation. Activities include identifying all other care units appropriate for the innovation and modifying the design of the innovation as necessary to accommodate larger numbers of patients and multiple care units. *Diffusion* involves as much or more planning as the trial. It is necessary to retrace many of the earlier planning steps in the context of implementing the innovation on a permanent and less reversible basis. Resistance, while present earlier and expected in any change effort, becomes a major issue as more staff (both nurses and others) are directly affected by the practice change.

Developing Mechanisms to Maintain the Innovation Over Time

An innovation, no matter how well planned and implemented, will not survive over time without institutionalizing mechanisms for its maintenance. Written procedures for the research-based practice must be developed, approved through regular channels, and accepted as standard practice. Patient outcomes need to be incorporated into the quality assurance program to ensure ongoing evaluation and monitoring. Plans are made for incorporating the new practice into the staff development program for newly employed nurses.

The above-described steps require that nurses synthesize and utilize their knowledge of research outcomes, research methodology, and planned change principles to ensure a precise definition of need, identification and transformation of solution, and adequate and accurate data on which to base decisions. The steps also address the need to effect change in a positive and productive manner, meaning that desired changes are accepted by those who are most affected by them and that the changes cause the least possible disruption to the ongoing activities of the department. The chapters that follow address each step in detail, discussing the necessary activities and potential problems in carrying them out.

REFERENCE

Horsley, J. A., Crane, J., & Bingle, J. D. Research utilization as an organizational process. *Journal of Nursing Administration,* 1978, *8,* 4—6.

Chapter 2
IDENTIFYING
THE CHANGE AGENTS
AND ORGANIZING FOR
ACTION

The approach to planning for research-based practice change adopted in this book is based on the following assumptions:

- Nursing interventions are general enough that any specific intervention will be useful on multiple nursing care units.
- Nursing service departments want nursing interventions delivered to all appropriate patients regardless of their nursing unit location, and
- Planning, implementing, and evaluating practice change across units is a complex activity requiring the joint efforts of personnel with a variety of roles, experience, and knowledge.

These assumptions lead us to define the research utilization process in this book as one that is group- rather than individual-directed. The change agents, functioning as a group or committee, provide a cadre of personnel to carry out the many activities involved in a research-based practice change. When an individual rather than a group is responsible for initiating the change, professional colleagues can be viewed as group members who would be consulted or otherwise involved on a task or functional basis as the change proceeds. Since research utilization is viewed as an organizational process, however, it is recommended that a committee be   **11**

designated as change agents to engineer the research utilization process within a given hospital.

GETTING STARTED: BASICS

The formation of a committee of change agents to direct a practice change effort should occur formally, and the committee should have a specific written charge and designated areas of responsibility and authority. The relationship between the committee and the formal administrative structure also should be clearly designated. Group membership, the formal charge for action, and the definition of lines of responsibility and authority usually will be determined by an administrator who is responsible for the delivery of care in a specific area. This administrator is likely to be the director or assistant director of nursing.

THE COMMITTEE

The process used to identify and select potential members should be designed to (1) maximize the chance that those selected have the complement of qualities, including knowledge and skills, necessary to carry out the task, and (2) be consistent with the organization's usual means for establishing such groups. In general, a process that identifies a pool of candidates who (1) have personal interest in the change effort, (2) enjoy the support of the various subgroups they represent, and (3) represent a variety of roles, types of influence, professional expertise, and subgroups, e.g., shift, ethnic group, will provide the administrator with ample opportunity to form a group with the necessary personal and professional resources to accomplish the work.

The committee selected should be small enough to ensure that members will be able to work together efficiently and large enough to ensure that it has the resources and linkages needed to carry out the required tasks. The chairperson should have the confidence of the director of nursing, and should have leadership capacity and experience.

The members should be interested in promoting research-based innovations in nursing practice and should represent a sound variety of personal and professional attributes. Attributes such as interest, time and energy, persistence, flexibility, interpersonal abilities, problem-solving skills, group skills, and experience within

the organization and/or with change are important. The members should provide a wide range of formal and informal relationships with key individuals and groups in their practice setting. Formal relationships within the practice setting are those that occur within the planned structure of designated organizational roles at various levels, such as staff nurse, head nurse, supervisor, staff development director, and assistant and associate directors of nursing. Informal relationships are those that occur outside the structure of organizational and administrative roles, in which something other than formal organizational linkage accounts for the sphere of influence of particular individuals. Often this is related to the respect one commands for particular skills or abilities or one's ability to be a good listener. The role of *opinion leader* is an example of informal leadership.

These formal and informal relationships become very useful as the group carries out its work because they represent channels of communication, power and influence, and resource allocation within the practice setting. Any change that depends upon the support or approval of others to carry it out requires effective use of formal and informal relationships within the system.

A typical committee might have the following members:

- Assistant or Associate Director of Nursing
- Patient Care Coordinator or Supervisor
- Staff Development personnel
- Head Nurses (2–3)
- Staff Nurses (1–2)
- Quality Assurance coordinator

The committee may well experience a need over time to replace members or create subgroups for special tasks. The same criteria should be used in selecting new participants. The requirements of the task and the interests and attributes of the people should be considered; new participants should complement the resources already present in the membership of the group.

REVIEW OF THE CHARGE

The first task of the newly formed group is to review the charge it has been given. This review is best done in the presence of the person who defined the charge, so that questions can be answered immediately and in the presence of all members. This will (1) minimize the possibility of misinterpretation of the task, and (2)

provide a means by which the members can arrive at a common understanding of what lies ahead of them. The review should include the following areas:

- The purpose and/or expected outcome of the committee's work
- The role and function of the leader and any other members whose roles or functions are specified in the charge
- The nature of the process and activities involved in accomplishing the charge
- The resources available to the members, e.g., time, materials, other personnel
- The lines of responsibility and authority that flow to and from the group
- The date by which the charge is to be fulfilled, and
- A means for seeking and receiving further clarification should that be necessary

The process of reviewing the charge should be as open as possible, with the members being encouraged to seek clarification of any aspect of the work as it relates to them and their regular employment role. The review should result in the members believing that the charge can be accomplished with the available resources and without creating unmanageable situations for any member vis à vis their regular work roles.

RESOURCES

Many types of resources are necessary to accomplish a reseach-based practice change. Some are general and necessary for any type of practice change; others are specific to changes based on scientific research. Necessary resources are presented below in outline form, to provide a context for the sections that follow.

Knowledge/Skills	**Personal Attributes**
Clinical practice	Interest
Research	Energy/enthusiasm
Planned change	Willingness to learn
Problem-solving	Persistance
Organizational analysis	Flexibility
Interpersonal	Creativity
Decision-making	

Materials

Literature

Experience

Practice change
Evaluation/research
Clinical practice
Leadership

Professional Attributes

Clinical judgment
Critical thinking
Formal influence
Informal influence

Support Services

Telephone
Secretarial support
Laboratory

The primary resource brought to bear on the task is the collective expertise, interest, experience, and energy of the group. It is therefore useful for the members to identify and share what each person brings to the group that will assist in accomplishing the work. This process of sharing should result in the identification of available resources and resources that must be acquired through other means, such as consultation, purchase, borrowing. It should also assist the process of the group by identifying the unique contributions each member can make and by establishing the interdependent nature of the group.

ESTABLISHING GROUND RULES FOR WORKING TOGETHER

Another early task facing the committee is the formulation of ground rules for working together. Things to be considered include

- *Meeting attendance:* Expected at all meetings?
- *Time:* How frequently will meetings be? How long will each meeting run?
- *Work assignments:* Will these be made according to individual interest, expertise, need?
- *Decision making:* Can subgroups be formed? Who decides? Consensus? Majority? What is the role of the leader?

Ground rules provide structure and decrease the chance that decisions made by individuals or the group will be arbitrary. Ground rules, when followed, help build trust.

UNDERSTANDING THE ORGANIZATIONAL CONTEXT FOR CHANGE

Up to this point, the committee has focused internally—on what it is charged to do, what general resources are necessary to accomplish the change, what resources are available within the committee membership and which need to be procured elsewhere, and how the committee will work together. Now the committee should be ready to focus attention on factors within the department or hospital that will influence or be influenced by it as the change project proceeds. This organizational review has two major aspects: First, how are the department and hospital organized and how do they operate? Second, how will the committee relate to the department and/or hospital to facilitate its work?

Understanding how the nursing department and hospital operate requires some knowledge of both the formal and informal organizational structure. The formal structure is represented on organization charts and shows the official relationships that exist among the operational units within the department. Knowledge of the formal lines of authority within the department is essential in order to facilitate the decision making and resource acquisition necessary to achieve change. Organizational charts should be available for the committee to review so that all members understand the formal structure.

The informal structure consists of relationships between members of the organization that are not formally recognized on the organization chart but that nevertheless play an important part in getting things done. For example, when a staff nurse has a new idea she (or he) would like to try in her practice, she shares it with a staff colleague who is known to be influential with the head nurse before she talks with the head nurse. The staff nurse is trying to get the support of this colleague so she can use her influence directly (have the colleague intercede) or indirectly (refer to the colleague's support) when she seeks the head nurse's approval to go ahead with her idea.

All organizations have people who are known to be able to influence the opinions of key groups within the organization. Such "opinion leaders" may hold formal positions within the organizational structure or be influential by virtue of special expertise, political acumen, longevity, or other informal bases. It is important to identify the opinion leaders in the organization so that they can be involved in the planning for change within the groups they influence.

Since the committee's charge is to produce research-based practice change, it is also useful to identify factors within the department that facilitate or hinder change projects. For example, how are changes communicated? Who is involved in decisions regarding changes? Are there suffficient resources? Are staff development resources adequate? Do people value change or do they feel the department functions very well the way it is? A discussion of current change processes in the department should assist the committee in identifying specific methods that are facilitativve.

COMMUNICATING WITH OTHERS IN THE DEPARTMENT

From the very beginning of a change project, the planning committee needs to identify those individuals and groups who will be affected by the change and (1) define how they are to be involved in the change process and (2) how to facilitate appropriate communication with them so they feel involved and are ready for the change when it occurs. Involvement may occur in many ways, such as simply being informed, offering structured input to the committee, consultation, or decision making. The following guidelines are useful in deciding what type of involvement a particular group or individual might have.

- Don't offer (or ask for) greater involvement than the committee is willing to accept. For example, don't ask for an opinion from someone when all you really want to do is inform that person.
- Ask only for information that you intend to use. This does not mean the committee has to act on the information, but it should be considered in the committee's deliberations.
- Give feedback to those who have offered information or advice so they know their efforts were meaningful.

Communication mechanisms should be appropriate to the level of involvement desired. An item in the department newsletter informs without inviting active involvement. A brief opinionnaire might be used to get broad input and then be followed by a newsletter item that informs respondents of the nature of the collective input and how the committee used the informaion. Generally speaking, the greater the involvement desired, the more likely it is that the communication will become interpersonal in nature. Thus, an opinion leader whose support is strongly desired by the committee might

act as a consultant or be taken to lunch by the chairperson to discuss aspects of the proposed change.

This chapter has reviewed a variety of activities in which a committee can engage to prepare for undertaking a practice change project. The purpose of the activities is to acquaint the committee members with the change, each other, and their organization, and in so doing assist them to develop a positive outlook about the work they will undertake together.

POTENTIAL PROBLEMS AND CONCERNS

If the goals and tasks of this type of project overlap with those of other established committees in the practice setting, it will be necessary to weigh the pros and cons of initiating a new committee versus asking an already established committee to take on a new task. Interest in and commitment to the task are key elements in carrying out an innovation project. A newly formed group is more likely to be committed to the task than one than adds this task to its established functions.

Practicing nurses generally are accustomed to short, efficient, task-oriented meetings. Therefore, they may not allow enough time to use committee meetings to clarify and consolidate new learnings. An important part of the task involves taking the time to learn about research-based innovations so that members can successfully communicate to their coworkers and foster their participation in the change project.

Case Example: Initiating a Research Utilization Effort

The Director of Nursing at North Central Hospital met with her associate directors and supervisory-level staff and shared interest in fostering improvement in nursing practice by using information from clinical nursing research to solve practice problems. She sought their support for this project and found them interested and willing to participate. She asked one of her associates to lead the project and work with the others to develop and carry out a plan. They all agreed that the following major ideas should guide their planning activities.

- The need for this project had been identified by nursing administrators and their continuing interest, involvement, and support would be essential to the success of the project.
- Interest, involvement, and support from various levels and groups

within the nursing staff were also essential to the success of the project.

- The project would require an ongoing commitment of time and energy by 6–8 nurses.
- The process of selecting the people to work on the project should foster wide interest and involvement in the goals of the project within nursing.

Having agreed to these statements, the nursing administrators developed and carried out the following plan:

1. All nurses were informed through the nursing department newsletter about the project and were invited to participate in it.
2. Nurses at various levels were asked to nominate themselves or others who they thought would be interested and who could contribute to the project.
3. The nursing administrators invited participation by staff development personnel, clinical specialists, or others whose involvement they wanted to assure.
4. A representative group of 6 to 8 individuals was recommended to the Director of Nursing, who made the final decision.
5. All nominees were thanked for their interest, and plans were made involve those not selected for the committee in other ways as the project proceeded.
6. Release time for participation was arranged for the committee members selected by the Director of Nursing.

At the first meeting of the committee, the Director of Nursing and the chairperson reviewed the committee's charge. They also discussed the goals of the project with the members and involved them in identifying and discussing the major ideas that they thought should influence their approach to their task. Questions were encouraged and the members gradually arrived at common general understandings of their task. A regular time and place for meetings was set and a tentative agenda was developed for the next meeting. Before the meeting ended, the chairperson reviewed what had gone on in this meeting and what she and the members would need to do to prepare for the next meeting.

CHECKLIST:
GETTING STARTED

This checklist provides questions that need to be addressed in implementing this step of the research utilization process. It is important to account for the issues and activities inherent in these questions before progressing to the next step.

Committee Characteristics

☐ Is the charge clear to the committee?

☐ Are the personal and professional resources that each member brings to the committee's work clear?

Organizational Factors

☐ Do the committee members understand the formal structure of the Nursing Department?

☐ Are the department's usual processes for producing change clear?

☐ Does the committee have a beginning plan for how it will communicate with nursing administration, nursing staff, and others?

Work Arrangements

☐ Are meeting times and places set?

☐ Are the decision-making process and other ground rules established and understood by all the members?

☐ Has release time or some other time arrangement been sanctioned for each member vis a vis their regular employment responsibilities?

☐ Has consideration been given to a plan and time line for providing feedback and progress reports to the Director of Nursing? to others?

Chapter 3
IDENTIFYING
PATIENT CARE
PROBLEMS

This chapter discusses the identification of patient care problems, why such identification is useful, and what needs to be done to make the process systematic and meaningful. Patient care problems are defined as difficulties or concerns experienced by patients or the nurses caring for them that are amenable to nursing intervention. They are patient care situations in which there is a discrepancy between current nursing practice and what is desirable.

Carrying out a process to identify patient care problems serves multiple purposes. First and foremost, it should provide accurate data to validate or invalidate the existence of suspected problems and establish whether they are of sufficient magnitude to warrant the costs involved in trying to solve them. Second, it should provide adequate data to guide decision making regarding the problem(s), for example, where the problem is located, the significance of the problem in terms of the number of patients who have it, and/or the seriousness of the problem. Finally, it can provide a means of helping staff members recognize problems of which they were unaware or about which they were previously unconcerned.

A useful side benefit of conducting a patient care problem assessment is that staff members whose opinions are sought become involved in the process of change at the outset. This is a common and relatively easy way to begin to decrease potential staff resistance to any change efforts that follow.

SOURCES OF INFORMATION ABOUT PATIENT CARE PROBLEMS

The selection of individuals who will provide information about patient care problems should be guided by the purposes to be served by the assessment. Therefore, if validation of suspected problems is desired, those staff members who would have accurate information regarding the presence or absence of the problem (e.g., staff who give direct patient care) should be involved in the assessment process. If the information gained is to be used to guide decisions regarding the nature and scope of the problem, other staff members with experience across patient care units or with special expertise in the problem area should also be involved. Finally, if staff awareness (or lack of awareness) is an issue, those staff who currently fail to recognize the problem may increase their sensitivity if asked to supply information about the existence, scope, and nature of the problem.

Patient records or quality assurance records may provide data to corroborate the information supplied by the staff. (e.g., information on the incidence of postoperative complications or decubitus ulcer formation). If such data are readily available, they should be included in the problem identification process. If they are not readily available, their use should probably be reserved for cases in which staff information is thought to be inadequate.

It usually is better to involve as many people as possible. Inviting nursing staff to participate in the assessment of patient care problems fosters their sense of involvement in decision-making processes and helps to build a potential base of support for future change efforts when a solution to the problem is introduced.

SELECTING A METHOD FOR COLLECTING THE INFORMATION

The next step in the process involves deciding how the information will be systematically collected from the staff. Two methods will be introduced: structured interviews and brief survey questionnaires. Structured interviews are carried out on a one-to-one basis, and the interviewer asks a predetermined set of questions. The set of questions is called an interview schedule and is used to structure

the interviews so they are similar across respondents. The questions may have predetermined categories for answers, similar to questions on a survey instrument. Generally, however, the interviewer will also invite or at least record any elaboration a respondent offers about a specific question and answer. This elaboration of answers produces the rich qualitative data for which the interview method is selected.

The structured interview method causes staff to be more likely to "respond" (to give the information that is being sought) and allows for much greater qualitative detail than a questionnaire usually produces. The disadvantages of the interview method are cost (in staff time) and difficulty in making adequate use of the qualitative data. In most instances, the use of the structured interview would prohibit the involvement of large numbers of staff in the assessment process.

A survey questionnaire provides the most cost-effective data when large numbers of people are involved. Survey questionnaires are usually designed to make use of forced-choice questions. Forced-choice/closed-ended questions structure the response obtained by designating the form of the response. This method also specifies the range of responses available. The following are examples of forced-choice questions because they identify the problem and offer a limited number of answer choices.

1. Are patients reluctant to:
   a. Breathe deeply postoperatively? Yes —— No —— (Check one.)
   b. Cough postoperatively? Yes —— No —— (Check one.)
2. To what extent do these problems occur among patients on your unit? (Circle the number that represents your response.)
   a. Postoperative patients are reluctant to breathe deeply.

1	2	3	4	5
Not at all	somewhat	moderately	considerably	great extent

   b. Patients are reluctant to cough postoperatively.

1	2	3	4	5
Not at all	somewhat	moderately	considerably	great extent

This format facilitates rapid data collection and easy summarization because the information has been precategorized. The information obtained from the respondent is easier to organize and interpret because the number of possible responses is limited. Designating and reducing the number of choices available can be either an

advantage or a limitation of this method. When knowledge concerning the subject is lacking, a more open-ended approach is best.

An example of a brief survey instrument designed for identifying patient care problems may be found in Appendix C. Our experiences in assisting nursing committees in the development of questionnaires would suggest that it is much easier to adapt an existing questionnaire than to construct an original instrument. When changes are made, it is important to test the adapted instrument to ascertain whether it is providing the information it was designed to produce. Testing is best done by having naive colleagues take the questionnaire and then carry out the necessary summary and interpretation to ascertain whether the new data are useful in fulfilling the purposes of the questionnaire, e.g., validation, decision making. The adapted questionnaire should not require much time to answer; 10 minutes or less would be optimal. The time requirement should be kept to under 15 minutes or the number of persons willing to answer it will decrease. (See References, p. 31.)

RESPONSE RATE

In the previous section it was pointed out that people are more likely to respond to an interview than a questionnaire. The term response rate refers to the number of persons who actually answer a questionnaire or who participate in an interview relative to the total number who were invited to respond. Response rates are important because they indicate what proportion of the selected persons actually reported their views regarding patient care problems. When the response rate is low, one has less confidence that the answers received represent the beliefs of those selected. This is particularly true if several groups of staff who might hold different views are selected and there is reason to question whether the groups are equally represented by the data from the questionnaires. If any of the groups are over- or underrepresented, the collective data are biased in the direction of the overrepresented group.

The following factors, which are known to influence response rates, should be considered when planning for a data collection effort such as a patient care problem assessment.

- The extent to which the respondent believes the data to be collected are important
- The amount of time required to answer the questionnaire
- Whether the respondent feels safe in revealing his or her views

- The amount of personal bother involved in completing the questionnaire, e.g., is it delivered and picked up?

Thus, a questionnaire that asks about important matters, takes 10 minutes to complete, is delivered and picked up, and that may be answered anonymously is more likely to be answered than one that is considered too long, mundane in orientation, etc. A response rate may be stated as the percentage of persons who actually responded in relation to all who were asked to respond. Generally, a response rate above 80 percent is considered adequate, whereas response rates of less than 70 percent may be considered inadequate or at least questionable.

ETHICS INVOLVED IN COLLECTING INFORMATION

Ethical concerns regarding the collection of research data are also applicable to data collected for administrative decision making and research utilization. Two areas of concern are particularly important. First, respondents should not be coerced into providing information they do not want to make known. Coercion can occur overtly or covertly. Overt coercion may take the form of requiring someone to participate or openly making fun of someone who has indicated a preference for nonparticipation. Covert coercion may take the form of having someone in a superordinate position deliver and pick up the questionnaire. Coercion is often used in an effort to increase response rate but ends up being self-defeating because a coerced respondent is more likely to try to give socially or professionally acceptable answers rather than express his or her true views.

Provision for anonymity of responses is the second area of concern. This is particularly important in situations when the data, if traced back to an individual respondent, might cause her or him embarrassment or harm. Anonymity can be protected by (1) not asking for information that is unique to an individual, e.g., name or position, and (2) controlling access to completed questionnaires so that unauthorized persons cannot read them.

PROCEEDING WITH DATA COLLECTION

At some point the committee will be faced with deciding whether the preparation for data collection is complete and the time has

come for proceeding with the data collection process. The checklist that follows can be used to determine whether the committee is ready to proceed.

- Have the patient care problems of interest to the committee been identified for inclusion in the questionnaire or interview?
- Has the method for collecting data been chosen?
- Is the instrument (interview schedule or survey questionnaire) ready for use? Are modifications completed? Has the instrument been pretested? Are sufficient copies available?
- Have the specific persons who are to answer the questions been identified?
- Have all persons who need to know about the data collection been notified? Do you have the necessary approvals to proceed?
- Are the arrangements for obtaining the data complete? How will respondents be approached? Who will deliver the instrument to respondents and answer questions? Will that individual remain or come back to pick up the questionnaire? When will respondents be approached to answer the survey (time of day, dates)? Who will follow-up respondents who do not respond? When will data collection end? Will end of data collection be determined by date? By response rate?
- Are ethical safeguards (anonymity, lack of coercion) provided?

If the committee has planned for all of the items on the checklist, it should be ready to collect the data.

PREPARING, ANALYZING, AND USING THE DATA FOR DECISION MAKING

Planning for how to handle the data from the interviews or questionnaires should begin before the data are actually collected. When such planning is inadequate, the sheer amount of information can be a shock to those confronted with trying to organize it. One approach that has been found to be useful is to assign the planning for this activity to a small subgroup. In a committee of 6 to 8 people there is usually at least one person who has some experience and/or interest in handling data. This person is a likely choice for leading the subgroup.

Specific tasks that require planning include:

- Preparing worksheets for recording and summarizing the original (raw) data. Extra questionnaires can be used for this purpose.
- Deciding what specific questions are to be answered by the data, and planning for/preparing the tables or graphs that will display the data and answer the questions.
- Identifying and specifying the way in which the data will be transformed from their raw state to a summarized form useful for decision making.
- Deciding who will be involved in tabulating the data.
- Establishing guidelines for how to record the data and what to do when information is missing.

It is useful to be ready to begin the recording and summarizing activities as soon as the first data become available. Immediate use of the data-recording and summarizing procedures provides a good test of the procedures and allows time for adjustments if necessary before large quantities of data are received.

Specific Steps in Preparing the Data for Analysis

1. Transfer the individual data to the summary worksheets.
2. Tabulate the data.
3. Have someone double-check the results for mistakes. When two people independently reach the same results, you can be more certain about the accuracy of the results.
4. Prepare a summary of all information collected. This should include the total number of problems identified for all units listed, in order of their frequency, and a list of the problems identified on each patient care unit, in order of their frequency.
5. Calculate the response rate for each patient care unit and for the total organization. Count the number of questionnaires returned for each group and divide by the number of persons in each group to whom questionnaires were distributed and then multiply by 100.

$$\frac{\text{Number returned}}{\text{Number distributed}} \times 100 = \text{Response rate}$$

An example of summary data from use of the Patient Care Problem Identification Guide (see Appendix C), displayed in graph form, may be seen in Figure 2.

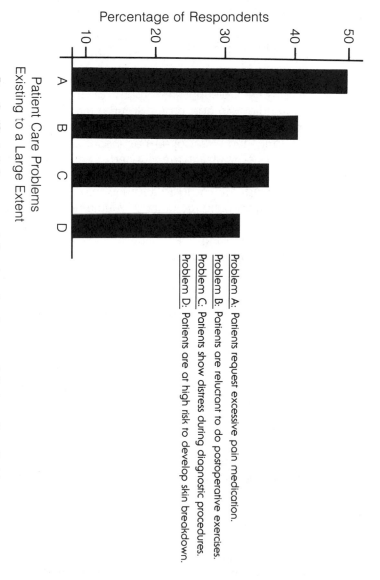

Percentage of Respondents

Patient Care Problems
Existing to a Large Extent

Problem A: Patients request excessive pain medication.

Problem B: Patients are reluctant to do postoperative exercises.

Problem C: Patients show distress during diagnostic procedures.

Problem D: Patients are at high risk to develop skin breakdown.

Fig. 2. (Partial) Summary of Results of a Survey of Patient Care Problems.

Analysis of the data begins when the summarizing procedures are completed. The analysis must include

- The response rate for each target group
- The results of the survey for each group
- An examination of similarities and differences of the results across groups

The analysis should result in answers to questions such as, What is the most prevalent problem? What patient care problems occur on which units? To what extent do the respondents view a particular problem as being serious? Do views vary among units or staff groups?

EXAMPLE

The analysis and subsequent decisions for the data displayed in Figure 2 might be as follows.

> The committee found that three patient care problems (which will be called problems A, B, and D) occurred on more than one unit and were related to the specific types of patients located on those units. Two of the problems (A and B) occurred on several of the surgical units. Problem D occurred on both medical and surgical units. After reviewing the results of the questionnaires, the committee had to decide which problem they would try to solve first. They considered the seriousness and the extensiveness of the identified problems. In this case, they decided to look for research-based solutions to problems related to the reluctance of patients to do postoperative exercises. Although this problem did not occur the most frequently, the committee decided it was serious enough and occurred frequently enough to warrant their attention first.

REPORTING THE RESULTS AND SUBSEQUENT DECISIONS

After the results of the questionnaire have been interpreted and the relevant decisions are made, it is important to provide feedback about the results to those persons who participated in the survey. This is important if the committee wishes to maintain the staff's interest in and cooperation with the change project being undertaken. The committee can anticipate interest in the results of the questionnaire related to each patient care unit as well as all the units combined. It is important to communicate to staff how the information was used in making a decision about the problem. When other

considerations outweigh the survey results, it is helpful to point out the reasons for this so that staff can see that their input was valued and used.

As discussed earlier, various strategies can be used to report the results of the survey. Written results of the survey provided via newsletters or memos can be used to describe and explain the findings. Reports or announcements at staff meetings allow for discussion and opportunity to clarify questions the staff may have about the results.

Ethical Issues Involved in Reporting Data

Safeguards should be provided wherever information is sought that may embarrass or endanger the person who supplies it. Patient care problem data could prove embarrassing to a nursing unit if the staff on that unit want to be perceived as providing excellent care and the data indicate otherwise. Similarly, an individual staff member who supplies negatively viewed data could be subjected to the anger of the unit administrator if the source of the data is known.

Several means can be employed to decrease the possibility of such negative outcomes and yet secure information that serves the intended purposes of the data collection effort.

- Making provision for individuals to answer questions anonymously. Lack of personal identification should help prevent negative responses directed at individual staff members.
- Reporting potentially embarrassing data to the involved nursing unit before it is reported to others. This gives the head nurse and unit staff an opportunity to "pave the way" for the data in ways that can minimize the potential for external criticism.
- Reporting data publicly without revealing the name of the unit(s).

POTENTIAL PROBLEMS AND STRATEGIES

Two potential problems that may arise when conducting a survey of patient care problems are *staff resistance* and *inaccurate data* upon which to base decisions. Staff resistance may lead to inaccurate data. Past experience with data collection, a lack of understanding about the survey's purpose, and low morale are some of the reasons staff may be resistant. By incorporating the principles of planned change into the method chosen for the survey, the commit-

tee can minimize staff resistance. While it cannot change the past, procedures can be implemented to demonstrate the committee's sensitivity to the issues involved in data collection.

The accuracy of the data is enhanced by careful planning and implementation of a consistent approach to data collection. A systematic approach to data collection means being organized and thorough. Another factor that affects the accuracy of data has to do with the nature of the data obtained. The survey may ask for the staff's perceptions of the patient care problems existing on the patient care units. This approach assumes that there is a high correlation between the perceptions staff have of patient care problems and the actual existence of such problems. It is safer to make this assumption when data are collected from groups of people, and it is more feasible to collect this information than to develop and conduct a survey concerned with the actual existence of each problem. However, there is a possibility that a discrepancy between perceived and real patient care problems may lead to a faulty decision. Whenever objective data about these problems are available from quality assurance or infection control programs, the information should be used to examine the correlation between perception (subjective data) and the facts, represented by data from quality assurance programs (objective data).

REFERENCES

Babbie, E.R. Survey research methods. Belmont, CA: Wadsworth Publishing Co., 1973, pp. 131–158, 171–186.

Polit, D.F., & Hungler, B.P. Nursing research: Principles and methods. Philadelphia, J.B. Lippincott, 1978, pp. 325–358.

CHECKLIST:
IDENTIFYING PATIENT CARE PROBLEMS

This checklist provides questions that need to be addressed in implementing this step of the research utilization process. It is important to account for the issues and activities inherent in these questions before progressing to the next step.

The Instrument

- ☐ Is the instrument ready for use?
    - ☐ Modified?
    - ☐ Pretested?
    - ☐ Sufficient copies?

Respondents

Have respondents been

- ☐ Identified?
- ☐ Notified regarding desired participation?

Data Collection Plan

- ☐ Have all necessary approvals been received?
- ☐ Are all arrangements complete? (see page 26)
- ☐ Do the data collection and feedback methods meet ethical requirements?

Data Analysis

- ☐ Are the members who will handle the data selected?
- ☐ Are the forms or tables on which the data will be tabulated and displayed ready?

Feedback to Respondents and Others

- ☐ Is the plan for informing others complete?
    - ☐ Nursing administrators
    - ☐ Respondents
    - ☐ Others

Chapter 4
IDENTIFYING AND ASSESSING RELEVANT RESEARCH-BASED KNOWLEDGE

The previous chapter focused on how to obtain valid and reliable information concerning patient care problems. This chapter focuses on where research-based knowledge can be found and how to assess this knowledge to determine its relevance for solving an identified patient care problem.

IDENTIFYING RESEARCH-BASED KNOWLEDGE

Scientific knowledge is generally found in the original reports of research studies. It is therefore important for the committee to locate original research reports regarding the patient care problem it is trying to solve.

Since clinical nursing research reports are not readily available, the committee must actively seek out resources to locate this information. In addition, there is need to discriminate between research-based and nonresearch-based solutions to patient care problems. Available sources of original research include:

33

• *Nursing research conferences.* Researchers who present papers at meetings usually cite their findings as well as the findings of other studies in this area. Description of the relationship between results of several studies is used to show how these findings build upon previously acquired knowledge.

• *Nursing journals.* Journals that publish research reports include: *Nursing Research, Research in Nursing and Health, Western Journal of Nursing Research,* and *Advances in Nursing Science.* These are excellent sources of research-based knowledge and include references to related studies. Other nursing journals, such as *Journal of Nursing Administration* and *Supervisor Nurse,* do not publish research in each issue of the journal but regularly include clinical applications that may provide leads to related research. It may be helpful to contact the author to determine whether a research base is available to support the practice ideas presented in the article and to locate the published research report.

• *Relevant research.* Nurses engaged in clinical research, expert practitioners, and nursing faculty members are likely to be familiar with research relevant to their interest areas and are often able to suggest where to look or whom to contact for research-based solutions to particular patient care problems.

• *Computerized retrieval services.* Universities and health care organizations usually have access to information systems in which computer searches of recent literature on health problems are printed as a bibliography. The user of such a service specifies the topic, and the computer retrieves titles of relevant articles or books. The bibliography then becomes a reading list to review for research-based knowledge in the field.

• *Using Research to Improve Nursing Practice,* a series of ten research-based practice protocols, developed during the Conduct and Utilization of Research in Nursing Project (CURN) and published by Grune & Stratton. The protocols are:

• *Preventing Decubitus Ulcers*
• *Structured Preoperative Teaching*
• *Clean Intermittent Catheterization*
• *Intravenous Cannula Change*
• *Reducing Diarrhea in Tube-Fed Patients*
• *Closed Urinary Drainage Systems*
• *Distress Reduction Through Sensory Preparation*
• *Preoperative Sensory Preparation to Promote Recovery*

- *Mutual Goal Setting in Patient Care*
- *Pain: Deliberative Nursing Interventions*

ASSESSING RELEVANT RESEARCH-BASED KNOWLEDGE

Finding and evaluating research studies is a time-consuming process requiring sophisticated technical skills and knowledge not yet widely available in nursing service settings. However, evaluation of identified research studies is essential to ascertain whether the resulting knowledge is scientifically sound, safe for use with patients, and the extent to which its use would be within the capacity of the available resources in the department of nursing. The evaluation process employed in reviewing research studies should decrease the potential for misutilization of clinical research. Misutilization occurs when either invalid knowledge is used as the basis for a practice change or valid knowledge is misunderstood by those using it and a proposed change in practice does not accurately reflect what is known.

It is our contention that no single study is sufficient to support a practice change and, therefore, evaluation of the research must also involve a synthesis of two or more studies that form a research base for the proposed change. A research base is a synthesis of the knowledge resulting from several studies whose findings corroborate, extend, or delineate the concept(s) investigated in the studies. Three sets of criteria for use in evaluating research bases for clinical utilization have been developed (Haller, Reynolds, & Horsley, 1979; see Appendix D). These criteria directly relate to the issues regarding misutilization.

The first set of criteria may be used to evaluate and integrate the scientific aspects of the studies that form the research base and result in a determination of the validity and generalizability of the knowledge. Included in this set are

- *Replication:* The research base must include more than one study.
- *Scientific merit:* Sample, design, methodology, results, and conclusions are examined.
- *Potential risk to patients:* This is used to mediate the stringency of the scientific merit and replication requirements.

The second set of criteria may be used to determine the practice-relevance of the research base. Bases with considerable practice-relevance are less likely to be misunderstood and inaccurately transformed into practice activities. Included in this set of criteria are

- *Clinical merit:* The extent to which the research base addresses a patient problem that is viewed as being significant by nurses.
- *Clinical control:* The extent to which nurses in practice settings can control the **independent variables** and **dependent variables** in the base.
- *Feasibility:* The extent to which nursing service agencies have the resources to implement the change suggested by the base.
- *Cost—benefit:* The costs involved in implementing the change do not outweigh the benefits to patients, the department, or both.

The third set of criteria may be used to determine whether the research base includes measurement instruments that can be used in conducting an evaluation of the practice change suggested by the research base. *Clinical evaluation* is used to determine whether misutilization has occurred in spite of the precautions taken to minimize its occurrence. The criteria in this set include

- *Availability of instrumentation:* Can nurses in clinical settings obtain evaluation instruments? Evaluation instruments are the same or similar to the instruments used by the researchers.
- *Clinical control:* Can nurses in the clinical setting make use of the evaluation instrument without the ongoing assistance of others?
- *Scientific merit:* Does the instrument produce valid and reliable data?

It is important for the committee to determine whether the research base being considered for use as the basis for a practice change meets these three sets of criteria. The review of research studies in relation to the criteria in sets one and three require advanced knowledge of research design and methodology. If an area of research for which there is no existing protocol is being reviewed, it would be advisable to secure the services of someone with such background to carry out that aspect of the review.

RESEARCH-BASED PRACTICE PROTOCOLS

The ten earlier-mentioned research-based practice protocols in the series *Using Research to Improve Nursing Practice* were developed from research bases that meet the previously stated criteria. In addition to meeting the criteria, these protocols provide a synthesis of the research comprising the base and transform the

research findings into clinically useful knowledge that is clearly defined for practice and yields an intervention with predictable patient outcomes. A protocol is directed toward the implementation and evaluation of a practice change and contains content pertaining to

- The need for change
- Description of the innovation
- Summary of the research base
- Limitations of the research base
- Research-based principle to guide the innovation
- Implementation of the innovation
- Evaluation of the effects of the innovation
- Summary
- References
- Suggested evaluation procedures and recording forms

When a new area of research meets the criteria for forming a research base, it would be useful to transform the findings into a protocol. This knowledge transformation forces those who develop the protocol to think through the issues involved in the subsequent change process and results in a written document that aids communication and understanding of the research.

Since this book is designed to be a guide for using the protocols in the series, *Using Research to Improve Nursing Practice,* it is assumed that the committee will have available for its use original research reports and a research-based clinical protocol to use in making a decision as to whether the identified patient care problem can be solved by the identified research. It is useful to review the protocol before the original reports are reviewed because the protocol should be easer to understand, provides a synthesis of the research, and identifies specific aspects of the individual studies that might be missed on first reading without the protocol's guidance.

CONSIDERING INNOVATION–ORGANIZATION FIT

After the protocol is reviewed and before the research studies are reviewed, it is useful for the committee to discuss whether the innovation as described in the protocol will solve the identified patient care problem. For example, a structured preoperative teaching program as proposed by Lindeman and Van Aernam (1971)

would not provide a solution for disorientation in postoperative patients. The discussion also should provide committee members with validating or corrective feedback regarding their individual interpretations of the protocol. When the committee members decide the protocol offers a potential solution for the identified problem, they should proceed with reading the original research.

Review of the research reports should be focused on (1) any areas needing clarification that were identified in the protocol discussion, (2) validating that the research provides an appropriate solution, and (3) the feasibility of implementing the potential solution within the department of nursing. Feasibility relates to how well the proposed innovation fits the department's values, structure, and resources. The question to be addressed is general—Is the proposed innovation feasible? This does not require that the committee decide on how the innovation would be implemented at this time. A guide to assist with the review of the research reports entitled Guide to Reading Research Critically, is provided in Appendix E.

Organizations vary in their values, structure, and resources. When considering a change in practice it is necessary to examine the characteristics of the department of nursing and the larger organizational context in which it exists to ascertain which organizational characteristics will facilitate a proposed change and which will impede it. Organizational variables that should be examined for their potential influence on the proposed change include

- *Administrative organization of personnel and departments:* decentralized or centralized structure, formal or informal lines of communication, interdisciplinary linkages.
- *Decision-making processes:* budget control, policy-making or revision, procedure development and approval.
- *Personnel:* number and availability of staff to assist with the process, interest in the proposed change, diversity of skills available among staff.

The initial review of the protocol and research base should focus on the fit between the innovation and the department. To facilitate examination of the fit between the innovation and the organization, an assessment instrument entitled the "Probability for Adoption Assessment Guide" was developed (see Appendix F). This guide assists change agents in nursing departments to assess the characteristics of potential nursing practice innovations that might affect their successful adoption. The use of the guide requires knowledge of the characteristics and requirements of the proposed innovation *and* the characteristics and resources of the nursing department.

At the completion of this step, the committee should be convinced that the innovation offers a feasible solution to the identified patient care problem. It is important that committee members work together in assessing the innovation protocol and research base so that they reach common understandings about the factors that contribute to the final decision regarding selection of the innovation. In addition, common understandings of the factors that facilitate or pose obstacles to the innovation will serve as a guide for subsequent activities related to planning and carrying out the change.

REFERENCE

Haller, K.B., Reynolds, M.A., & Horsley, J.A. Developing research-based innovation protocols: Process, criteria, and issues. *Research in Nursing and Health,* 1979, *2,* 45–51.

CHECKLIST:
IDENTIFYING AND ASSESSING RESEARCH-BASED KNOWLEDGE

This checklist provides questions that need to be addressed in implementing this step of the research utiliization process. It is important to account for the issues and activities inherent in these questions before progressing to the next step.

Research Base

☐ Is there any reason to question the scientific basis of the clinical protocol to be implemented?

☐ Has someone who can assist with the review of the research base been identified?

☐ If yes, have they agreed to assist with the review?

Innovation—Organization Fit

☐ Does the clinical protocol potentially solve the identified patient care problem?

☐ Is there any reason to question whether the innovation is feasible within the department of nursing?

☐ If yes, what specific areas are of concern?

Chapter 5
ADAPTING AND DESIGNING THE RESEARCH-BASED PRACTICE INNOVATION

This chapter focuses on designing a nursing innovation and its evaluation that are within the limits (requirements) of the research base and that fit the unique requirements of the department of nursing. Understanding the limits of the research base simply means identifying specifically what has been studied so that it can be discriminated from what has not been studied. For example, if the research of interest has been conducted only on adult subjects, its use is limited to adult patients until new research extends the finding to children.

The idea that research bases have limits is very important. The value of research-based knowledge rests in its capacity to predict that a specific intervention delivered to a specific patient population should produce specific patient outcomes. If the innovation does not reflect what is known or exceeds what is known from the research, we can no longer accurately predict the patient outcomes. Some preoperative teaching programs offer excellent examples of situations in which the requirements of the research base are not met or, on the other hand, the intervention as designed exceeds the limits of what has been studied. Lindeman and Van Aernam (1971), Lindeman (1972), and others have demonstrated that a structured preoperative teaching program that teaches patients to cough, **41**

deep-breathe, and exercise and that requires them to practice these activities preoperatively can affect their postoperative function. Today most departments of nursing offer some form of preoperative instruction for patients; however, upon examination, many of these programs do not accurately reflect what is known to work. For example, some programs teach patients about coughing, deep breathing, and exercise but do not include a supervised practice-component. These programs do not meet the requirements of the structured preoperative teaching research base. Other programs include additional information such as descriptions of preoperative procedures, preoperative medications, or transfer to a stretcher. The effects of providing this information were not studied within the research base, and its inclusion in the structured preoperative teaching program would therefore exceed the limits of the base and should not be delivered with the teaching program until it is known whether this addition interferes with the learning the research-based program is designed to facilitate.

UNDERSTANDING THE REQUIREMENTS AND LIMITS OF THE RESEARCH BASE

The protocol provides information regarding the specific requirements and limits of the research base. However, it does not offer detailed operational information regarding the ways in which individual investigators defined their populations, interventions, and patient outcomes. Since most investigators vary the way in which they design their studies, research reports offer not only more operational detail, but also detailed descriptions of various ways of defining population, intervention, and outcome. A critical review of the original research articles is essential for identifying and understanding the variety of approaches to be considered when designing the innovation and its evaluation. This is accomplished by reviewing each article separately to identify how the researcher defined the study population, the independent variable, and the dependent variables, and what measurement tools were used to measure the effects of the independent variable. These components of a research study are directly related to the components of the nursing process: the study population and patient population, the independent variable and nursing intervention, the dependent variable and patient outcomes, and finally, the research measurement

tools and tools to assist in evaluating the effects of the nursing intervention.

The critical review of the original research is carried out by re-examining the information collected through use of the *Guide to Reading Research Critically* during the previous step (pp 130–134). If there is reason to question the adequacy or accuracy of the information collected, committee members should reread the articles at this point. Table 1 shows one way to summarize the information from each study and across multiple studies. A summary table such as this will facilitate the later work of the committee members as they decide how they will define each component of the innovation, because it displays the range of options available for each component.

After the range of options regarding the components of the innovation has been identified and is understood, the next step involves thinking about how the characteristics of the potential innovation interact with the characteristics of the department of nursing. During an earlier step, the committee determined that the potential innovation fit the requirements of the department sufficiently well to proceed with its planning. The "Probability for Adoption Assessment Guide" (Appendix F) was used in making this initial determination. At this point, the committee needs to re-examine the data from this guide to identify whether potential problem areas exist (items with low scores) and to determine whether they can design the innovation in a way that will minimize the impact of any identified problem areas and maximize the innovation's potential for adoption.

Innovations vary in their potential for adoption because of characteristics inherent in the innovation that are known to facilitate or impede acceptance by organizations. Nine characteristics of innovation that influence probability for adoption have been identified (National Institute of Mental Health, 1971). These characteristics are relevance, compatibility, relative advantage, observability or communicability, complexity and feasibility, reversibility, divisibility, trialability, and credibility. Understanding the relationship between these characteristics and an innovation's potential for adoption is important because most innovations can be designed in a variety of ways, and if the various designs alter the characteristics of the innovation, the innovation's potential for adoption can be increased or decreased by the way it is designed. The nine identified characteristics of innovations are briefly discussed below, with attention

Table 1
Critical Review of Original Research: Summary

Components	Detailed Description of Components		Summary across Articles
	Article 1	Article 2	
Population: Patient population	≥ 15 yrs, non-emergency, non-ENT surgery requiring general anesthesia.	Generally same as Article 1.	≥ 15 yrs, non-emerg, non-ENT surgery requiring general anesthesia.
Independent variable: Intervention	Structured teaching of stir-up regime: coughing, deep-breathing, leg + foot exerc.	Group vs individual teaching mode.	Structured teaching of stir-up regime; plus group-individual instruction.
Dependent variable: Patient outcome	Length of hospital stay, analgesic use, ventilatory function.	Same as Article 1 plus length of learning time (control for age, smoking, incision ×).	LOS, analgesic use, vent. funct., length of learning time
Measurement tools: Evaluation	Spirometer: vital capacity, expir. flow rate.	Same as Article 1.	
Findings	Ventilatory function enhanced. Length of stay shorter for experimental group. Analgesics: no difference.	Group teaching is as effective as individual teaching in relation to vent. func., LOS, and analgesic use. Length of learning time shorter with group teaching.	Structured teaching of stir-up regime enhances vent. func. ↓ shortens LOS. Group teaching is as effective as individual instruction; learning occurs in less time.

focused on how they relate to adoption potential and how the committee can alter an innovation or use information to enhance the positive qualities of each characteristic.

RELEVANCE.   The more an innovation addresses a difficult problem or potentially offers benefit to many, the more likely it is to be adopted (referred to earlier as clinical merit). Since the determination of relevance rests in part on the perceptions of the staff, the committee can influence their perceptions of the solution by using patient problem-identification data to clarify the scope of the problem and therefore the relevance of the solution.

COMPATIBILITY.   The more an innovation fits the department's established values, norms, and procedures, the more likely it is to be adopted. The structured preoperative teaching innovation can be designed to be delivered by a small group of clinician-teachers or by all relevant nurses, depending on the norms of a given department.

RELATIVE ADVANTAGE.   The more an innovation is viewed as presenting a relative advantage over existing practice, the more likely it is to be adopted. The advantage may relate to patient outcomes, cost, public relations, satisfaction, or other similar factors. The determination of relative advantage may be enhanced by collecting evaluation data that specifically demonstrate differences between the innovation and existing practice that are known to be important to the organization, e.g., cost, patient- and/or staff-satisfaction data.

OBSERVABILITY OR COMMUNICABILITY.   The more tangible the outcomes of the innovation, the more likely it will be adopted. Technological innovations generally are adopted faster than interpersonal innovations. Reporting positive outcomes (data) of the evaluation of the innovation to staff members who are targeted to deliver it in the future increases the potential for its adoption.

COMPLEXITY AND FEASIBILITY.   The easier an innovation can be understood and implemented, the more likely it will be adopted. Materials are prepared to assist the staff to understand and deliver a complex innovation, e.g., slide-tape shows, flip-charts used for the structured preoperative teaching innovation.

REVERSIBILITY.   An innovation that is viewed as being reversible is more likely to be adopted. Designing the structured preoperative teaching innovation so a few clinician-teachers deliver it is more reversible than having all the relevant nurses deliver it.

TRIALABILITY.   Innovations that can be tried on a pilot basis are more likely to lead to adoption than those that cannot be initiated on a pilot basis. Instead of trialability per se, what is important here is making the trial as simple as possible, e.g., trying to confine the pilot to one nursing unit.

DIVISIBILITY.   An innovation that can be broken into parts that are introduced in stages is more likely to be adopted than one that cannot. When an innovation includes both an assessment device and an intervention, the two parts can be introduced in stages.

CREDIBILITY.   The more an innovation is viewed as arising from a credible source, e.g., research, or is espoused by a credible source, e.g., a person or committee, the more likely it is to be adopted. The deliberate use of opinion leaders who favor the innovation can be planned by the committee.

Clearly, characteristics such as compatibility, complexity, reversibility, and divisibility should be considered when designing the innovation, while characteristics such as relative advantage, observability, and trialability should be considered when designing an evaluation of the innovation. At this point, the committee members should be in a position to use the information in Table 1: Critical Review of Original Research: Summary, and Appendix F: Probability for Adoption Assessment Guide, to assist them in deciding how to design the innovation for their nursing department.

A written description of the innovation should now be developed, and it should have as much detail as possible in relation to what the components of the innovation to be implemented in that hospital will look like. Specifically, it answers the following questions:

- What patient population will participate in the trial (defining characteristics)?
- Where (name of service/unit) are the patients located?
- What is the intervention? The structured preoperative teaching program description would include form (e.g., individual versus group teaching method), content (e.g., coughing, deep breathing, exercise, information, demonstration, and practice) technology (e.g., slide tape, flip-chart).
- Who is going to carry out the intervention? All nurses? Some nurses? If not, are ancillary staff involved? If yes, who?
- When and where will the intervention occur?

When the written description is completed, it should again be

reviewed to decide whether it in fact still meets the requirements and limits of the research base. When the intervention design creates a need for alteration in the basic philosophical or structural components of the department or when it will require the acquisition of costly equipment, administrators should be apprised and sanction for these changes sought before planning activities begin.

EVALUATION OF RESEARCH-BASED INTERVENTIONS

The previous section discussed how an evaluation of the innovation can provide data to demonstrate the relative advantage of the innovation vis a vis existing practice and to make the outcomes of the innovation visible for the nurses who will be expected to deliver it. An even more important reason for conducting an evaluation is to provide a safeguard against the possibility of misutilization. In Chapter 4 misutilization was described as occurring when either (1) invalid knowledge is used as a basis for the intervention, or (2) Valid knowledge is misunderstood and an intervention does not reflect accurately what is known.

Evaluation of the innovation, if properly conducted, will provide data to assist in making a decision to adopt, alter, or reject the new practice. An evaluation can be designed so it includes the three components of quality assurance programs: process, outcomes, and structure. Process and outcome evaluations provide data for misutilization considerations, while cost—benefit considerations are provided for by structural evaluation.

In some respects evaluating a research-based innovation is easier than evaluating an innovation that does not have a research base. The "ease" arises from two places. First, there is a known predictable relationship between the nursing intervention and the patient outcome. Therefore, if patient-outcome data deviate from what is expected (predicted), something is wrong. It is also possible to try to establish whether it is a matter of inaccurate implementation, by collecting process data that describe the nature of the intervention as it is delivered (which may be different from what was designed). If the process data demonstrate inaccurate implementation, the cause of the "misutilization" is identified and corrective action can be taken. However, if the process data show the intervention was accurately delivered, the cause of the misutilization cannot be discerned. Misutilization arising from invalid knowledge cannot be demonstrated directly. Logic is used to conclude that

something other than inaccurate implementation interfered in the predicted relationship, and one possible explanation is that the original relationship was not valid.

The research base also makes evaluation easier by providing specific direction about what variables are evaluated (measured) and how to measure them. In other words, patient outcomes (dependent variables) are operationally defined, and in many instances the measurement instruments used by the original investigators are available for use in a clinical evaluation.

Structural evaluation is usually not addressed in the research base. The most cogent type of structural variable is cost. Cost data should be separated into two types: those costs arising from the initial change and those that are ongoing if the change is adopted.

THE NATURE OF EVALUATION: WHAT MUST BE CONSIDERED

In many respects, evaluation is similar to research in that it requires the utilization of scientific methods just as research does. It differs from research because it has a different purpose, i.e., the purpose of evaluation is to produce data for local, departmental decision making, while the purpose of research is to produce data that permits decision making of a much more generalizable nature, i.e., across all people in the relevant population not just those patients cared for in one hospital.

Evaluation requires consideration of a number of factors such as sample, design, measurement, and analysis. Analysis will be addressed in Chapter 7; the other components are addressed below.

Variable Selection

The variables to be included in the evaluation come from the research base. The independent variable to be used for the process evaluation is the intervention as it is designed for use in the department of nursing. The dependent variable(s) or patient outcomes also are identified in the original research. At least one, and preferably more, of the variables in the base should be selected for the evaluation. Other dependent variables such as patient satisfaction may be added if they are judged to be important to the department, but additional new variables should not substitute for

one or more of the original research base variables. The original dependent variables are essential to test the expected relationship between the intervention and patient outcome.

Sample

The sample consists of the patients who will participate in the evaluation. It is important that these patient's accurately represent the population sampled in the original research. The characteristics (diagnosis, age, sex, etc.) of the selected population should have been defined when the intervention was designed. Sampling refers to the use of procedures that assure that the patients selected for the sample do represent the specified population. A *convenience sampling* procedure is adequate for the purposes of most clinical evaluations. A convenience sample is made up of subjects who are easy to access for the purpose of evaluation i.e., they are in the hospital and located on the nursing unit to be used for the evaluation. This means that readily available patients who have the required population characteristics will be "selected" until the desired number is reached. The desired number is always as many as budget and time will allow. Usually 20 patients per group would be a good size sample. The sample size should not be less than 10 patients per group.

Design

Outcome evaluation as it is used here requires that the patient outcomes produced by the innovation be compared with the patient outcomes that are produced by existing practice. Such comparisons are made possible by the collection of a set of data taken when existing practice is being delivered and the collection of a different set of data taken when the innovation is being delivered. One aspect of design relates to the way the evaluator arranges the collection of the two sets of data. The collection of data may be arranged temporally so that one data set (baseline: existing practice) is collected first; after the innovation is implemented another data set (postimplementation: innovation) is collected. The collection of data also may be arranged so that it comes from different groups of patients; in this case, one group (comparison) receives the existing practice and the other group (intervention) receives the innovation. These two sets of data are then compared. The type of arrangement chosen for a given evaluation depends on the nature of the

intervention and the nature of the questions the data are supposed to answer. The protocols in the series *Using Research to Improve Nursing Practice* include a specific discussion of the evaluation design suggested for use with the innovation. The committee should review the suggested evaluation designs and follow them as closely as possible.

Measurement

When measurement is considered, two issues are of paramount importance: is the measurement instrument valid, i.e., does it measure what it is supposed to measure, and is the instrument reliable, i.e., if the measurement was repeated in the same patients, under the same conditions, would the same results be obtained? For example, when measuring the variable temperature, validity would be addressed by asking whether a thermometer produces a true measure of temperature; reliability would be addressed by determining whether the same thermometer would produce the same temperature readings if the measurements were repeated in the same patients and under the same conditions. When the measurement consists of an observation made by a single person, e.g., a patient's pulse, the reliability issues are similar to those for a mechanical instrument. However, when the observation system requires that multiple persons carry out the observation, a different reliability issue is of concern. In this instance, we must be confident that different people observing the same event at the same time will produce the same measurement. This type of reliability is referred to as interrater reliability. Interrater reliability is also a concern when a measurement device requires that a person and a mechanical device interact to produce a measurement (e.g., blood pressure). Guidelines and procedures for establishing interrater reliability may be found in Appendix G.

Another issue is whether the instruments used by the researcher are available and/or useful to nurses in clinical settings. For example, the Minnesota Multiphasic Personality Inventory (MMPI) is a commonly used and accepted research instrument for psychological studies. However, one must meet special requirements to use it and have special training to interpret the data. As a clinical evaluation tool for most nursing situations, therefore, it is essentially useless.

Developing Data-Recording Devices

The committee also must develop forms on which to record the collected data. When possible, the recording forms should be designed so that all the relevant data for a particular patient can be entered on a single form. The recorded data should include relevant demographic data (diagnosis, sex, unit, age) as well as the specific evaluation variables identified for the trial. Sample data-recording forms may be found in Appendix H.

Designing an Evaluation

Each of the components discussed above must be considered when designing the evaluation for the practice change. As with the design of the intervention, the research base also provides useful information relevant to the evaluation. The chart in Table 1 can be used to identify the range of options available for defining the sample, the dependent variables, and the measurement tools. In addition, the committee should consider how the evaluation can be designed to enhance the relative advantage of the innovation and make the patient outcome highly visible.

A written description of the evaluation plan should also be developed. It should be as detailed as posssible and should cover

- The specific dependent variables (e.g., patient outcomes, staff outcomes) to be measured. One dependent variable must come from the research base.
- The specific instruments to be used to measure the selected dependent variables.
- Who is going to collect the evaluation data and how they will be trained (see Appendix I).
- The number of patients to be included in the intervention group and the comparison group.
- The specific nursing unit(s) from which the patients will be selected.
- The design to be used in producing the two sets of data to be compared.
- How the evaluation data will be collected.

When the evaluation description is completed, it should be reviewed to determine whether it reflects the evaluation components

in the research base. The descriptions of the innovation and the evaluation plan form the basis for the planning activities discussed in the next chapter.

REFERENCES

Lindeman, C. Nursing intervention with the presurgical patient: Effectiveness and efficiency of group and individual preoperative teaching—
phase two. *Nursing Research,* 1972, *21,* 196–209.
Lindeman, C., & Van Aernam, B. Nursing intervention with the presurgical
patient—the effects of structured and unstructured preoperative teaching. *Nursing Research,* 1971, *20,* 319–322.
National Institute of Mental Health. *Planning for Creative Change in Mental
Health Services: A Distillation of Principles on Research Utilization.* Vol.
1. U.S. Department of Health, Education, and Welfare, 1971.

CHECKLIST:
ADAPTING AND DESIGNING THE RESEARCH-BASED INNOVATION

This checklist provides questions that need to be addressed in implementing this step of the research utilization process. It is important to account for the issues and activities inherent in these questions before progressing to the next step.

Description of the Innovation

☐ Is it completed?

☐ Is it written?

☐ Does it meet the requirements and limits of the research base?

Description of the Evaluation

☐ Is there at least one outcome variable from the research base included in the evaluation?

☐ Is it completed?

☐ Is it written?

☐ Does it meet the requirements and limits of the research base?

Chapter 6
CONDUCTING A CLINICAL TRIAL AND EVALUATION OF THE INNOVATION

O nce the innovation has been adapted for use in a particular department of nursing, the committee must focus on its introduction to the others who will be expected to participate in its implementation on a trial basis. The focus of this chapter is on how to plan for the introduction of the innovation so that is continues to meet the requirements of the research base and yet causes the least amount of disruption possible to the ongoing activities of the department. The key to the attainment of such change lies in the use of planned change principles, including the use of a clinical trial.

A clinical trial is a pragmatic way to introduce a practice change. It simply means that the innovation will be tried on a small scale, e.g., one nursing unit, before a decision is made to introduce it in all appropriate locations within the organization. It is interesting to note that dictionary definitions of the term *trial* range from "an examination" to "an affliction or trouble" (Random House, 1967). It is the examination aspect of a clinical trial that makes it important and pragmatic in relation to the introduction of the change. On the other hand, careful use of the principles of planned change should minimize the sense of affliction and trouble experienced by those who direct and experience the change.

54 The purposes of using a clinical trial are threefold:

- It makes reversibility of the change easier by involving fewer people and resources at the outset. Reversibility refers to the ease with which the practice can be returned to its previous state, if necessary.
- It provides experience with the innovation as it occurs under actual practice conditions and therefore permits the identification of operational problems and modifications of processes and procedures before wide-scale implementation occurs.
- It provides data on which to base a decision to adopt as originally designed, modify or redesign, or reject the innovation. A successful trial provides an examination of the effects of the practice change with as little bias as possible. Success rests on the lack of bias in the examination, not on the outcomes of trial vis a vis adoption of the innovation. Thus, a trial that shows that an innovation should be rejected will be considered as successful as one that supports adoption of the change, as long as there are sound data on which to base the decision.

PLANNING FOR IMPLEMENTATION OF THE INNOVATION

Planning means to think out, *before the fact,* the purposes of introducing the innovation and the activities necessary to attain these purposes. In addition, it requires that materials necessary for implementation of the plan be acquired or developed before initiating a clinical trial of the innovation.

The importance of planning and the amount of time required to develop an adequate master plan are often underestimated. An adequate plan needs to address all aspects of the proposed change in considerable detail and in written form. It ensures that the sanctions needed are secured, that the required resources are on hand, and that staff who need to perform in some explicit way during the trial are well prepared to do so. Recording the plan in writing is essential if the committee is to effectively coordinate all of the detailed activities that must be carried out according to a time schedule. In addition, a written plan will facilitate the achievement of consistency in the implementation of the plan. Inadequate planning can doom to failure an otherwise important and potentially effective change because problems occur that could have been avoided or minimized. When this occurs, it irritates personnel whose support is

essential to the project and causes frustrating (and often costly) delays.

Purpose of a Master Plan

A master plan for implementing a trial of the innovation should do the following:

- Specify and organize required activities around a projected timetable.
- Account for all activities to be carried out, including specification of who will do them, and when, where, and how they will be done.
- Be flexible enough to allow for the unexpected, for example, loss of a key person because of illness; broken equipment; or changes in the hospital census. Alternative or contingency planning should be done where appropriate and feasible.
- Include consideration of potential sources of resistance to change and the identification of strategies for dealing with it when it occurs. For example, what if staff members do not come to a retraining program that is essential to orient them to the new practice?

The master plan evolves over time; it is not predetermined and static. Later stages in the plan are dependent on the successful course of early stages, while decisions made in early stages are often reworked later to take into account events and information that were unknown at the time the initial decisions were made. For example, a committee decided to deliver a preoperative teaching innovation using a sound-on-slide program developed by the researcher. They determined that they could afford to purchase three copies of the program. Later in the planning process, however, they found the department had only one sound-on-slide machine available for use and no funds available to purchase additional equipment. At this point, the committee needed to review their objectives regarding implementation and consider the following alternatives:

- Convert the cost of one sound-on-slide program into a sound-on-slide machine and cut back the number of sites for delivery of the teaching program from three to two
- Change the teaching methodology from sound-on-slide to flip-charts, which could be made at the hospital within the current budget limitation
- Adjust the projected timetable by slowing down the planning

process and staging the implementation of the innovation so that the budget for the next year would be available to continue with the original plan for securing three sound-on-slide programs

Considerations in Developing the Master Plan

The section that follows will outline in detail the things that need to be considered in developing the master plan. The outline is set to demonstrate the normal flow of the planning sequence. However, it should be recognized that the actual planning process often flows backwards as well as progressively forward, as was illustrated in the example cited above. A comprehensive master plan should include the following components.

1. An exhaustive list of the activities that must be completed to implement the innovation and to conduct an evaluation of the trial:

- A written description of the innovation and evaluation to facilitate the identification of the major tasks to be addressed.
- The major tasks should then be reviewed to identify specific activities that comprise and support the implementation and evaluation of the innovation on a trial basis. For example, if all nursing staff are expected to deliver the new practice, they must have some type of educational program to prepare them. The development of a staff development program is an important support activity that becomes part of the master plan. Training observers and obtaining interrater reliability estimates are similar types of support activity directed toward the evaluation aspects of the trial.

2. A comprehensive list of the resources necessary to implement and evaluate the innovation. Of particular importance are:

- Personnel involved in each activity, e.g., identification of those who will conduct the teaching program, as well as those who will assist with evaluation
- Equipment, e.g., sound-on-slide machines, laboratory tests
- Facilities and space, e.g., classrooms for educational programs, a cabinet to store equipment or data.

3. A time schedule that organizes the sequencing of activities and resource acquisitions necessary to conduct the trial.

- The schedule should always represent the best estimate of time required for each activity and should remain flexible enough to adapt to erroneous estimates or unanticipated events.
- The time schedule should be planned in a backwards flow, i.e., start with a target date for completion of the trial and work backwards toward the present time.
- A timetable helps the committee anticipate greatest periods of activity and plan for them. It also is a useful means of gauging progress. Timetables are always approximate and may need to be revised.
- Plotting activities on a timetable from the outset may shorten the time it takes to accomplish the innovation because it organizes activities and highlights the need for effective delegation of responsibility for tasks.
- A calendar can be used to make the master plan clear. Necessary activities can be entered on it in sequence with notes made of who is responsible for accomplishing the activity. Copies of this information can be made for all members.

4. *Securing the sanctions and approvals* and local resources necessary to carry out the plan.

- Plans for the trial need to be approved by those groups or individuals who have authority over the decisions involved in conducting the trial and in changing nursing practice within the institution. Frequently these persons are the director of nursing, and staff development director, supervisors, and the head nurse of the unit where the trial will be conducted.
- The materials, resources, and administrative cooperation needed for a trial must be negotiated during the planning process.
- Maintaining communication with these policy makers throughout the trial also encourages their continued support and is likely to facilitate their willingness to continue the innovation on a more permanent basis if warranted by the trial.

5. *Acquiring resources* that are not available in the local hospital environment.

- Resources, e.g., equipment, that are unavailable and require purchase from external sources can pose severe problems for the planning process.

- It is important to identify unavailable resources as early as possible and to initiate the purchasing process immediately, beginning with approval to purchase, selection of the equipment and final ordering.
- If possible, an estimate of the normal time required for delivery of purchased items should be identified and included in the master plan.

6. *Developing materials and procedures* required for implementation of the innovation and its evaluation. At this point, the committee should have at its disposal (or on order) all of the resources that need to be acquired from sources external to the committee in order to conduct the trial. The next steps in the planning process are to identify the materials that need to be developed or adapted for the innovation and evaluation, and develop the procedures that will organize the utilization of the resources into patterns of activity necessary to produce the innovation and evaluation.

Whenever possible, materials developed by others, e.g., researchers, other nursing departments, should be adapted for use rather than beginning anew, in order to reduce personnel time, costs, and frustrations involved in material development. Rarely will the materials developed by researchers be usable without some adaptation. The circumstances of a given practice setting may be very different from the setting in which the research was conducted; in addition, the researchers may have had more elaborate equipment, trained personnel, or resources than those available in the average practice setting.

Material and procedure development is a time-consuming process that must be completed before the trial begins or the trial is very likely to be interrupted, with resulting undue costs and irritation to those involved.

MATERIAL ADAPTATION AND DEVELOPMENT.   An example of material adaptation might consist of taking new slides for use in the structured preoperative teaching program so the actors in the program represent the predominant ethnic groups represented in the hospital's patient population.

- The following materials are usually developed for an innovation:
    Assessment forms
    Patient teaching materials
    A written description of the procedures
    Staff-development materials

Devices to record assessment and intervention components (see Appendix H)
- The following materials are developed for an evaluation:
  Data collection instruments (see Appendix H)
  Data summary forms (see Appendix H)

PROCEDURE DEVELOPMENT.   Procedure development almost always is department specific and would involve such considerations as whether as assessment form is part of the patient's permanent record and should be filed directly on the patient's charts and who will file it.

- If equipment is used in the innovation, the procedure should specify where it is stored, how it can be signed out, how to use it, etc.
- A procedure might be developed to designate communication mechanisms. For example, if the assessment shows the patient is at risk for developing a decubitus ulcer, then a nursing order for the small shifts intervention should be written and an orange circle attached to the patient's bed to clearly designate the patient as being at risk.
- The following types of procedures are developed for an intervention:
  Delivery of the intervention
  Communication (when multiple staff, departments are involved)
  Specific instructions for use of equipment
- The following types of procedures are developed for an evaluation:
  Patient identification—communication of availability
  Training evaluators (see Appendix I)
  Establishing interrater reliability (see Appendix G)
  Data collection (who, when, where)
  Data recording (how, where)
  Reporting interruptions in data collection activities
  Data tabulation—analysis

7. Staff development. Before beginning the trial, the committee will need to be sure that the staff development requirements of the innovation have been carefully accounted for. This may involve the introduction of new knowledge and skills or the review and reorganization of old knowledge and skills.

Any practice innovation requires nurses to learn or review certain

knowledge and skills. It is necessary to identify the new knowledge and skills required by the research-based innovation and to plan for ways in which they can be taught to those who will be involved with the innovation. The intravenous cannula change regimen *(Intravenous Cannula Change, 1981)* for example, requires knowledge of the bacterial and physiochemical sources of infusion-associated venous reactions. The structured preoperative teaching *(Structured Preoperative Teaching, 1981)* requires nurses who will conduct the patient classes to understand the principles underlying effective teaching of skills.

- All who participate directly in the delivery of the intervention will need to undergo some staff development.
- It is also necessary to offer staff development programs to others who are less directly involved but who have a supportive role in the intervention, e.g., supervisors, nurses' aides.
- Each hospital will have different resources available to support staff development, and the committtee will need to identify needed resources specifically relevant to their innovation.
- Planning for staff development involves assuring that the knowledge and skills required by the innovation are provided by qualified persons and that all those involved in implementing the innovation have the opportunity to learn the knowledge and skills before they are expected to use them.
- During the trial, only staff who will be involved with the trial units should be involved in the staff development program. Later, if the innovation is adopted, large-scale staff development effforts will need to occur.
- In a way, the staff development teaching program developed for the clinical trial can be a "trial" for the large-scale staff development program needed if the innovation is adopted on a permanent basis. Certainly the small program used in the trial should be evaluated as to its strengths and weaknesses before large-scale efforts are undertaken.

8. *Communicating with others* about the plan and its proposed implementation.

- Communicating effectively with others about the plans for the trial is essential to its success.
- Informing others about the plan for a trial serves two purposes: (a) it provides accurate information to those participating in the trial about what is being done and helps to elicit their coopera-

tion; (b) by communicating with those not directly involved in the trial, the committee is laying the foundation for their support during the later stages of the change project.

- The information provided should correct misunderstanding and satisfy curiosity expressed about the trial; in the absence of information, people may speculate about the trial and misinterpret its intent.
- Deciding who should be informed requires an assessment of the formal and informal communication and decision-making linkages between people in the practice setting. The committee should "touch base" with various groups of staff and individuals who will influence later full-scale adoption of the innovation.
- There are several potential communication problems the committee should consider in relation to planning for an evaluation. Evaluation tends to imply a negative attitude toward the quality of care currently being delivered. This may make some individuals hesitant to cooperate with the evaluation. It should be emphasized that the purpose of the evaluation is not to single-out individuals for criticcism but to improve the overall quality of care delivered, first on the trial unit and later on all appropriate patient care units.
- Sometimes the knowledge that evaluation is being done makes people self-concious and alters their usual way of doing things. If practice is altered during the baseline evaluation period, the results of the evaluation will not reflect typical care. For this reason, it may be necessary to plan a longer evaluation so that the initial effects of measuring performance can be overcome.
- Maintaining communication throughout the trial with those who have authority over decisions involved in its conduct will be likely to facilitate their continued support through the trial and their subsequent willingness to continue the innovation if warranted by the trial.
- It also is important for the committee to invite feedback from the nursing staff during the trial and particularly to provide feedback about the results after the trial. These strategies not only serve to reduce resistance but also enhance the staff's sense of involvement in bringing about research-based practice changes.

Resistance to Change

Resistance to the proposed changes can and should be anticipated in the planning process. Resistance is most likely to occur

when people are experiencing change in something that is important to them, for example, their values, position in the organization, self-esteem, personal capacity to fulfill their role obligations, the cohesiveness of their reference (work) group, and their personal influence. Identifying sources of resistance (people) and the reasons for the resistance can occur naturally during .the planning process if committee members are sensitive to their own descriptions of how others will respond at a future time. Even though committee members are committed to the change and have accepted the personal alterations it will cause, each member may still experience times of thinking "I don't want to do this." These personal exclamations are likely to forecast what others will experience and, if shared and examined, will be useful in identifying reasons for resistance. The responses of others to future events are often anticipated in off-the-cuff comments such as "Mrs. Smith will retire if she has to do this." Again, such thoughts are worthy of examination not only as a means of identifying sources of resistance (Mrs. Smith) but also, if taken a step further (why would this be troublesome to Mrs. Smith?), as a means of identifying the reasons for the resistance.

Once the sources and reasons for resistance have been identified the committee can plan strategies for dealing with it. Zaltman and Duncan (1977) have identified four types of strategies that can be used to reduce resistance.

FACILITATION.   This strategy is used when people are aware of the need for change and are receptive to information regarding the change. It involves supporting their receptivity by offering information about the change in pleasant, stimulating, and easily obtainable ways, e.g., staff meetings, newsletters.

RE-EDUCATION.   This strategy is used when people are in need of and want information regarding the change. It may involve classes, workbooks, and/or staff-development programs.

PERSUASION.   This strategy is used when people are not committed to the change for straightforward, rational reasons. It emphasizes values as a way to induce change and is the most common approach for reducing resistance.

POWER.   This strategy is used when people have little or no commitment to the change. It requires that those in power be in a position to deliver rewards and punishments to those who resist. It results in compliance to, rather than acceptance of, the change.

During the change effort the committee may employ all four types of strategies. It is useful, however, to resist the use of power strategies if possible, in that their use may lead to more subtle resistance in the future.

Finally, as the others within the organization become involved, the presence or absence of resistance may prove useful to the committee if it is read as a signal regarding the effectiveness of the planning effort. If resistance is high, this may signal the need for further (rapid) planning and/or alterations in the activities already under way.

Walking Through a Trial

"Walking through" a set of planned activities before implementing them is a technique for identifying the need for additions or modifications that were not fully anticipated in earlier stages of planning. When the committee members believe that their plan is reasonably complete, they should imagine themselves carrying out each action step in the plan sequence. As they do this, they should imagine what they are doing, where they are doing it, why they are doing it, and the people and materials involved as if the plan were actually happening. In addition, it may be helpful to role-play or rehearse certain aspects of the plan. Walking through a plan in this manner usually stimulates its realistic appraisal and allows for additions or modifications before the actual trial is under way.

Selection of a Trial Unit

The selection of a setting for the trial is an important step in the planning process because it requires committee members to integrate their understanding of the limits and requirements of the research base, the characteristics of the setting, and the principles of planned change. Factors that affect the choice of the trial site include patient availability, personnel interest and involvement, timing, and diffusion implications.

Patient Availability

Where are appropriate patients located? Are sufficient numbers of these patients likely to be available on one unit in the time period

planned for the trial and its evaluation? Are there any obstacles to nurses having access to these patients for purposes of conducting a clinical trial and evaluation of this innovation at this particular time on this particular unit? If so, can these obstacles be overcome?

Resources such as admitting and operating room scheduling records and hospital census data for comparable time periods help committee members more accurately predict patient availability on certain units. Preliminary exploration with groups or individuals who have authority over access to patients in the setting being considered also may provide information that will affect the selection of a trial unit.

Personnel Involvement

Nursing staffing patterns and staff relationships on potential trial units should be such that staff are likely to be willing and able to cooperate with the trial of this practice innovation. Early exploration with nursing administrators such as supervisors or head nurses associated with potential trial units can serve the purposes of locating likely settings and engaging the interest and support of relevant nursing administrators. The head nurse on the trial unit is a key person who must be involved early in the planning process and whose cooperation and support are needed and should be actively sought.

Timing

Is there anything else going on at this particular time on the proposed unit that might interfere with implementation and evaluation of the nursing practice innovation? Sometimes potential trial units are undergoing other major changes that would make it difficult or impossible to undertake another at the same time with the same degree of enthusiasm and effort. Renovations of the physical plant, relocation of units to another floor or building, institution of primary nursing, or major changes in leadership are examples of changes that might deter a trial on a particular unit. If these conditions exist, it might be useful to consider delaying the trial until a later, more convenient time. In the interest of time, however, it may be necessary to select a different, less-satisfactory patient care unit for the trial.

Diffusion Implications

If the evaluation of the trial is favorable, the innovation will likely be extended to other relevant hospital units. A factor in the initial selection of the trial unit is the perceived likelihood that other relevant units will be willing and able to institute the innovation and achieve similar results following the trial. An "ideal" unit—well staffed with enthusiastic and well-prepared individuals—might not be the best trial unit if it is anticipated that staff on other relevant units might reject the innovation because their working environments and situations are perceived so differently from those of the trial unit. On the other hand, such a unit might be perceived as the best setting to conduct a fair and successful trial. Diffusion is a long-range concern but worthy of careful consideration in the choice of a trial unit.

There are many interdependent issues to consider in the selection of a setting where the innovation can be accurately and successfully implemented and evaluated on a trial basis. The committee is required to weigh the information that has been gathered about the innovation, the setting, the patients, and the staff and to determine where, in its opinion, a fair test of the innovation can be facilitated within a realistic time period.

The following criteria might be considered in making the final selection of a pilot unit:

- Unit has an adequate number of patients who would qualify for receiving the innovation.
- Staff are receptive and interested.
- Unit has adequate staffing to support the trial.
- Unit problems are such that they are not likely to preclude a successful trial.
- Unit is similar enough compared to other units that diffusion potential is maximized.
- Unit staff are able to tolerate the temporary nature of the trial.

It is useful to establish comparable criteria for selection of a trial unit prior to actually considering specific units.

CONDUCTING AND EVALUATING A TRIAL

When it has been ascertained that the planning phase has been completed with sufficient care to assure a reasonable test of the innovation, it is time to implement the trial and its evaluation. To keep

the trial running smoothly and to accomplish its purposes, the committee should establish some means of monitoring the effort once implementation has begun. In spite of careful planning, there are always some unanticipated events and obstacles encountered while implementing the plans that have been made.

Monitoring the Trial

Monitoring the progress of the trial and evaluation makes it possible to respond in a flexible manner to unanticipated events and to make mid-trial adjustments so that the process is not halted or greatly delayed. Without monitoring the process, events such as equipment failure, loss of data collectors due to illness, changes in patient population or census, or incomplete data collection can bog down or halt the trial and interfere with the progress of the master plan.

Selection of a coordinator who is responsible for troubleshooting and overseeing the trial is a useful strategy. This coordinator should have knowledge of the entire process and should have actively participated in the planning phase. The coordinator should regularly review plans and procedures in order to discover and overcome unanticipated obstacles. Minor revisions often can be made in trial activities to accommodate changes occurring in other parts of the system that could be ultimately disruptive. The coordinator should be able to make these adjustments without interfering with essential features of the trial. In spite of the need for adjustments, the limits and requirements of the research base must be considered when any changes are made. When necessary, the coordinator can discuss the problem and potential solutions with the committee.

The following example emphasizes the importance of having a coordinator available during a trial to handle unanticipated events. In a hospital where structured preoperative teaching was selected as an innovation, the location designated for preoperative classes for surgical patients was a patient lounge. Although administrative clearance was obtained, the committee had forgotten to inform patients on the ward that the lounge would be used for classes for one-half hour each evening. Once the classes began, the teachers were surprised to find patients regularly wandering into the lounge and interrupting the class. A solution was easily found for this problem: The coordinator arranged to have chairs moved to a temporary sitting area for patients during the time the lounge was unavailable for general use and posted a sign on the door indicating

that preoperative classes were scheduled each evening from 8:00 to 8:30 and that a temporary sitting area was available during this time.

Implementing the Trial

The following discussion outlines the responsibilities of the coordinator for each phase in the trial: baseline data collection, implementation of the innovation, and postimplementation data collection.

When the evaluation of the trial is designed to make use of a baseline data collection, followed by implementation of the innovation and postimplementation data collection, the trial begins with a baseline evaluation of care as it is currently administered.

Implementation of the innovation itself does not occur until the baseline data collection period is completed. The coordinator will need to become a communication center for all aspects of the implementation activity. This individual must be able to monitor and make adjustments in case the following events occur as the trial proceeds.

1. Inconsistencies with planned procedures. These need to be analyzed to ascertain whether they are resistance-related and participants need to be interviewed accordingly.
2. Interruptions. The coordinator needs to fix whatever is causing the interruptions and determine the extent to which interruption may interfere with staff motivation and cooperation. One interruption may precipitate others.
3. Unanticipated unusual events (example: unanticipated staffing changes or a precipitous unit closing). These need to be recorded and plans adjusted as needed or the trial discontinued if necessary.
4. Missing or inaccurate data. This can be prevented by reviewing Data-recording forms regularly during the trial.
5. Need for support for unit staff and evaluators.

Implementing the Innovation

It should be noted that those staff members who actively participate in the evaluation components of the trial should not be actively involved with implementing the innovation; it is important to maintain the independence of the two aspects of the trial.

The coordinator should be sensitive to staff responses as they attempt to implement the innovation. The staff may suggest modifications in the practice innovation that they think would make it easier to use or more effective. It is important for both the coordinator and the committee members to remain open to feedback from staff regarding the innovation and its implementation. The coordinator should analyze any suggested changes and decide if the modifications can be made without exceeding the limits of the research base from which the innovation was derived. Minor adjustments in the innovation, those that do not exceed the research base, can be made readily and are likely to influence the staff's willingness to use the innovation. When major redesigning of the innovation is indicated, however, it may be necessary to discontinue the trial until the changes are made or a decision is made to terminate the trial effort.

During the implementation phase, the coordinator should monitor the following:

1. Inconsistencies with planned procedures. Analyze to see whether they are resistance-related and intervene accordingly.
2. Staff preparation. Determine if the staff development program was adequate and the extent to which staff are developing themselves in the midst of the trial.
3. Discrepancies between plans and reality. Evaluate resources required, projected time line, and rate at which patients are identified.

Postimplementation Evaluation

The events monitored during the postimplementation evaluation period should be similar to those monitored during the baseline period. In addition, there is a higher chance that bias may be introduced into the data collection at this point due to enthusiasm or disappointment resulting from the innovation. Such potential sources of bias should be noted by the coordinator so it can be accounted for in the analysis of the data.

The End of the Trial

When postimplementation data collection is complete, the committee should allow the trial unit to decide whether it will continue with the new practice while the data are being analyzed and decisions regarding adoption are being made. Rapid data analysis

is of utmost importance to minimize the amount of time the unit is in limbo regarding the decision to adopt, modify, or reject the innovation.

A case study entitled "Conducting a Trial of a Preoperative Teaching Program" has been included in Appendix J to illustrate the activities that are carried out during this stage of the research utilization process.

REFERENCE

Zaltman, G., & Duncan, R. *Strategies for Planned Change.* New York: John Wiley & Sons, 1977, 90–165.

CHECKLIST:
CONDUCTING A CLINICAL TRIAL AND EVALUATION OF THE INNOVATION

This checklist provides questions that need to be addressed in implementing this step of the research utilization process. It is important to account for the issues and activities inherent in these questions before progressing to the next step.

☐ Are all resources required for implementation on hand? On order?

ITEM	DATE EXPECTED	HAS ARRIVED
_____	_____	☐
_____	_____	☐
_____	_____	☐

☐ Are all materials adapted or developed?

MATERIALS	PROJECTED COMPLETION DATE	DONE
_____	_____	☐
_____	_____	☐
_____	_____	☐
_____	_____	☐
_____	_____	☐
_____	_____	☐

☐ Are all procedures designed?

PROCEDURES	PROJECTED COMPLETION DATE	DONE
_____	_____	☐
_____	_____	☐
_____	_____	☐
_____	_____	☐

☐ Is the staff development program ready?
    ☐ Are the educational materials developed?
    ☐ Who is to attend?
    ☐ When and where will it be offered?

☐ Are the evaluators prepared to begin data collection?
    ☐ Time schedule set?
    ☐ Release time (flexible time) for evaluators arranged?
    ☐ Evaluation training complete?
    ☐ Interrater reliability established, if applicable?

☐ Are the nursing units prepared for the trial to begin?
    ☐ Know when the trial will begin?
    ☐ Understand the general process that will occur on the unit?
    ☐ Know how to reach the committee if they feel they need to?

☐ Has the person who will monitor the trial been selected and flexible or release time arrangements made?

Chapter 7
DECIDING WHETHER TO ADOPT, MODIFY, OR REJECT THE INNOVATION

The data collected during the trial should be used to decide whether to recommend adoption, modification, or rejection of the innovation for permanent use, and to assist others in the organization to understand the rationale for the recommendation.

A decision to adopt the innovation is made when the data indicate that the new practice is better in some way than the old practice. A decision to modify before adoption is made when the trial has indicated the need for a specific change in process that should not influence the outcomes as observed during the trial. A decision to reject the innovation should occur when the data indicate that the new practice did not produce the expected results and offers no gain over the existing practice. The committee should use the data to help others understand the process used in arriving at the decision, regardless of its exact nature. Allowing others to understand the data-based process used in arriving at the decision will help establish a positive climate for future change.

The quality of the decision to adopt, modify, or reject the innovation is dependent upon the adequacy (amount) and accuracy (reliability) of the collected data and the quality of the interpretation of the data. The major determinant of adequacy is simply the number of patients included in the groups to be compared, i.e., the

baseline and postimplementation groups or the comparison and intervention groups. The reader should recall that the larger the group size, the more confidence one can have in the meaning of the data. What is at issue is the extent to which any single patient's data can influence the total group score. In small groups, a single patient's data are much more influential than in large groups. For example, in a group of 10 patients, each patient's data represent 10 percent of the total group score, while in a group of 20 patients, a given patient's data represent only 5 percent of the total group score. When the group size is small (10–15 patients), it is very important to examine the individual patient data to ascertain whether 1 or 2 patient's data are exerting undue influence on the group score. If this should occur, the comparisons might be better carried out at the individual rather than the group level or by using statistics such as the median, which does not require summing the scores.

The adequacy of the data base may be negatively affected by reductions in the planned number of patients or subjects in each group. Such reductions may be necessary when the data collection period is prolonged well beyond the original time projection. This problem is best handled during the early stages of the trial when reductions can occur evenly in all groups. For example, if the initial trial plan called for 60 patients, 30 in each of two groups, a decision to reduce the total number of patients to 40 could result in very different outcomes depending on when the change in plans occurred. If the change occurred during the baseline period, it would be possible to maintain two equal groups of 20 patients each. If the decision to reduce the number occurred after completion of the baseline period, the groups might be quite unequal, e.g., 30 patients in the baseline group and only 10 patients in the intervention group. The committee should carefully guard against such unequal outcomes in reductions because the resulting data base is only as adequate as the smallest group, in this case, 10 patients.

Missing data also negatively influence the data base. Data are considered "missing" when the scores regarding a specific variable on a given patient were either not collected or not recorded and are therefore unavailable for the analysis. For example, if a patient had stool frequencies recorded for the day shift and the night shift, but not for the evening shift, the missing data for the evening shift must be noted and handled in some way. The way in which this problem is handled is dependent upon the adequacy of the rest of the data collected for the variable. If the rest of the data are considered adequate, they can be used to generate a score for the data that are

missing. In the case outlined above, the data for the day and night shifts might be considered adequate, and the evening score could be generated by obtaining an average score for the two recorded shift scores and using this average score for the missing data. When the other data are.considered to be inadequate, e.g., scores are available for one shift and unavailable for two shifts, the patient and all of his or her data may have to be removed from the data base, thus reducing the overall number of patients in the group.

The accuracy of the data base is dependent upon the extent to which the data are consistently collected. The committee should review the procedures used to ascertain interrater reliability, review the degree to which reliability was originally assured, and identify any conditions that might have negatively affected reliability over the course of the trial, such as a prolonged data collection period without re-establishment of reliability estimates after 2 months.

Another important issue for the committee to address before analyzing the data is the comparability of the two groups on factors that are known to affect the outcome of the intervention. The test of the effectiveness of the intervention vis à vis existing practice rests on the assumption that the two groups are similar on all influencing factors except the intervention. If the groups are in fact dissimilar in some regard, it will be difficult to ascertain whether the intervention or the other factor is responsible for differences in outcomes between the groups. The committee should ascertain any differences that might exist in the characteristics of the groups before analysis of the data occurs.

ORGANIZING AND SUMMARIZING DATA TO ASSIST WITH THE DECISION-MAKING PROCESS

Raw data need to be summarized and displayed in a manner that assists the decision-making process. In order to assure that the data are in a useful form, it is helpful to identify both outcome and process questions for which the data are to provide answers before the summarization process begins. For example, if incidence of diarrhea, patient satisfaction, and nurse satisfaction were the outcome variables that were measured, then the data should be arranged so the committee could determine whether there were differences in these outcomes that corresponded with the presence or absence of the innovation. Questions to be answered might include (1) What was the average stool frequency in the comparison

group and in the intervention group? (2) What was the average score on the patient-satisfaction questionnaire for each patient group? (3) What was the average score on the nurse-satisfaction questionnaire before and after the trial of the innovation?

When the process data are summarized, questions regarding the nature of the intervention as it was delivered need to be formulated. For instance; (1) To what extent was the intervention actually delivered? (e.g., What tube-feeding preparations were actually given to the patients in each group)? (2) Was the intervention administered similar to the intervention designed for the trial? (e.g., Did patients attend the whole preoperative teaching program or did they leave before the practice session occurred)? (3) If the actual intervention was different from the one planned in the trial, what actually occurred, and did it meet the requirements and limits of the research base?

Raw data collected during an evaluation are not very useful because there are simply too many pieces of information to be able to give meaning to them. It is therefore important to manipulate these raw data so they become more manageable and intelligible. This can be accomplished by reducing or summarizing the data using statistical procedures such as averages and percentages. These processes reduce the total number of numbers that one must think about (deal with) when trying to ascertain whether a specific innovation was effective. For example, if the raw data regarding number of stools per patient for the patients in the baseline and postimplementation groups were as follows:

Baseline	Postimplementation
Patient A = 8	Patient A = 8
Patient B = 7	Patient B = 8
Patient C = 7	Patient C = 6
Patient D = 9	Patient D = 6
Patient E = 9	Patient E = 7

It would be more difficult to deal with 10 numbers than if the data for each group were added to provide the number of stools per group (baseline = 40, postimplementation = 35) or the average number of stools per patient per group was calculated (baseline = 8, post-implementation = 7). This process of reducing data makes data analysis much easier. The techniques used to reduce the raw data should be those necessary to answer the questions posed for the analysis. The most common procedures include simple addition,

Table 2
Summarized Data Form

| | Trial Conditions | |
Patient Outcomes	Baseline	Postimplementation
Total number of stools	360.0	120.0
Average number of stools per patient per day	6.0	2.0
Average stool consistency rating	2.0	6.2
	N = 20	N = 20

averages, percentages, medians, and frequency distributions. References for calculating each of these statistics may be found in Appendix K.

The data summary process begins with individual data and moves through the various groupings of data of interest to the committee. In other words, the first summary might produce data regarding the number of stools per patient, the next summary might address average number of stools per patient by nursing care unit, and, finally, the third summary might yield the average number of stools per patient per group (intervention and comparison). It is useful to develop forms or tables to use during the summarization process. Often the original data-recording form can be used to assist in summmarizing individual data; sample data-recording forms can be found in Appendix H. New forms will have to be developed for the later stages in the summarization process; a sample summary form can also be found in Appendix H.

When the data have been summarized and organized, they should be in a form that will facilitate the analysis. The individual categories of summarized data should be displayed as in Table 2 to answer specific questions, e.g., what are the scores of the two groups in respect to total number of stools, average stools per patient per day, and stool consistency ratings?

ANALYZING THE DATA AND MAKING A DECISION

When the data for each variable of interest have been summarized and displayed on tables, the analysis of the data can take place. The purpose of the analysis is to give meaning to or interpret the results of the trial as indicated by the summarized data and the

committee's experience with the innovation. Analysis begins with a comparison of the results for each variable between the two groups, e.g., was the stool consistency rating higher in the postimplementation group than in the baseline group? Did postimplementation group patients have fewer stools per day than patients in the comparison group?

The next step in the analysis is to examine whether the differences between the two groups fit or match what was predicted from the research base for all variables selected from the base. New variables that were added in the trial should be examined in relation to what the committee expected or hoped to find, e.g., higher patient and staff satisfaction postimplementation. When this analysis shows that the results match the prior predictions or expectations and the intervention delivered met the requirements and limits of the research base, it can be assumed that misutilization has not occurred and the committee should proceed with the decision-making process regarding adoption. At this point the committee should review other factors, such as costs and convenience, that might negatively influence a decision to adopt even though the outcomes met expectations.

If the analysis shows that the results do not match prior predictions or expectations, the committee must look for possible explanations for these unanticipated results. The process data should be carefully reviewed to look for discrepancies in the actual versus the planned implementation of the intervention. A re-examination of the comparability of the two groups also would be in order at this point. This analysis continues until the committee can explain the results or determines that they cannot explain the results.

DECISION TO ADOPT THE INNOVATION

A decision to recommend adoption of the innovation rests not only on the match between predicted and actual outcomes, but on other considerations such as cost, ease of operation, and staff morale. These other factors are important enough that they might argue against adoption even though the trial data support it *or* they might persuade the committee to recommend adoption even though the trial data are equivocal. The first case might occur when the costs involved in full-scale implementation exceed the available funds or when the trial has in some way heightened staff resistance to the

intervention to such an extent that full-scale implementation would be too costly vis à vis staff morale. Other factors that might impede further implementation can be identified by redoing a probability-for-adoption assessment (Appendix F). Committee members have considerably more information available to them regarding the innovation and the organization than when the initial assessment was completed, and a reassessment can be used to confirm their current thinking regarding adoption. If this aspect of the analysis supports full-scale implementation, the committee is in a position to recommend adoption of the innovation on a permanent basis.

Once the decision to recommend adoption is made, the committee members should organize the summary tables and the other information they considered into a logical written report that demonstrates the decision-making process they followed. The specific information included in a report will vary depending on the intended audience. For example, the director of nursing service would be interested in cost considerations and they would be included in her report. However, a report prepared for the staff on the trial units and other units to be added later might be more interested in patient outcome and staff satisfaction data than in cost data. The reports should be written to support future goals, i.e., to convince the director to adopt the innovation or enhance future acceptance of the change should full-scale implementation occur.

DECISION TO MODIFY THE INNOVATION

A decision to modify the innovation before full-scale implementation occurs is indicated whenever the trial outcomes do not match the predicted outcomes and the process evaluation data pinpoint a specific discrepancy in the administration of the innovation that can be remedied. In such a case, the innovation would be redesigned and another trial conducted. Modification can occur without another trial if the modification will not cause a substantive change in the innovation, e.g., using TV rather than sound-on-slide methods in delivering the structured preoperative teaching program.

Reports written to communicate a modify-before-adoption recommendation should clearly indicate the reason(s) for the suggested modification and how it would remedy the situation. If a new trial is suggested, the reasons for this should be explicitly stated.

DECISION TO REJECT THE INNOVATION

A decision to recommend rejection is difficult to make. Every way to explain the results should be reviewed and the results recorded before the recommendation is forwarded to the decision makers. Such a recommendation arises when:

- Evaluation outcome data do not support the predicted outcome, *and*
- There is no identified process problem that can explain the outcome, *and*
- Other factors such as enhanced staff morale do not override the negative outcome.

The committee must construct a report that not only justifies the decision but that can also be used to help those who participated in the trial understand why their efforts did not lead to a decision to adopt the innovation. The clarity of this communication may well influence the staff members' willingness to participate in future clinical trials.

CHECKLIST:
DECIDING WHETHER TO ADOPT, MODIFY, OR REJECT THE INNOVATION

This checklist provides questions that need to be addressed in implementing this step of the research utilization process. It is important to account for the issues and activities inherent in these questions before progressing to the next step.

Data Summary: Display

☐ Are the outcome data summarized and displayed so they answer the relevant questions?

☐ Are the process data summarized and displayed so they can show whether the intervention was adequately carried out?

Deciding to Adopt the Innovation

☐ Do the trial outcome data match what was

    ☐ predicted from the research-base?

    ☐ expected (variables not covered in research base)?

☐ Was the intervention implemented as planned?

    ☐ Were there any deviations from the requirements and limits of the research base?

☐ Are there any organizational factors that will impede large-scale implementation of the innovation?

☐ Are the reports prepared and plans for communicating the decision completed?

Deciding to Modify the Innovation

☐ What is to be modified?

☐ Does it constitute a substantive change in the intervention?

    ☐ Does the modified intervention meet the requirements and limits of the research base?

    ☐ Are plans for another evaluation ready?

☐ Are the reports and plans for communicating the decision completed?

Deciding to Reject the Innovation

☐ Is there a mismatch between the trial outcome data and what was predicted from the research base?

☐ Did the trial outcome data for any of the other variables match expectations?

☐ Did the process evaluation indicate any specific problem(s) with the way the intervention was implemented?

☐ Are there any other factors that might override the decision to reject?

☐ Are the reports and plans for communicating the decision completed?

☐ How will the staff on the pilot units be notified? How will they be assisted to understand that they should stop the new practice?

Chapter 8
DEVELOPING THE MEANS TO EXTEND OR DIFFUSE THE ADOPTED INNOVATION

The decision to adopt an innovation, with or without modification, moves the change process into a different sphere: diffusion. Diffusion is the process by which the acceptance of ideas, practices, and technologies spreads and crosses natural boundaries within an organization (such as patient care units and divisions) or between one organization and another. During the trial, the innovation was viewed as a reversible change; during diffusion, the change becomes permanent. Careful and sustained effort is needed when putting the innovation into wider use throughout the nursing department. The process becomes more complex, involving more and different staff members and patient care units than were involved in the trial. Because of the permanent nature of the change, new mechanisms that ensure continuity over time will need to be identified and/or developed. At the same time, it is important to make the diffusion process as easy as possible for those involved with it in order to facilitate its acceptance and operationalization. It is also imperative to involve others who will work with the committee in planning for diffusion of the innovation to additional patient care units. This is necessary to increase the sense of ownership of the new practice change among those who will be responsible for implementing it, and to minimize the potential for resistance at the **83**

time when the change will have an impact on the largest number of nursing staff.

The timing of the diffusion effort merits careful planning, and adequate time should be provided in which to implement it. Further, the change should not be introduced unless the staff and the organization have the capacity to accept and sustain the innovation. For this reason, diffusion may be delayed to avoid competition with previously introduced changes that are currently placing unusually heavy demands on the nursing staff. Consideration should also be given to other factors that might influence timing: an impending JCAH accreditation visit; periods when the greatest turnover of staff can be expected; and vacation and holiday schedules. An example of poor timing occurred in one situation where an innovation that required a vigorous staff development program was implemented at the same time that a large group of newly registered nurses was scheduled for intensive orientation to the hospital. In this situation, the staff development department was unable to meet all the demands required to prepare staff for mutually setting goals with patients. Later, as nursing staff were required to assist patients with establishing health care goals, they became frustrated with their own lack of skill in doing this and soon reverted back to the original system in which nurses set goals for patients independently. This innovation was doomed because of poor timing.

The evaluation component that was carried out during the trial is dropped at this point unless there are identifiable reasons to believe that the earlier condition would not generalize to other units during diffusion. It it is felt to be necessary, a time-limited evaluation can be designed and implemented when diffusion occurs. Generally, however, once a trial has been conducted and a decision to adopt an innovation has been made, there is no need to continue the evaluation process. Monitoring the innovation through usual quality assurance mechanisms becomes the norm for ongoing evaluation of its effectiveness.

INVOLVING OTHERS

During the trial, one nursing unit was involved in implementing the innovation; however, for the purposes of diffusion it is necessary to identify the target patient care units where the tested innovation will be introduced for permanent adoption. One way to approach this is to identify the types of patients for whom the innovation can be

expected to be effective and then determine where these patients are located in the hospital. In some instances the location of patients to be affected by the change will be obvious; in others it may not be readily apparent. For example, the majority of surgical patients are hospitalized on surgical units. However, some patients are sent to surgery from medical units or from the outpatient department. In a hospital where the structured preoperative teaching innovation is to be diffused to all appropriate units, it will be necessary to consider the diffusion process in relation to patients located in these three settings. The nursing staff on the identified units will be directly involved with the implementation of the new research-based practice.

In addition to the staff on the targeted patient care units, it is necessary to identify others who will be affected by the increased scope of the change. These individuals may include nursing administrators, hospital administrators, physicians, laboratory personnel, those providing transportation services, and others. It is important to communicate with those who are relevant to implementation of the innovation on the larger scale required for diffusion purposes in order to secure required resources as well as approval and sanctions.

At this time consideration should be given to extending the committee's membership to include key individuals from the targeted patient care units to assist with planning and implementing the diffusion activities. Those individuals identified as "key" include head nurses and opinion leaders. Involving such individuals is important so that they can be instrumental in promoting the adoption of the innovation on their respective units. As they become committed to the change, they will communicate this to others, who are likely then to be more receptive to the change. Planned change literature documents the importance of involving others at this point so they feel they have some control or influence over the innovation process.

New members who are added to the committee should be assisted to understand the protocol, the research base, and the process that has occurred so far. Also, they need to understand the relationship of the innovation to the identified need for the practice change; the data obtained from use of the "Patient Care Problem Identification Guide" should be shared with them. Similarly, results of the evaluation of the trial should be made available, along with the rationale for the decisions made regarding adoption of the innovation. All of this information is needed by those engineering the

diffusion process for two reasons: (1) it serves as essential background information for making decisions relevant to diffusion, and (2) explanations made to staff on the targeted units can be made on the basis of full knowledge of the innovation and the process and outcomes to date.

The committee needs to identify ways to communicate with the newly identified nursing units to which the innovation will be diffused. If the committee has representatives from each unit, these representatives can serve as a vital link. The staff on the targeted diffusion units are likely to have some knowledge concerning the innovation from prior general communications about the trial. It is important to understand what they already know and how they came to know it. Prior knowledge of the innovation and its trial can serve to make the staff more receptive or more resistant; for this reason, the response of the staff to prior exposure to the innovation would be useful in the planning process.

PLANNING FOR DIFFUSION

While there is a natural tendency to view the trial plan as sufficient for the purposes of diffusion to additional patient care units, in actuality *the diffusion process requires as much or more planning than the trial.* Some aspects of the trial plan may transfer directly to the diffusion plan, e.g., assessment materials, teaching plans, and permanent recording forms; however, much of the trial plan was directed toward evaluation, an activity that does not usually occur during diffusion.

The extended committee will need to go through many of the same activities carried out in planning for the trial because the permanent, large-scale nature of the diffusion process will require some modifications in the procedures worked out for the small-scale trial. The basic differences in the nature of the trial and diffusion activities necessitate the development of a new master plan for the diffusion process. The preparation of this plan should proceed in a manner similar to the trial master plan. The reader is referred to pages 56 to 62 where master plan development is discussed. Points relating to evaluation planning should be disregarded unless an evaluation of the diffusion activity is to take place.

New approvals and sanctions will need to be secured at this point in the planning process and resources must be secured for long-term adoption. If many nursing units are to be involved in diffusion,

the plan may be constructed to facilitate phasing in the implementation process in stages on one or two units at a time as opposed to changing all units at the same time. The decision to phase-in the implementation of the innovation or begin on all units at once should be made prior to the beginning of the planning activities, as it will influence planning decisions at all points.

Implementation of the innovation beyond the trial setting may require participation of groups that need to be more actively involved than they were during the trial. For example, the extended committee should not assume that because the chief of surgery was in support of the trial of structured preoperative teaching, he will not need to be contacted about the wider implementation of this innovation. He or she might have suggestions about how the innovation could be presented to the surgical residents or staff physicians to enhance their full acceptance of its diffusion.

In the planning phase, it is often necessary to make modifications in the procedures to facilitate larger-scale adoption and to adjust for problems encountered during the trial. Modifications made at this point are usually minor and are primarily directed at adapting the process to accommodate larger numbers of patients and multiple nursing units. For example, the structured preoperative teaching program may need to expand so that it can handle three times as many patients. This in turn may necessitate limiting the number of patients who can attend any given session and may require a previously not needed scheduling mechanism for both patients and teachers. Other necessary modifications identified during the trial would also be designed at this time. In one hospital, patients in the trial group suggested that the time and place of the structured preoperative teaching presentation be changed so they could more easily involve their visiting family members. This kind of modification can readily be made without departing from the research base.

In some cases, it may be necesssary to make differentiated implementation plans to meet specific needs of certain patient care units. For example, if the structured preoperative teaching program is to be used with all presurgery patients regardless of their location within the hospital, it will be imperative to develop differentiated plans for those patients who are initially located in the outpatient department or on medical units. The procedures for these patients will necessarily differ in some respects from the procedures for those patients who start out on surgical units prior to surgery.

Finally, all written materials need to be reviewed and revised to account for the modifications, wider scope, and permanent nature

of the innovation. For example, assessment instruments might now be printed and new procedures developed regarding the entry of that data into the patient's permanent record.

When all of the modifications have been identified and designed, the revised innovation should be reviewed carefully to determine whether the requirements of the research base are still met. This also gives new committee members an opportunity to match the diffusion plans with the research base underlying the practice innovation and to understand both of these thoroughly.

STAFF DEVELOPMENT TO FACILITATE DIFFUSION

A well-conceived plan for staff development is crucial to the success of the diffusion effort. Re-educative strategies are essential to the implementation of any innovation, but this is particularly true when the change is a major departure from past practices. It is important for the nursing staff members who will be responsible for implementing the innovation to perceive that they have, or will be provided with, the necessary knowledge and skills to implement the change. Otherwise, it is quite likely that resistance will be encountered as staff members feel increasingly inadequate to implement the change.

The effectiveness of the staff development program used in he trial should be reviewed and modifications made accordingly. Modifications will also be needed to accommodate larger numbers of nursing staff in the teaching programs. Strategies such as delivering the staff development program on each of the designated units might be useful to ensure that all personnel have acquired the necessary knowledge and skills to implement the innovation.

Finally, the staff development program should make staff members aware that the innovation is research-based, and the original research articles and protocol should be made available to those interested in reviewing them. This will serve to help nursing staff members distinguish scientifically based practices from those that are not—an important first step in changing values and norms regarding nursing practice.

MONITORING THE DIFFUSION EFFORT

Once implementation of the diffusion process is under way, it will need to be monitored just as carefully as the trial was. A coordinator or coordinating committee should be designated to serve this

function for an extended period of time until the innovation is accepted and well stabilized on all target patient care units. Monitoring the implementation of the innovation during diffusion is important and serves a number of purposes. First, it provides a mechanism for assisting those who need help in handling implementation problems as they arise. Second, it is a way of providing support to those involved, even when there are no major problems. Third, through monitoring of the diffusion process it is possible to detect breaks in the implementation plan and to become aware of sources of resistance in time to intervene to save the diffusion effort. Finally, the person(s) responsible for monitoring the implementation of an innovation across units can provide useful liaison to the committee and can assist the members in understanding the realities (the problems and pleasures) of bringing about large-scale research-based practice changes.

CHECKLIST:
DEVELOPING THE MEANS TO EXTEND OR DIFFUSE THE ADOPTED INNOVATION

This checklist provides questions that need to be addressed in implementing this step of the research utilization process. It is important to account for the issues and activities inherent in these questions before progressing to the next step.

Revising the Committee Membership

☐ Have new members been identified and asked to join the committee?

☐ Do the new members provide communication links to all the nursing units that will now become involved in implementing the innovation?

    ☐ If not, is there a plan for communicating with all involved units?

☐ How will the new members be oriented to what has occurred thus far and to what is yet to come? Do they understand the research base?

Reviewing the Innovation in the Context of Full-Scale Implementation

☐ What adjustments are necessary in

    ☐ Materials _____

_____

_____

    ☐ Procedures _____

_____

_____

    ☐ Staff development program _____

_____

_____

Use relevant sections from the checklist on planning for a trial to assist you with planning for the diffusion effort (see pages 56–62). Remember that in planning for diffusion it is not usually necessary to include the evaluation component.

Chapter 9
DEVELOPING MECHANISMS TO MAINTAIN THE INNOVATION OVER TIME

INSTITUTIONALIZING A CHANGE

Planning, implementating, evaluating, and diffusing a research-based practice change represent a substantial investment on the part of the nursing department. Unfortunately, it is also true that many well-planned and implemented changes diminish over time because organizations fail to build mechanisms to assure ongoing maintainence of an innovation. Mechanisms for maintainence may be people-related or structure-related and result in institutionalization of the change. Zaltman and Duncan (1977) define *institutionalization* as the "development of a set of shared, learned norms among members in the system that define the new change or innovation as a legitimate aspect of carrying out their roles. . . ." Institutionalization means that the new practice has become an accepted and expected part of the appropriate nursing staff members' roles.

Havelock (1973) used the term *stabilization* to address these issues and suggests six areas needing consideration: continuing

rewards, routinization, structural integration, continuing evaluation, maintainance, and continuing adaptation capability. Each of these areas will be discussed in relation to changes in nursing practice.

REWARDS.   Rewards are people-directed and should be visible to those who adopt the new practice. They may arise from the actual performance of the practice, e.g., improved patient outcomes, or be mediated by others, e.g., gain them approval or recognition.

ROUTINIZATION.   This means that the new practice becomes a part of the routine professional repertoire of the nurse and is automatically carried out in the appropriate situation.

STRUCTURAL INTEGRATION.   This means that the innovation becomes a part of the everyday behavior in the system. It includes such things as providing time to carry out the new practice, providing policies and procedures that support the change, acquiring the resources required for the new practice, and preventing other tasks from interfering with the use of the new practice.

CONTINUED EVALUATION.   Continued evaluation of the innovation should provide a way to monitor for lapses in its use; it also supports the innovation by making clear the organization's interest in its maintenance. For most nursing practice innovations, continued evaluation can take place within the context of the quality assurance system. The trial data can be used to establish both process and outcome standards for the quality assurance program.

MAINTENANCE.   This means that mechanisms such as staff development are available to assist when there is an indication that the practice is not being adequately carried out. In departments with high staff turnover rates, the innovation may be incorporated in orientation programs for new employees.

CONTINUING ADAPTATION CAPABILITY.   This refers to the potential need to alter the innovation because circumstances have changed. This is particularly true with research-based innovations, in which new research is likely to alter the basis for the practice. Basically this requires the organization to act as if the change is permanent while always looking for and valuing new practices that will eventually replace the "old" innovation.

One department of nursing developed the following mechanisms to support its structured preoperative teaching program:

- The process and outcome evaluation data were used to define criteria and standards for the intervention and patient outcomes.
- New nursing staff members were oriented to the basis for the program and how they were expected to support the change through the performance of their roles.
- A cost analysis was done and specific charges were identified and billed for patients who received this service.
- A place to record attendance at the preoperative teaching programs and follow-up practice activities was incorporated into the permanent patient record system.

The committee's role regarding institutionalization is twofold: first, to make key persons within the organization aware of the need for mechanisms to support institutionalization, and second, to encourage and support deliberate action in this regard by identifying specific mechanisms to support the change efforts.

REFERENCES

Havelock, R.G. *A Change Agent's Guide to Innovation in Education.* Englewood Cliffs, N.J.: Educational Technology Publications, 1973, 133–139.

Zaltman, G., & Duncan, R. *Strategies for Planned Change.* New York: John Wiley & Sons, 1977, 221.

CHECKLIST:
DEVELOPING MECHANISMS TO MAINTAIN THE
INNOVATION OVER TIME.

This checklist provides questions that need to be addressed in implementing this step of the research utilization process. It is important to account for the issues and activities inherent in these questions before progressing to the next step.

☐ Is there a need to educate new staff regarding the innovation during their orientation period?

☐ Are departmental policies and procedures adjusted so they support the new practice?

☐ Are all forms, billing procedures, etc. printed and distributed to persons who need them?

☐ Has the new practice been incorporated into the quality assurance system?

☐ How will staff members who continue to support the innovation be rewarded?

☐ Have job descriptions been altered if necessary?

APPENDICES

APPENDIX A
GLOSSARY OF TERMS

T he following terms appear throughout this guide. They are defined here to clarify the context in which they have been used to discuss the research utilization process.

CLINICAL EVALUATION A strategy used to determine whether a specific nursing intervention has produced predicted or expected outcomes when implemented in a clinical practice setting.

CLINICAL PROTOCOL Transformation of the research base into clinically relevant knowledge that is precisely defined for practice and that specifies an intervention with predictable patient outcomes and recommended procedures for its evaluation.

DEPENDENT VARIABLE The measured effect that is thought to result from or depend on the independent variable; the effect in a cause-and-effect relationship; may become the patient outcome.

DIFFUSION The process by which the acceptance of ideas, practices, and technologies spreads and crosses natural boundaries within an or-

ganization, such as patient care units, divisions, or departments, or between one organization and another.

INDEPENDENT VARIABLE

The variable that comes first in time and is assumed to cause the effect that is being studied; it is often a nursing intervention, patient characteristic, or patient behavior that is studied to determine its effect; the cause in a cause-and-effect relationship; may be the innovation tested or the intervention used to produce the desired outcomes.

INNOVATION

A change in nursing practice that is perceived as new by those adopting it and that represents a significant alteration in the status quo.

INTERRATER RELIABILITY

The extent of agreement among observers regarding specified events.

OPINION LEADER

An individual who has the ability to influence informally other individuals' attitudes or behavior with relatively high frequency and whose acceptance of an innovation lends it credibility; one who exerts informal leadership within an organization.

PATIENT CARE PROBLEM

A difficulty or concern experienced by patients or the nurses caring for them that is amenable to nursing intervention; a patient care situation in which there is a discrepancy between what is desirable and what currently exists.

PLANNED CHANGE

A rational and deliberate effort to bring about change in the process and/or structure of an organization, which is directed toward a stated

goal and carried out in such a way as to make the changes more acceptable and beneficial to those involved.

RESEARCH

Application of the scientific method of inquiry for the purposes of producing knowledge and discovering solutions for practical problems that are generalizable beyond the population directly studied.

RESEARCH BASE

A synthesis of the knowledge resulting from two or more related studies whose findings delineate, corroborate, and extend the concepts investigated; a single study cannot provide a research base because even "statistically significant" findings can result from accidental (uncontrolled) factors or from unintentional oversights in methodology.

RESEARCH-BASED PRACTICE

Practice that reflects the characteristics of the research base from which it is derived and within which the components of the nursing process (assessment, planning and intervention, and patient outcomes and evaluations) are precise and linked in predicted relationships.

RESEARCH UTILIZATION

A process directed toward the transfer of specific research-based knowledge into practice through the systematic use of a series of activities that include (1) identification and synthesis of multiple research studies that are related within a common conceptual base (research base); (2) transformation of the research-based knowledge into a clinical protocol that

specifies nursing actions to meet specific patient care problems; and (3) implementation and evaluation of these nursing actions within nursing service organizations through the use of a planned change approach.

RESISTANCE TO CHANGE Any response or behavior that serves to keep things as they are in face of the pressure to change; protective action to guard against the consequences of a proposed change that threatens beliefs, values, attitudes, and behavior central to those affected; a response to change which can be protective and even beneficial and should be seen as a signal to proceed with caution after reflection.

APPENDIX B
RESEARCH UTILIZATION AS AN
ORGANIZATIONAL PROCESS

Jo Anne Horsley, Joyce Crane, and Janet D. Bingle

D uring the past decade, multiple internal and external forces have resulted in accelerating pressure for nursing to demonstrate the scientific basis for its practice. The nursing profession has responded to these pressures by increasing the number of research-prepared nurses, the funds allocated for the conduct of research, and, as a result of these two tactics, the research base on which the practice of nursing rests. Yet, the pressure still exists and will continue to do so as long as the knowledge derived from research is not transferred into nursing practice activities.

To date, there is minimal evidence to suggest that such transfer is occurring or that research findings are directly influencing the quality of patient care. As research-generating activities multiply,

Jo Anne Horsley, R.N., Ph.D., professor of nursing at The University of Michigan School of Nursing and principal investigator of the Michigan Nurses Association project to study the conduct and utilization of research in nursing. Joyce Crane, R.N., M.S.N., associate professor of nursing at The University of Michigan School of Nursing and program director of the MNA project. Janet Bingle, R.N., M.S., was assistant professor of nursing at The University of Michigan School of Nursing and faculty associate on the MNA project at the time this article was written.

The project described here is funded by the Division of Nursing.DHEW Grant R02 NU 00542.

the utilization of research-based nursing knowledge becomes an increasingly important issue for the profession.

This article describes a research utilization (RU) project under investigation in Michigan. In 1975, the Michigan Nurses Association (MNA) sought and received funds to develop and test a method to transfer research findings into viable nursing practice activities. This project, CURN (Conduct and Utilization of Research in Nursing), is being conducted by faculty and graduate students at the University of Michigan School of Nursing and the Institute for Social Research and also at the Michigan State University School of Nursing. A subcontracting mechanism is used by MNA to employ these institutions to accomplish the scientific work of the project.

During the five-year funding period (1975–1980), departments of nursing in approximately 40 hospitals in southern Michigan will participate in the project. Of these 40 hospitals, 20 will serve as intervention (experimental) sites and 20 will serve as comparison sites. In the intervention situations, the RU model to be tested will use both on-site (consultant) and off-site (workshop) training methods. The model described is designed to investigate research utilization in JCAH accredited nonpsychiatric hospitals with more than 99 in-patient beds. The sample has been stratified on the basis of metropolitan versus nonmetropolitan location and bed size (100–219, 220–399, and 400 or more beds). This target nursing population was selected in recognition of the fact that research utilization models will vary in relationship to the context in which nursing practice occurs. The RU model being tested was selected in part because it allows for the flexibility in decision making that is required by any variance in types and levels of resources across settings.

RESEARCH UTILIZATION IS NOT RESEARCH CONDUCT

Our brief experience with research utilization has demonstrated that there is considerable confusion among nurses about the differences between the *conduct* of research studies and the *utilization* of the knowledge resulting from such studies. For example, when asked to describe how they might use research findings in their practice, nurses often cite a process of replication. It is important to differentiate the goals and therefore the persons, knowledges, and contexts relevant for the conduct of research from those that are relevant for research utilization.

Research conduct is directed toward the production of knowledge that is generalizable beyond the population directly studied. Undertaking a study occurs largely in the academic context where persons with specialized knowledge and skills in the methods of scientific inquiry can obtain the resources and control of conditions necessary. The process of research utilization, then, is directed toward transferring specific research-based knowledge into actual practice. Research-based techniques should be developed and tested in the practice contexts where persons with particular knowledge, skills, and experience in the methods of nursing practice can examine the relevance, means, and utility of any innovations. In reality, these defined differences between conduct and utilization become blurred because neither set of activities can succeed in isolation from the other.

GUIDELINES ESTABLISHING THE PARAMETERS OF RESEARCH UTILIZATION

Professional or societal guidelines defining the parameters of safe nursing research utilization do not currently exist. Our guidelines establish the following parameters:

• No single research study can provide sufficient, valid research evidence to justify ethically its use with health care clients. Research utilization should be based only on a series of replicated studies.

• When direct replication is minimal, indirect replication may be used to validate and extend a defined area of nursing research. Indirect replication exists when a generic principle can be derived from a group of sound clinical research studies which investigate relationships among similar variables. The empirical findings from these studies must corroborate, extend, or define the results of each other. The principle derived can then be translated into a clinically validated nursing intervention. The group of studies related to preoperative teaching and its effect on postoperative recovery is an example of research which has been indirectly replicated. The term indirect replication relates to the same processes inherent in systematic and constructive replication.[1,2]

• The nursing practice innovation which is developed from a research base must be evaluated. The evaluation measure must include at least one of the dependent variables used by the original investigators, and as many more as are clinically reasonable.

The first two guidelines are directed toward eliminating areas of nursing research where the findings are insufficient or inconsistent enough to question the validity of the resulting knowledge. The third guideline addresses the fact that sound research utilization should result in the client outcomes predicted by the research base. Failure to achieve those outcomes should raise questions regarding the design and implementation of the practice innovation and/or the research base.

THE RESEARCH UTILIZATION PROCESS

We view the research utilization process as an enduring set of organizational functions which can positively influence the quality of care delivered in nursing service settings. The organization, and particularly the nursing service department, must be committed to the process in order for it to have an impact on nursing practice. In this case, commitment means structuring visible, potent, *enduring mechanisms* (standing committee(s), policies, and procedures) to carry out the basic functions. It also means providing the *substantive resources* (personnel, equipment, time, funds) necessary to adequately maintain these functions. The research utilization process requires the input of nursing personnel who are (1) knowledgeable and experienced regarding the formal and informal organizational structure of the nursing service department and hospital; and (2) interpersonally potent, influencing others and accepting attempts by others to influence them.

There are six distinct phases in the research utilization process—each directed toward a different function. The first phase involves two interrelated activities: identifying nursing practice problems which need solution and assessing valid research bases to utilize in practice. Generally speaking, people tend to identify problems and then seek solutions. However, the reverse can also occur. For example, new knowledge can alter one's perception of events so that a specific practice, previously judged as satisfactory, now becomes questionable or problematic. Thus, nursing service departments must structure mechanisms which (1) identify and evaluate current nursing practice problems existing within the department and (2) provide access to persons, organizations, and written materials as sources of valid research bases. Note that we are *not* suggesting that the nursing service department is or should be responsible for evaluating the validity of the research base. At

this point in time, that function should rest with academe, research consultants and organizations, or professional associations.

The second phase of the research utilization process is directed toward evaluating the relevance of the research-based knowledge as it pertains to the identified clinical practice problem, the organization's values and current policies, and the potential costs and benefits to accrue from its use. A set of probabilities should be established concerning the potential for organizational adoption of a practice innovation which will be derived from the research base under consideration. The second phase ends when the probability for organizational adoption has been determined.

The major activity during the third phase is to design a nursing practice innovation which meets the needs of the clinical problem and does not exceed the scientific limitations of the research base. The innovation describes the intervention as it is to be carried out and prescribes the clinical limitations to be imposed. The design also contains a plan for implementation. The plan should include the following: a time frame; identification of a single unit on which a trial of the innovation will be implemented; identification of all key personnel related to the actual implementation; means for identifying and acquiring adequate resources (personnel, equipment, time, money); provision for staff training if necessary; and finally, provision for adequate evaluation of the effects of the innovation.

The fourth phase comprises an actual clinical trial and evaluation of the innovation on an individual nursing unit. The trial should include baseline measures of the predicted outcomes. Adequate monitoring must be provided to ascertain the occurrence of unanticipated events. The evaluation should be structured so it is a natural part of the innovation—not an artificial, added activity without relevance. As mentioned previously, the evaluation measures should include as many dependent variables from the research base as are clinically reasonable. Divergence between the research base and the innovation trial data concerning these variables should be treated as a serious problem which needs resolution before the meaning of the evaluation can be fully ascertained.

The fifth phase, occurring after completion of the trial and evaluation, is directed toward making a decision to adopt, alter, or reject the innovation under consideration. The quality of the decision is totally dependent upon the adequacy and accuracy of the evaluation measures carried out during the clinical trial. A decision to reject the innovation completes the cycle of the process and it

begins again at phase one with a new research base. A decision to alter the innovation returns the process to phase two, three, or four depending on what the evaluation data indicate as the cause for the faulty trial. A decision to adopt the innovation leads to phase six—the development of means to extend the innovation to other appropriate nursing units within the hospital. This requires additional consideration of the issues involved in phases two, three, and four. The total process may recycle, to begin review of another research base before, during, or after the initial innovation is fully implemented on the appropriate nursing units.

The research utilization process outlined above is relatively elaborate, and it is appropriate to question its cost/benefit ratio. On the cost side, considerable expenditure of staff time is required to maintain access to new research-based knowledge; to develop, implement, and evaluate new practice innovations; and to provide for necessary staff development. The process may also require expenditure of funds for equipment and measurement devices currently unavailable in most nursing service departments.

On the benefit side, the functions involved in the research utilization process complement quality assurance programs, and the patient benefits that result from new practice innovations should serve to balance some of the cost of their development. The process is both a data-consuming and data-producing system. This characteristic is beneficial in two ways. First, it provides a rationale for practice activities that can be meaningfully understood inside and outside the profession. Second, it moves clinical practice into a vital role in nursing research activity by evaluating knowledge generated under relatively controlled conditions and producing systematic clinical data which can be used to validate current findings. Finally, the clinical data produced by this system should provide direction for future nursing research studies.

REFERENCES

1. Sidman, M. *Tactics of Scientific Research*. New York: Basic Books, 1960, 110–139.
2. Lykken, D. Statistical significance in psychological research. In *Statistical Issues: A Reader for the Behavioral Sciences*. R. Kirk (Ed.) Monterey, Cal.: Brooks Cole Publishing Co., 1976, 155–157.

BIBLIOGRAPHY

Becker, M.H. Factors affecting diffusion of innovations among health professionals. *American Journal of Public Health,* 1970, *60,* 294–304.

Emery, F.E., & Trist, E.L. Socio-technical systems. In *Management Sciences, Models and Techniques,* Völ. II. Churchman, E.W., & Vehulst, M. (Eds.). London: Pergamon Press, 1960.

Havelock, R.G. *Resource-User Linkage and Social Problem Solving.* Ann Arbor, Mich.: Center for Research on Utilization of Scientific Knowledge, Institute for Social Research, 1972.

Havelock, R.G. & Benne, K.D. An exploratory study of knowledge utilization. In *The Planning of Change.* Bennis, W.G., Benne, K.D. & Chin, R. (Eds.). New York: Holt, Rinehart and Winston, 1969.

Werley, H.H. This I believe . . . about clinical nursing research. *Nursing Outlook,* 1972, *20* (11), 718–722.

APPENDIX C
PATIENT CARE PROBLEM
IDENTIFICATION GUIDE

This questionnaire has been developed to assist nursing service departments to collect information from nursing personnel about the perceived extent of patient care problems for which there are specific research-based solutions. These research-based solutions are available in the form of nursing practice protocols that can be used to institute research-based practice changes (see list of research-based protocols on pages 34–35).

GUIDE FOR USE

Those responsible for the distribution of this questionnaire will wish to maximize responses from appropriate personnel. Only then can they be sure that they have gained enough information to reliably gauge the perceived extent of the identified patient care problems. Ensuring response from appropriate personnel involves consideration of several issues. Each is discussed below.

Selecting the Potential Respondents Who Will Receive the Questionnaire

A survey of patient care problems is best directed toward those nursing personnel who provide or supervise direct patient care and/or are accountable for patient care on specific units in the hospital. Various types and levels of nursing personnel can be

included (registered nurses, licensed practical nurses, nursing assistants). It is desirable to obtain as complete a picture as possible of the problems as they are perceived by those best qualified to assess the problem situation. Some personnel may not be included because they do not directly encounter the problem situations identified in the questionnaire. The standard questionnaire has a place for respondents to indicate the unit on which they work. Those distributing the questionnaires may decide to broaden or narrow the extent of the identifying information requested, as discussed below.

Informing and Gaining Cooperation of Potential Respondents

Once the potential respondents have been identified it is necessary to consider how to inform them of the effort to identify current patient care problems and to enhance their willingness to complete and return the questionnaire. The return rate of questionnaires significantly affects the reliability of the information gained from the questionnaires. Careful planning for informing the respondents, encouraging their cooperation, facilitating their completion and return of questionnaires, and providing feedback about results can greatly increase the response or return rate. It is well worth the extra effort that may be needed initially to attend to these factors. A return rate of 80 percent or better should be the expected outcome. At the least, a majority or 60 percent of the potential respondents should complete the questionnaire. Otherwise, the reliability of the information regarding incidence of problems comes into question.

Organizing the Survey

Identifying and delegating the tasks to be accomplished, establishing the time frame involved, and obtaining the needed resources are all important to the success of the survey. A plan for distributing and retrieving the questionnaires within a specified time frame will facilitate the survey. This plan should clearly indicate what is to be done, when it should be done, and by whom. Sufficient questionnaires and return envelopes will be needed to cover all potential respondents. Extras should be available for recording and organizing the results or for unanticipated needs. If different information regarding respondents is sought than is asked for on the standard questionnaire, plans will need to be made for making this modification in advance.

Recording and Organizing the Results of the Survey

Recording and organizing the information from the questionnaires is best done by as few people as possible and by those who enjoy working with numbers. The time involved will depend upon the total number of responses and the number of categories into which responses will be organized. For example, if 100 questionnaires are returned and there is no plan to subcategorize responses by unit or type or personnel, the questionnaire data can be recorded and organized relatively quickly. However, subcategorizing the information so that response trends can be identified across units, types of personnel, or both will slow down the recording process. Those responsible for the survey need to decide whether it is valuable to subcategorize the responses. In doing so, they should determine what use will be made of this information and whether it justifies the extra effort involved.

PATIENT CARE PROBLEM IDENTIFICATION GUIDE

Date _____

Nursing Unit _____

RN _____ LPN _____ Nursing Asst. _____

This questionnaire has been developed to assist nursing service departments in identifying patient care problems for which they would like to find solutions. For the purpose of this questionnaire, *patient care problems are defined as difficulties or concerns experienced by patients or the nurses caring for them that are amenable to nursing intervention; they are patient care situations in which there is a discrepancy between what is desirable and what currently exists.* The first section focuses on patient problems that have specific research-based solutions available. The last section focuses on questions about general problems. The answers to this section can be used to provide direction for the development of solutions to the identified patient care problems.

PATIENT CARE PROBLEM IDENTIFICATION GUIDE
(continued)

Section I

For each patient care problem listed below, please check the response in the right-hand column that best indicates the extent to which you believe it is a problem *on your nursing unit(s)*.

PATIENT CARE PROBLEMS	INSIGNIFICANT	MODERATE	RELATIVELY LARGE	DO NOT HAVE PATIENTS WITH THIS PROBLEM	DON'T KNOW
			EXTENT OF THE PROBLEM		
1. Patients are reluctant to cough and deep-breathe and/or engage in postoperative exercises.	☐	☐	☐	☐	☐
2. Postsurgical patients request excessive amounts of pain medication.	☐	☐	☐	☐	☐
3. Cholecystectomy patients stay more than 6 days postsurgery (count from day following surgery through day of discharge).	☐	☐	☐	☐	☐
4. Patients show signs of distress during the following types of diagnostic and therapeutic procedures:					
a. Cast removal	☐	☐	☐	☐	☐
b. Endoscopic exam	☐	☐	☐	☐	☐
c. X-ray procedures, minor (e.g., GI, GU, IVP)	☐	☐	☐	☐	☐
d. X-ray procedures, major (e.g., cardiac catheterization, arteriogram).	☐	☐	☐	☐	☐

PATIENT CARE PROBLEM IDENTIFICATION GUIDE
(continued)

Section I (continued)

PATIENT CARE PROBLEMS	EXTENT OF THE PROBLEM				
	INSIGNIFICANT	MODERATE	RELATIVELY LARGE	DO NOT HAVE PATIENTS WITH THIS PROBLEM	DON'T KNOW
e. Pelvic exam	☐	☐	☐	☐	☐
f. Lumbar puncture	☐	☐	☐	☐	☐
g. Other (please specify) ———	☐	☐	☐	☐	☐
——————————————— ———————————————	☐	☐	☐	☐	☐
5. Patients have high risk of developing skin breakdown (e.g., diabetics, elderly).	☐	☐	☐	☐	☐
6. Patients develop skin breakdown during hospitalization.	☐	☐	☐	☐	☐
7. Patients with chronic voiding disorders develop urinary tract infections.	☐	☐	☐	☐	☐
8. Patients with acute voiding problems develop urinary tract infections while using indwelling catheters.	☐	☐	☐	☐	☐
9. Patients on IV therapy develop phlebitis and/or venous infections.	☐	☐	☐	☐	☐
10. Patients who receive tube feedings have diarrhea.	☐	☐	☐	☐	☐
11. Patients do not experience adequate relief from pain interventions.	☐	☐	☐	☐	☐

PATIENT CARE PROBLEM IDENTIFICATION GUIDE
(continued)

Section I (continued)

PATIENT CARE PROBLEMS	EXTENT OF THE PROBLEM				
	INSIGNIFICANT	MODERATE	RELATIVELY LARGE	DO NOT HAVE PATIENTS WITH THIS PROBLEM	DON'T KNOW
12. Adequate relief from pain occurs too slowly following the intervention.	☐	☐	☐	☐	☐
13. Patients do not participate as much as they should in setting goals for their own health care.	☐	☐	☐	☐	☐
14. Patients do not make the amount of progress toward goals that they are expected to make in the following general areas:					
a. Physical recovery	☐	☐	☐	☐	☐
b. Learning from patient education programs	☐	☐	☐	☐	☐
c. Socio-emotional recovery	☐	☐	☐	☐	☐

PATIENT CARE PROBLEM IDENTIFICATION GUIDE
(continued)

Section II

Please describe any other patient care problems that are particularly important on your unit(s) and for which you would like to find new solutions.

1. _____
   _____
   _____
   _____

2. _____
   _____
   _____
   _____

3. _____
   _____
   _____
   _____

APPENDIX D
DEVELOPING RESEARCH-BASED INNOVATION PROTOCOLS: PROCESS, CRITERIA, AND ISSUES*

Karen B. Haller, Margaret A. Reynolds, and Jo Anne Horsley

The criteria and issues involved in a process of transferring research-based knowledge into innovation protocols for nursing practice are discussed. Three sets of criteria are identified: (a) criteria that pertain to evaluating and integrating studies that constitute a base, (b) criteria that address the issue of how relevant the base is for nursing practice, and (c) criteria related to the potential for evaluation in the clinical setting. The format of the innovation protocol is presented. It is suggested that the protocol may be seen as a form of methodological approximation between research and practice. It is also noted that the process involved in identifying research bases for utilization can serve to identify needs for the conduct of nursing research in the future.

*Ms. Karen B. Haller and Ms. Margaret A. Reynolds are doctoral students in clinical nursing research at the University of Michigan and research assistants for the Conduct and Utilization of Research in Nursing (CURN) Project. Dr. Jo Anne Horsley is professor of nursing at the University of Michigan School of Nursing and principal investigator of the CURN Project. Requests for reprints may be addressed to the CURN Project, School of Nursing, The University of Michigan, Ann Arbor, Michigan 48109. This paper was received August 10, 1978, was revised, and was accepted for publication February 15, 1979.

This research is supported by Division of Nursing, DHEW, Grant NU00542 awarded to the Michigan Nurses Association. The scientific work of the project is conducted by faculty and graduate students at the University of Michigan School of

This paper deals with the criteria and issues involved in a process of transferring research-based knowledge into innovation protocols for nursing practice. Content for the paper developed from work on a funded project titled the Conduct and Utilization of Research in Nursing (CURN). Now in its fourth year of activity, CURN is addressing a widespread and critical problem in the nursing profession. The amount of sound nursing research has been increasing steadily, but often this research has had little appreciable impact on nursing practice (Aydelotte, 1976; Ketefian, 1975; Krueger, 1978). Project staff are investigating ways in which scientific knowledge may be transferred to the practice of nursing and ways in which clinical practice might influence nursing research so that it more closely approximates the clinical setting's methods and goals.

Requisite to this work is the identification and evaluation of nursing research that is suitable for transfer to practice settings. This process has involved retrieving, reviewing, and organizing studies into areas of conceptually related research, followed by an evaluation of each area's potential for use. The final step in this sequence is the development of "innovation protocols" for nursing care interventions based on the identified research. Although specific criteria have guided the process of transforming clinical research into such protocols several issues of concern have emerged. It is our intent in this paper to describe the process and the criteria used and to delineate the issues that have arisen.

PROCESS

The project staff's experience with research utilization to date has demonstrated that considerable confusion exists among nurses regarding the differences between the conduct of research and the

Nursing and the Institute for Social Research and at the Michigan State University School of Nursing.

This paper was presented under the title "Developing research-based practice innovations; Criteria, processes, and issues" at the Eleventh Annual Communicating Nursing Research Conference, Western Society for Research in Nursing, Portland, Oregon, May 4, 1978.

The authors acknowledge the contribution of Ms. Janet Bingle, former associate on the CURN Project, to early development of ideas embodied in this paper.

Reprinted from Haller, K.B., Reynolds, M.A., & Horsley, J.A. Developing research based innovation protocols: Process criteria, and issues. Research in Nursing and Health, *1979, 2, 45-51. Copyright © 1979 by John Wiley & Sons. Reprinted by permission of John Wiley & Sons, Inc.*

utilization of the knowledge resulting from such research. For example, when asked to describe how they might use research in their practice, nurses often cite a process of replication. It is important to differentiate the goals and, therefore, the people, knowledge, and context relevant for research conduct and research utilization, respectively. Research conduct is directed toward the production of knowledge that is generalizable beyond the population directly studied. The process of research utilization, on the other hand, is directed toward transferring specific research-based knowledge into actual practice. The conduct of research generally occurs in the academic context where people with specialized knowledge and skills in the methods of scientific inquiry can obtain the resources and control of conditions necessary. To be effective, however, research-based knowledge should be implemented and evaluated in a practice context where people with knowledge, skills, and experience in the methods of nursing practice can examine the relevance, means, and utility of new techniques (Horsley, Crane, & Bingle, 1978).

A key dimension on which the conduct of research varies from research utilization is methodology. The tenets of scientific methodology can be contrasted with those of the methodology of practice. Nurses in settings where research is conducted rely on scientific methodology that is systematic, controlled, and generally inflexible. Research methods are relatively rigorous and attempt to minimize personal bias. The researcher takes a logical approach and attempts to discover common patterns in a population. In nursing practice, however, skill is a paramount concern and methods are individualized. Clinical measures are relatively flexible, may rely on precedent, and call on clinical judgment. The clinician takes an intuitive approach and views each case as unique. These methodological differences are important because they affect the interactions that occur between the research and practice settings. Such differences have tended to preclude the use of research in practice as well as to inhibit the conduct of practice-relevant research. A process of methodological approximation, or a systematic effort to close the gap between research methods and practice methods, is essential to research utilization. Both researchers and clinicians need to assume responsibility for approximating one another's methods. The innovation protocol may be viewed as one step in a series of methodological approximations that are necessary for utilization. Later approximations can occur when nurses in a practice setting transform the protocol for their own particular needs and again when the change is implemented. The process used to

develop innovation protocols will demonstrate this notion of methodological approximation.

The approach used to identify research-based knowledge with potential for use in nursing practice is based on the idea that there are areas of research in which studies can be related to one another by common variables and by relationships between those variables. Studies contributing to a particular area of research form the base from which nursing knowledge and nursing activities may be derived. When the activity suggested by the research base is different from traditional practice, that is, it either adds to practice in some way or calls for the extinction of a practice, it is an "innovation." Innovations in nursing imply changes in practice that are new to those using them and that are intended to benefit clients. Once a potential practice innovation has been identified, an attempt is made to "package" the information into an "innovation protocol"; this represents a methodological approximation of research to practice. An effort is made to write the protocols in a form that will be useful to nurses interested in implementing research-based planned change in nursing practice. An innovation protocol, therefore, is research-based knowledge put in the form of a product; the product is nursing knowledge that has clearly definable parameters for use in practice.

THE PROTOCOL

At this point it might be useful to describe the form and content of an innovation protocol. Each protocol begins with a section on the need for change, documenting the extent of the clinical problem and the relevance of the problem to nursing practice. The second section gives a description of the innovation, including information on the types of patients most likely to benefit from the innovation. The protocol then provides a summary of the research base and identifies "research-based principles" to guide the implementation of the innovation. Although the use of the term "principle" is not scientifically accurate, CURN Project staff have persisted in using the term because it was found to communicate the appropriate intent to nurses who use the protocols. It is more accurate, however, to say that what are extracted from the research bases are empirical generalizations.

The remainder of the protocol deals with implementation of the innovation and systematic evaluation of its effects. With regard to both of these processes, the protocol describes the materials that

will be required, the personnel development that may be necessary to carry out the activities suggested, and the costs that are likely to be incurred. Finally, each protocol is summarized by a discussion of the benefits that can be expected to result from a successful trial of the innovation. Additional materials may be appended to the protocols as they are available or can be developed. These materials always include the primary sources of the research base. They may also include an annotated bibliography, an evaluation procedure designed by the author of the protocol, and any additional tools or resources that are available from the original researchers.

Ten research-based practice protocols have been developed by project personnel and are being field tested. These include:

1. Structured preoperative teaching
2. A lactose-free diet
3. Sensation information: distress reduction
4. Sensory information: recovery rate
5. Nonsterile intermittent urinary catheterization
6. Prevention of catheter-associated urinary tract infections
7. Intravenous cannula change regimen
8. Prevention of decubiti by means of small shifts of body weight
9. Mutual goal setting: goal attainment
10. Deliberative nursing: pain reduction

CRITERIA FOR UTILIZATION OF RESEARCH IN NURSING PRACTICE

When project staff began the search and retrieval process for research bases, a number of well-known nursing researchers were asked to identify areas of clinical research which they felt were sufficiently developed to merit use in practice. Responses indicated a wide range of opinion; for example, some felt that "anything may be utilized; the determination rests with those who want to incorporate the ideas in any given study into their clinical work." Others responded toward the opposite end of the continuum: "No area of clinical nursing research is currently adequate for utilization in practice." Clearly such a range of answers suggested that different processes, criteria, and issues were considered by the respondents. The nursing literature also offered little assistance in defining how or with what criteria one may determine the adequacy of clinical research bases. Therefore, CURN Project personnel established criteria for selecting the research that is used in the development of

protocols and in the utilization efforts of the project. The criteria were organized into three major categories: (a) criteria that pertain to evaluating and integrating studies that constitute a base, (b) criteria that address the issue of how relevant the base is for nursing practice, and (c) criteria related to the potential for evaluation in the clinical setting. Each of these will be discussed.

Evaluation and Integration of Studies

REPLICATION. The first criterion for identifying studies that constitute a research base is replication. Ideally there is more than one study in a research base to provide greater assurance against committing a Type 1 error, thereby inferring an effect where none exists. Some researchers criticize this approach by noting that the Type II error can be just as costly in inferring a lack of effect when there actually is one. Certainly, postponing implementation of a valid study is of concern; however, the possibility of implementing an innovation based on a "false positive" has legal and ethical ramifications that project personnel were unwilling to risk. Therefore, when developing protocols in any given area of research, an effort is made to establish that the conceptual and constructive propositions have been confirmed in more than one study; this is a process of construct replication. According to Lykken (1968), construct replication tests that validity of the "relation between meaningful constructs, generalizable to some broad reference population, which the [original author] claimed to have established" (p. 156). Construct replication is achieved when a second investigator begins with a similar problem statement but formulates original methods of measurement and design to verify the first author's findings. The advantage of construct replication over literal or operational replication is that it validates previous work, extends the findings, and offers great utility because it builds knowledge efficiently.

In order to obtain a solid research base for an innovation, it has been necessary to organize studies according to the concepts tested and to actively seek instances of consturct replication. For example, numerous investigators (Felton, Huss, Payne, & Srsic 1976; Fortin & Kirouac, 1976; Johnson, Rice, & Endress, 1975; Lindeman & Van Aernam, 1971) studied structured preoperative teaching and its postoperative effects. At the time the literature search was done, it was clear that these studies did not directly replicate one another. Yet the studies did demonstrate—in varied settings, using different populations, and a number of me-

thodologies—that structured preoperative teaching does have a positive postoperative effect on clients. In other instances such replication has not been found. For example, numerous investigators studied various treatment modalities for decubitus ulcers (for a review of the literature, see Berecek, 1975). In these studies, to date, the findings are not corroborated: therefore, in spite of the extensiveness of the research, no base is available from which to develop a particular nursing innovation for treating decubitus ulcers.

SCIENTIFIC MERIT.   The second criterion for studies constituting a research base is scientiffic merit. Each study with potential for contributing to the base is reviewed in terms of its design and methodology. Validity and reliability are key issues. The appropriateness of the sample for the clinical problem is also considered; generalizability is at issue here. At least one study in the research base must be conducted in a practice setting. Finally, the study's assumptions, findings, and conclusions are examined. The value of a study to the conceptual base is not determined entirely by the statistical significance of the findings; rather, an attempt is made to understand the functional relationships between variables in a base. The conclusions and implications of each study are evaluated in terms of their power to corroborate, extend, or delineate the conceptual base.

In the process of evaluating individual studies and comparing each with other studies in the base, conflicting findings may be found. Attempts are made to resolve contradictory findings either through identification of methodological weakness or through a theoretical explanation for the discrepancy. It is also recognized that in a series of replications of the same study, a nonsignificant difference may be expected to occur a certain number of times on the basis of chance alone. For example, the research base underlying the regimen for changing intravenous cannula consists of some 20 studies (e.g., Collin, Collin, Constable, & Johnston, 1975: Thomas, Evers, & Racz, 1970). Collectively, these studies support the proposition that duration of cannulization is positively related to local venous infection and infusion phlebitis. The findings of one study (Crossley & Matsen, 1972), however, resulted in a departure from this generalization. Closer scrutiny revealed that only intravenous infusions of greater than 24 hours' duration were included in the calculations. In truncating the data at one end of the scale, the significant effect of time on the dependent variables of infection and phlebitis may have been lost. Theoretically, this suggested that the

findings were not necessarily contradictory to the research base but that there was probably a maximum time beyond which duration of the intravenous infusion does not correlate significantly with complications. Further search and retrieval was indicated to confirm this suspicion and to define what the maximum time might be. The example demonstrates that each study in a conceptual area is evaluated on its own scientific merit as well as on its power to contribute to a research base for practice by corroboration or extension.

RISK. The third criterion used to identify clinical research bases is risk. The concept of risk is used to mediate the stringency with which the criteria of replication and scientific merit are applied. Where the risk to the client is small, a generalization is made more readily than in those instances where risk is great. For instance, studies exist that can be grouped conceptually into an area; yet, considered together, these studies do not deal fully with the functional relationships among the variables. There may be some weaknesses in methodology; there may be conflicting findings; or perhaps the case for construct replication is not strong. If there is little potential harm to the client, the practice action suggested by the research base may be tentatively implemented *pending clinical evaluation*. Such is the case in the decubitus prevention protocol. The nursing innovation derived from the base calls for unscheduled small shifts of body weight in addition to routine, scheduled turning. Although this research base has some weaknesses, implementation of the innovation requires little time or training on the part of the staff and does not jeopardize the client in any way. In other protocols where risk to the client is greater, the criteria have been applied more stringently.

Relevance to Practice

Once it has been established that a research base exists, the second major category of criteria needs to be considered; these criteria deal with the issue of practice relevance. When applied to an innovation, practice relevance means that the innovation derived from the base meets the demand of a nursing problem in a clinical setting. To state it another way, a research-based innovation that is practice relevant means that it has approximated the practice setting's goals and methods. The degree to which this approximation has occurred may be judged by four criteria: (a) degree of

clinical merit, (b) extent of clinical control over the variables, (c) feasibility and (d) cost.

CLINICAL MERIT.   Clinical merit is the degree to which the research base addresses a problem of significance to the practice setting or the degree to which the suggested innovation will be potentially useful. Clinical merit represents an approximation of the research problem to the clinical goal.

CLINICAL CONTROL.   A second consideration is clinical control. It is essential that nursing has, or is able to achieve, clinical control of the independent and dependent variables in the research base. If nurses are to use the research base, they must be in control of the events required for implementation and evaluation of the innovation. Control is problematic for two reasons: (a) the outcomes of nursing practice are often influenced by multiple factors external to the nurse-patient relationship; and (b) the instruments used to measure the effects of the innovation may not be available for use by nurses in the practice setting.

In the first instance, control over the outcomes of nursing practice is the concern. Occasionally, the variables in the research base fall clearly within the purview of nursing and control becomes almost automatic. An example of this occurs in the decubitus prevention protocol where the independent variable is small shifts of body weight and the dependent variable is occurrence of pressure sores. Clearly both variables are within the purview of nursing with minimal input from other professionals. In most of the protocols, however, clinical control of the variables must be achieved through the development of collaborative decision making with other practitioners. For instance, implementation of the nonsterile intermittent catheterization protocol requires cooperation with physicians. Input by physicians is necessary in making the decision to use nonsterile intermittent catheterization with individual patients, in prescribing drugs used in conjunction with the innovation, and in ordering laboratory studies to determine the effectiveness of the innovation. Clearly, securing the involvement of physicians is crucial to clinical control over implementation and evaluation of this innovation.

The second control problem relates to measurement. The protocols require the use of some of the dependent variables from the research base for evaluation of the innovation. Frequently, however, the methods that the researchers used to measure the dependent variables are not immediately available in the clinical setting. In some cases, an approximation to practice can be made by the

substitution of valid clinical measures for the research instruments. In other cases, the clinical setting may approximate the researchers' methods by acquiring the new knowledge or skill needed to use the research tools. When the preoperative teaching protocol was implemented in two different Michigan hospitals, one setting chose to substitute tape measurement of chest expansion and auscultation for spirometry as measures of respiratory status. This particular substitution was adapted from work done by Horn and Swain (1977) and demonstrates an approximation to practice. The second setting chose to work with the respiratory therapy department to gain access to the knowledge and skills needed to do spirometry; in this case, a clinical approximation to research methodology was made.

FEASIBILITY. Feasibility is the next factor that is considered in determining practice relevance. Given the constraints of the environments in which nurses practice, is it feasible to implement the innovation? Feasibility varies from institution to institution because it is related to the availability of resources (e.g., time, personnel, expertise, and equipment) and to the dominant feeling about change in the clinical setting. Each of these factors will vary in turn by the nature of the innovation, such as the degree of change it implies, the relative compatibility of the innovation with current nursing practice, the number of clients who will be affected, or the number of staff nurses to be involved.

COST BENEFITS. Closely related to feasibility but treated as a separate factor is cost. The financial cost of implementing and evaluating the innovation suggested by the research base is balanced against the potential benefit to clients. Since this type of analysis is rarely documented in the research literature, an estimate is made. Estimates most frequently balance the costs of materials, laboratory expenses, personnel development and staff time against such benefits as reduced incidence of complications and patient or staff satisfaction.

Potential for Clinical Evaluation

Each research base must be reviewed in relation to its potential for permitting adequate clinical evaluation of the proposed practice change. A key distinction between research utilization and replication of research points to the importance of clinical evaluation. Utilization implies that the practitioner transforms the new knowledge for use in the practice setting. Even under ideal conditions of

clinical control, utilization of research in the clinical setting constitutes a change in the independent variable. To assure that this change or transformation has not extended beyond the limits of the research base, it must be possible to evaluate clinically the effects of the innovation once the protocol has been implemented. More specifically, the criterion states that there must be one or more dependent variables in the original research base that can be reliably measured by clinicians in practice settings. There are actually two components to this criterion: (a) the clinical knowledge and skills of the general nursing staff necessary to measure reliably the dependent variable and (b) the clinical control of the variable, which was discussed earlier. Using this criterion, project staff found that many of the dependent measures in the research base are not useful for clinical evaluation. Further, those measures that do meet the demands of the criterion are often the weakest in the research base in terms of validity and reliability.

PURPOSES OF INNOVATION EVALUATION. Evaluation of an innovation serves multiple purposes. Clinical evaluation moves practitioners to approximate research methodology more closely since such evaluation requires a systematic and controlled process involving measurement, data collection, and analysis. Evaluation can also be used to assess the extent to which research knowledge is applicable to practice settings. This information can then provide useful feedback to the original researchers. In addition, clinical evaluation questions whether the innovation is relevant to a practice problem, that is, whether or not it produces an outcome that justifies its use. The data base provided by clinical evaluation can serve to justify the new practice to others and is useful in meeting legal and ethical concerns related to accountability.

CHARACTERISTICS OF INNOVATION EVALUATION. Initially, it was anticipated that the research base would identify the outcome variables and also assist in the development of appropriate measurement procedures for use in evaluation. This has not always been true, and as a result greater flexibility has been required in the design of evelation procedures to accompany the innovation. For instance, the original work on nonsterile intermittent catheterization was done by physicians. Some of the dependent variables, such as cystoscopy results, were not felt to be appropriate as nursing outcomes. On the other hand, some of the variables of keen interest to nursing were not accounted for in the research base; these included patient satisfaction, patient mobility, and degree of social

interaction. Therefore, an evaluation procedure was devised that included variables from the research base and also drew on introspection about clinical practice.

Evaluation of the innovation is structured into a process component and an outcome component, providing a format that parallels current efforts in quality assurance. Independent variables from the research base are measured in terms of process to assure that the innovation has been implemented accurately and consistently; dependent variables are measured as outcomes. Once such an evaluation has been designed, it is easily placed into the ongoing quality assurance system.

To date, all evaluations use a pre- and postimplementation design. Baseline data and postimplementation data are usually summarized by frequency tables, ranges, rates, or means for purposes of comparison. Differences in the data are not tested for statistical significance. Again, a process of clinical evaluation rather than replication is advocated.

CONCLUSION

Development of research-based practice innovation protocols begins with a search for conceptually related studies that have potential for utilization in clinical nursing settings. Each potential practice area is then appraised according to the three major criteria that have been established by the CURN Project staff. If the area has an established research base, is practice relevant, and can be reliably evaluated by clinicians, it is judged sufficient for utilization in practice settings. An innovation protocol is subsequently developed, serving as a form of methodological approximation.

In many instances, potential practice innovations fail to meet the criteria and thus do not merit utilization in practice. Perhaps a replication of the original study is all that is necessary to permit its utilization, or it may be that a more valid and/or reliable tool is required in order to evaluate clinically the effects of the innovation. Through the process of subjecting each area to the demands of the criteria, missing links and deficiencies that preclude utilization become apparent. The identified deficiencies are of major importance, for they point to areas that need further research. Therefore, the process can also serve to guide future research efforts in nursing.

REFERENCES

Aydelotte, M.K. Nursing research in clinical settings: Problems and issues. *Sigma Theta Tau Reflections,* 1976, 2, 3–6.

Berecek, K.H. Treatment of decubitus ulcers. *Nursing Clinics of North America,* 1975, *10,* 171–210.

Collin, J., Collin, C., Constable, F.L., & Johnston, I.D.A. Infusion thrombophlebitis and infection with various cannulas. *Lancet,* 1975, *2,* 150–153.

Crossley, K., & Matsen, J.M. The scalp-vein needle: A prospective study of complications. *Journal of the American Medical Association.* 1972, *220,* 985–987.

Felton, G., Huss, K., Payne, E.A., & Srsic, K. Preoperative nursing intervention with the patient for surgery: Outcomes of three alternative approaches. *International Journal of Nursing Studies,* 1976, *13,* 83–96.

Fortin, F., & Kirouac, S. A randomized controlled trial of preoperative patient education. *International Journal of Nursing Studies,* 1976, *13,* 11–24.

Horn, B.J., & Swain, M.A. Development of criterion measures of nursing care. Unpublished manuscript, School of Public Health, University of Michigan, 1977.

Horsley, J.A., Crane J., & Bingle, J.D. Research utilization as an organizational process. *Journal of Nursing Administration,* 1978, *8* (7), 4–6.

Johnson, J.E., Rice, V.H., & Endress, M.P. Making psychological concepts concrete for medical education. *Proceedings of the 14th Annual Conference on Research in Medical Education.* Washington, D.C.: Association of American Medical Colleges, 1975, 125–130.

Ketefian, S. Application of selected nursing research findings into nursing practice. *Nursing Research,* 1975, *24,* 89–92.

Krueger, J.C. Utilization of nursing research: The planning process. *Journal of Nursing Administration,* 1978, *8* (1), 6–9.

Lindeman, C.A., & Van Aernam, B. Nursing intervention with the presurgical patient—The effects of structured and unstructured preoperative teaching. *Nursing Research,* 1971, *20,* 319–332.

Lykken, D.T. Statistical significance in psychological research. *Psychological Bulletin,* 1968, *70,* 151–159.

Thomas, E.T., Evers, W., & Racz, G.B. Postinfusion phlebitis. *Anesthesia and Analgesia,* 1970, *49,* 150–159.

APPENDIX E
GUIDE TO READING RESEARCH
CRITICALLY

This guide was developed to assist in the review of original research reports. Its intended purpose is to guide the reader in identifying specific content that is critical to developing the knowledge necessary to implement research-based practice changes. It is not intended to provide guidance for a review of the scientific merit of reported studies.

The guide is an essential tool for the research utilization process described in this book. A separate guide should be filled out for each research article that comprises the research base. This provides basic information to be considered in carrying out the steps in Chapters 4 and 5, and serves as a convenient reference for use throughout the research utilization effort.

RESEARCH ARTICLE/REPORT

Title and Author:

Journal in Which Reported:

QUESTIONS TO BE CONSIDERED

1. What was the problem that was studied?

2. Does this study help solve a clinical problem which you face currently? If so, describe the problem.

3. To what extent does the solution investigated in this study solve the clinical problem you have identified?

4. In what setting was the research conducted? Be specific and describe in detail (For example, was it in a laboratory or clinical setting? What type of institution? What type of unit? Was there anything about the setting that makes you think that it is not typical of clinical settings?)

5. In what ways is your practice setting similar or different from the setting in which the research was conducted?

6. What patients or clients were studied?

   a. primary diagnosis or condition

   b. sex

   c. age

   d. other

7. Is there anything about these patients or clients that makes you think they are atypical? How do they differ from the patients or clients you might involve in a trial of the research-based practice?

8. What was the total number of patients or clients studied? Is there any reason to question the adequacy of this number?

9. What is the independent variable that was studied? (An independent variable is the variable that comes first in time and is assumed to cause the effect that is being studied. It is often a nursing intervention, patient characteristic, or patient behavior that is studied to determine its effect.)

10. Is this independent variable a nursing intervention? If so, describe the intervention as it was carried out by the researcher.

11. What are the dependent variables in the study? (A dependent variable is the measured effect that is thought to result from, or depend on, the independent variable.)

12. How were these dependent variables measured in the study?

13. Which of these measurement methods are familiar to you? Which can be used in your setting?

14. What effects were seen in patients or clients that the author attributed to the independent variable (intervention)?

15. Do you agree that the independent variable (intervention) was responsible for the changes in patients/clients as stated by the author?

16. Based upon your knowledge and experience, what other rationale might explain the results of this study?

17. To what extent does the author discuss the reliability of the data collected? How was reliability achieved? At what level? (The concept of reliability suggests that if the measurement was repeated on the same patients, under the same conditions, the same results would be obtained.)

18. To what extent does the author discuss the validity of tools used in collecting the data? How was validity determined? (The concept of validity suggests that the instruments used to measure the effects of the interventions measure what they were supposed to measure.)

19. Does the author state that the conclusions reached are based on results that are statistically significant?

20. Based upon this report, can you ascertain whether or not the researcher has carried out other studies in this area? Does this study expand on prior research?

21. Are you familiar with other studies which address the same problem and/or the same intervention? How were the results similar or conflicting?

22. After critically examining this study, are you interested in using the intervention in your clinical practice? Why?

23. After reading this article, what additional information is needed to evaluate these findings?

24. How would you go about obtaining the additional information if needed?

APPENDIX F
PROBABILITY OF ADOPTION
ASSESSMENT GUIDE

Innovation: _____
_____

Date: _____

This guide was developed to assist change agents in nursing departments in assessing the characteristics of potential nursing practice innovations that might affect their successful adoption. The use of the guide requires knowledge of the characteristics and requirements of the proposed innovation and the characteristics and resources of the nursing department.

Guide for Use

1. On a separate sheet of paper, briefly describe the characteristics and requirements of the innovation you wish to assess. Note what would be involved in carrying it out, and identify staff, materials, patients, equipment, budget, etc., that would be needed.

2. Keeping the characteristics and requirements of your innovation in mind, answer each question in the guide and give your innovation a score, which you record in the right-hand column.

(Continued)

3. When you have finished answering the questions, add up the scores for subscales I and II, and record a total score. Compare these scores with the probability scales on the last page of the guide. These scores will give you a working estimate of the likelihood that your innovation can be successfully implemented in your nursing department.

4. Go back and review the questions in the guide to see if there are some that you think are more important and that should be weighted more heavily in this assessment. Examine the scores from these questions separately. If they have been scored 1–3, you may consider the probability of this innovation's adoption questionable.

QUESTIONS TO CONSIDER	SCORE
I. Factors Affecting Ease of Implementation	
a. How tangible (technological/material) or intangible (interpersonal/nonmaterial) is this innovation? 1 2 3 4 5 Very intangible; Has both Very tangible; involves change tangible and only involves in attitudes, intangible using new communication, features equipment etc.	___
b. How much change in current nursing function(s) would this innovation require? 1 2 3 4 5 Extensive Moderate No change change change	___

(Continued)

QUESTIONS TO CONSIDER	SCORE

c. To what extent does this innovation address a relevant nursing practice problem or need in your hospital?

1	2	3	4	5

There is little or no concern by anyone | There is moderate concern by some | There is great concern by many

_____

d. Would this kind of practice change be acceptable to you and others on your unit?

1	2	3	4	5

Not acceptable at all | Acceptable to me and half or more of the others | Highly acceptable by all

_____

e. To what extent is nursing in your hospital free to decide to carry out this innovation?

1	2	3	4	5

Requires hospitalwide approval and cooperation | Requires some other group's approval and cooperation | Requires no other group's approval or cooperation

_____

f. To what extent would this innovation fall under the control of nursing in your hospital?

1	2	3	4	5

Nursing would have no control | Control would be unclear; other departments also involved | Nursing would have clear control

_____

(Continued)

QUESTIONS TO CONSIDER	SCORE
g. To what extent do nursing staff have to be involved in implementing the innovation?	

	1	2	3	4	5	
	Entire nursing service must be involved		Small group of nurses plus some nursing administrators need to be involved		Small group of nurses need to be involved	___

h. To what extent are the patients to whom the innovation is directed available on one unit or spread across many units?	

	1	2	3	4	5	
	Many units with small numbers of patients		Several units with moderate number of patients		Few units with large numbers of patients	___

i. To what extent would this innovation require changes in staffing patterns for nursing personnel?	

	1	2	3	4	5	
	Substantial change required		Some change required		No change required	___

j. To what extent can the innovation be divided into separate phases that can be implemented one step at a time?	

	1	2	3	4	5	
	Complex and not divisible		Probably divisible		Easily divisible or not necessary	___

(Continued)

QUESTIONS TO CONSIDER	SCORE
k. To what extent can the innovation be stopped if it does not prove desirable? 　　　1　　2　　3　　4　　5 Very difficult to stop　　Stopped with some difficulty　　Stopped without any difficulty	＿＿＿
l. To what extent would a trial of this innovation disrupt or interfere with the way nurses currently function? 　　　1　　2　　3　　4　　5 Would be very disruptive　　Would cause some disruption　　Would not interfere or disrupt	＿＿＿
m. What length of time would be required to carry out this innovation, considering needed training, materials, staff, etc.? 　　　1　　2　　3　　4　　5 A long time; 6 months or more　　A moderate time; about 3 months　　A short time; 2 weeks to 1 month	＿＿＿
n. How difficult would it be to demonstrate that this innovation has had an effect on patient care? 　　　1　　2　　3　　4　　5 Very difficult　　Moderately difficult　　Easy	＿＿＿
o. How difficult would it be to get appropriate staff (or others) involved in collecting evidence that the innovation is effective? 　　　1　　2　　3　　4　　5 Very difficult　　Moderately difficult　　Easy	＿＿＿
	(Continued)

QUESTIONS TO CONSIDER	SCORE

p. What length of time would be required to evaluate the benefits?
 	
  1 2 3 4 5
 	
  Long time   Reasonable time   Short time (few
  (several months)   (few weeks)   days)
 	
Subtotal
	____
	
	____

II. Cost–Benefit Factors
 	
a. To what extent would the benefits derived from the innovation be visible?
 	
  1 2 3 4 5
 	
  Intangible and   Visible but not   Highly visible.
  not obvious   very tangible   Obvious to all
 	
b. To what extent would the benefits of the innovation affect the physical and emotional well-being of the patients?
 	
  1 2 3 4 5
 	
  Minimal   Modest   Major
  improvement in   improvement in   improvement in
  patient   patient   patient
  well-being   well-being   well-being
 	
c. To what extent would this innovation facilitate or interfere with the work of nurses in your hospital?
 	
  1 2 3 4 5
 	
  It will interfere   It will neither   It will facilitate
  with their work   facilitate nor   their work
    interfere with
    their work
 	
(Continued)
	____
	
	____
	
	____

QUESTIONS TO CONSIDER	SCORE

d. To what extent are the materials required by this innovation currently available in your hospital?

1	2	3	4	5

Not at all available	Available but controlled by others	Readily available to nursing

_____

e. To what extent would personnel require specialized training in order to implement the innovation?

1	2	3	4	5

Extensive training and re-education required	Some training and re-education required	Little or no special education or training required

_____

f. To what extent would the benefits support the time and energy involved in implementing the innovation?

1	2	3	4	5

Takes months to implement and benefits are obscure for a long time	Takes reasonable amount of time and benefits occur within a few weeks	Takes limited time and benefits readily felt

_____

g. How costly would it be to start this innovation?

1	2	3	4	5

Requires extra staff and costly materials/ equipment	Requires some extra staff and materials/ equipment	Requires no additional staff, materials/ equipment

_____

(Continued)

QUESTIONS TO CONSIDER	SCORE

h. How costly would it be to <u>maintain</u> this innovation once it were started?

	1	2	3	4	5

_____

Requires ongoing budgeting for several additional staff plus costly materials/ equipment, etc.	Requires ongoing budgeting for some staff, materials, equipment, etc.	Requires no additional staff, materials, equipment, etc., to maintain

i. To what extent would the monetary cost of nursing care (or costs of other aspects of hospital care) be altered by implementing this innovation?

	1	2	3	4	5

_____

Increased costs per patient-day	Some savings per patient-day	Major savings per patient-day

j. To what extent would the benefits of the innovation be proportional to <u>all</u> the difficulties inherent in implementing this innovation?

	1	2	3	4	5

_____

Difficulties totally outweigh any benefits	Benefits are balanced by difficulties	Benefits totally outweight any difficulties

I.   Cost–Benefit Subtotal _____

II. Ease of Implementation Subtotal _____

III. Combined Total Score _____

PROBABILITY OF ADOPTION SCALES

Total Score	Probability of Adoption	Explanation of Scores

I. Ease of Implementation (16 items)

64–80	*Very* good	
48–64	Good	
Below 48	Questionable	

II. Cost–Benefit Factors (10 items)

40–50	*Very* good	
30–40	Good	
Below 30	Questionable	

III. Combined Total Score

104–130	*Very* good	The average score is between 4 and 5, indicating high estimates of ease of implementation and a favorable cost–benefit ratio.
78–104	Good	The average score is between 3 and 4, indicating that there are some obstacles but that the chances of successful implementation and adoption are good.
Below 78	Questionable	Too many questions have been scored 1–3, indicating that there are many obstacles to successful implementation and adoption.

APPENDIX G
INTERRATER RELIABILITY

DEFINITION

The concept of *reliability* suggests that if a measurement were repeated on the same patients under the same conditions, the same results would be obtained. While there are many types of reliability, the one of concern here is *interrater* (interobserver) reliability. It is the extent to which different nurses can independently arrive at the same judgment. It can be expressed as percentage of agreement.

PURPOSE

The purpose of achieving high interrater reliability (IRR) is to ensure that nurses are measuring the same phenomenon (variable) and coming to the same conclusion or agreement about that phenomenon. For example, in many clinical settings nurses might have different methods of measuring whether or not phlebitis is present. Nurses may look for redness, pain, swelling, etc.; they may use any one or a combination of these symptoms to make a clinical judgment about the presence or absence of phlebitis; (Nurse A may use redness alone, Nurse B may use all three symptoms). In evaluating practice, the important point is that the two nurses come to agreement about whether or not phlebitis is present or absent when observing the same phenomena. Achieving high interrater reliability establishes the fact that the nurses can come to the same

conclusion and lends credibility to the clinical judgments being made in relation to a given phenomenon.

In many instances, nurses cannot agree about their clinical judgments; in such instances, interrater reliability would be low. Definitions and procedures describing how to make clinical judgments are often used to help nurses come to the same conclusion and thus improve the interrater reliability. Again using the phlebitis example, a procedure describing the symptoms of redness, pain, and swelling in combination and how each is measured would assist nurses in coming to the same conclusion about whether or not phlebitis is present.

When different nurses can agree on the measurement, greater confidence can be felt about the conclusion or judgment. When nurses attempt to evaluate the effects of their practice, having confidence in the evaluation measures lends credence to the evaluation process itself.

GUIDELINES

The following are several guidelines for the establishment of interrater reliability.

Timing of IRR

For use with CURN protocols, interrater reliability should be established just prior to data collection. It can be assumed that once a level of interrater reliability is established, the level will be maintained throughout a data collection period lasting approximately 2 months. If data collection exceeds this time limit, interrater reliability should be re-established. It is essential, however, that nurses continue to use the tool exactly as they were trained. Otherwise, interrater reliability will be reduced when the tool is used for actual data collection.

Selection of Observations

When establishing interrater reliability, it is important to use a wide range of observations. For example, on a distress rating scale observations would include patients with a wide variation in the symptoms of distress; e.g. some with no distress, some with moderate distress, and others with great distress; this would offer a

more adequate testing of whether or not nurses can come to the same conclusion.

Generally, the more ratings one has in the determination of interrater reliability, the better the reliability is likely to be. More confidence can be placed in a larger number of ratings, and by using a larger number of ratings, each disagreement is less costly. A minimum of 10–15 ratings is usually considered essential.

Selection of Raters

A minimum of two raters is required. While one nurse can serve as the only rater during actual data collection, a second nurse is always needed for purposes of establishing the initial level of interrater reliability. In most instances, however, one rater will not be sufficient to cover all of the observations that need to be made during a data collection period. More than likely, 4 or 5 nurses will be required to assure that observations will be made on the needed shifts and units. It is suggested that the number of raters be kept to a minimum to reduce the amount of effort required for training and testing.

In making the observations required to determine interrater reliability, it is best for each rater to rotate with as many partners as possible. In this manner, each rater will have an opportunity to compare results with every other rater and work toward overall agreement.

Defining Agreement

In most instances it will be obvious whether or not different nurses "agree" in their judgment on a specific measure. In other instances it will not be obvious, but perfect agreement between raters is probably not necessary. Agreement may be defined anew for each situation. If pulse rate is the observation, for example, agreement may be defined as "within 4 beats per minute." When multiple-point scales are used, agreement may be defined as being "within 1 scale point."

Adequate Levels of Interrater Reliability

Determining an adequate level of interrater reliability is sometimes an arbitrary decision; however, for use in clinical evaluation, a level of 80 percent is considered sufficient. An interrater reliability of 90 percent is very good.

Training

Training activities should be conducted to increase interrater reliability. Basic training activities include the following:

(1) An initial orientation to the measures to be used in data collection and a discussion session to clarify the procedures, terms, and issues.
(2) Practice sessions in which nurses actually make independent observations and/or ratings. It will be helpful to practice in pairs, compare individual ratings, and discuss instances of disagreement.
(3) Determination of interrater reliability (see discussion below).
(4) If interrater reliability is not adequate, additional training and discussion sessions prior to determining interrater reliability a second time.

After the training period, staff need to determine interrater reliability before proceeding with data collection. All raters should perform a rating in tandem with all other raters. The ratings made by each member of the rater pair should be done at the same time, and it is essential that they be done *independently,* i.e., the raters should not state or discuss their individual ratings until each has privately recorded his or her own rating.

Example

The following is an example of how 4 nurses completed training on two scales measuring effectiveness and satisfaction. Agreement was defined as being within 1 scale point. Tabulation of the sample data is shown in Table 1.

In this example, notice that 4 raters and 6 patients were observed. All possible rater pairs (6) were used, and every pair completed a rating of 2 patients, so that an adequate number of ratings (12) were done. Each patient in the example was rated by two pairs of nurses. It should be noted, however, that a single nurse made only one rating on a given patient. That is, it would have been inappropriate for both pair A and B and pair A and C to have done ratings on patient 1, since nurse A's rating would have been counted twice. One alternative to doing four single ratings on a patient (two pairs per patient) would be to observe 12 patients, i.e., one rater pair per patient.

Table 1
Interrater Reliability

PATIENT	NURSE PAIR	EFFECTIVENESS RATING	SATISFACTION RATING
1	A & B	A	A
	C & D	D	A
2	A & C	A	A
	B & D	A	A
3	A & D	A	A
	B & C	D	A
4	A & B	A	D
	C & D	A	A
5	A & C	A	A
	B & D	A	A
6	A & D	A	A
	B & C	A	A
6 Patients	12 Ratings	83.3% Agreement	91.7% Agreement

(A = Agreement; D = Disagreement)

Interrater reliability was calculated as follows, and expressed as a percentage:

$$\frac{\text{Interrater}}{\text{Reliability}} = \frac{\text{Number of agreements}}{\text{Number of ratings}} \times 100 = \frac{A}{N} \times 100 = \underline{\hspace{1cm}}\%$$

With the sample data shown for the tension scale, an interrater reliability of 83.3 percent was achieved.

$$\frac{A}{N} \times 100 = \frac{10}{12} \times 100 = 83.3\%$$

An interrrater reliability of 80 percent is considered sufficient for purposes of evaluation here. A low interrater reliability may suggest

a need for further training. For instance, 1 or 2 raters may have reduced the overall reliability, and these individuals may need additonal practice. In the example, rater C was involved in two "disagreements" with the effectiveness scale and may need more training. It is also possible that all raters may have difficulty with a certain section of a scale. In the latter case, clearer decision rules for rating may be needed. After additional training, interrater reliability may be determined again.

APPENDIX H
DATA RECORDING AND
SUMMARIZING TOOLS

The data recording and summarizing tools in this appendix are intended to serve as examples and models that can be adapted to serve other purposes or projects.

Data Collection Form

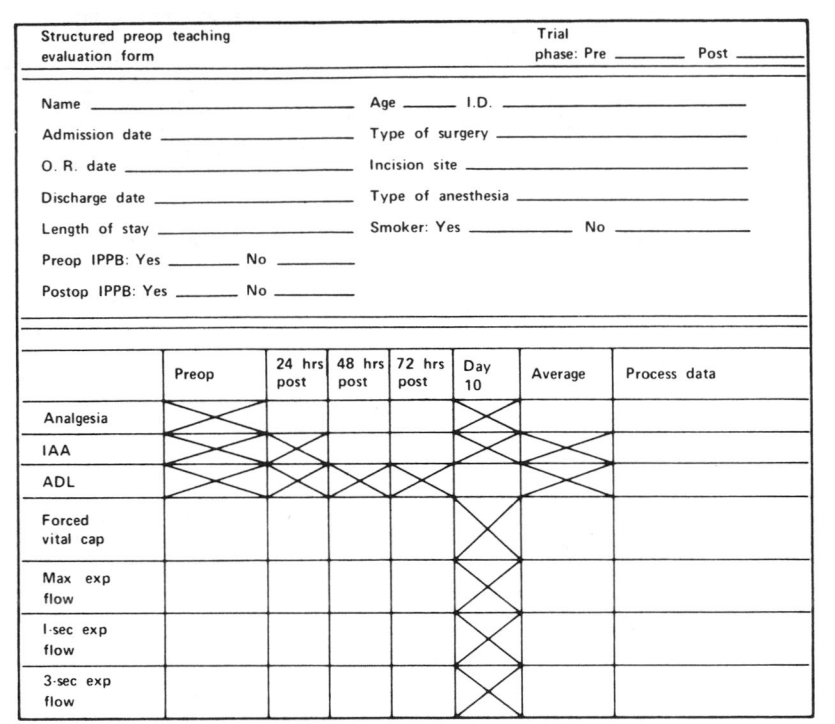

	Preop	24 hrs post	48 hrs post	72 hrs post	Day 10	Average	Process data
Analgesia							
IAA							
ADL							
Forced vital cap							
Max exp flow							
1-sec exp flow							
3-sec exp flow							

Structured preop teaching evaluation form

Trial phase: Pre _____ Post _____

Name _____ Age _____ I.D. _____

Admission date _____ Type of surgery _____

O. R. date _____ Incision site _____

Discharge date _____ Type of anesthesia _____

Length of stay _____ Smoker: Yes _____ No _____

Preop IPPB: Yes _____ No _____

Postop IPPB: Yes _____ No _____

Reprinted from CURN Project: *Structured Preoperative Teaching.* New York, Grune & Stratton, 1981, p. 34.

Intervention Recording Instrument: Example A

Decubitus Prevention Protocol: Small Shifts of Body Weight Intervention

NAME/I.D. *John Doe 654321*			
DATE	WEIGHT SHIFTS (√)	DATE	WEIGHT SHIFTS(√)
(Adm.) **9-9**	Days: Afternoons: Nights:	(1 week postadm.) **9-16**	Days: ✓✓✓ Afternoons: ✓✓✓✓✓✓✓ Nights: ✓✓✓✓
	Days: Afternoons: Nights:	**9-17**	Days: ✓✓✓✓✓ ✓✓✓ Afternoons: ✓✓✓✓✓✓ Nights: ✓✓✓✓
	Days: Afternoons: Nights:	**9-18**	Days: ✓✓✓✓ Afternoons: ✓✓✓✓✓ ✓ Nights: ✓✓✓✓
	Days: Afternoons: Nights:	**9-19**	Days: ✓✓✓✓✓ ✓ Afternoons: ✓✓✓✓✓ Nights: ✓✓✓✓
	Days: Afternoons: Nights:	**9-20**	Days: ✓✓✓✓ ✓✓✓✓✓ ✓✓ Afternoons: ✓✓✓✓✓ Nights: ✓✓✓✓
	Days: Afternoons: Nights:	**9-21**	Days: ✓✓✓✓✓ ✓✓✓✓✓ ✓✓ Afternoons: ✓✓✓✓✓ ✓ Nights: ✓ ✓✓✓
	Days: Afternoons: Nights:	**9-22**	Days: ✓✓✓✓✓ ✓ Afternoons: ✓✓✓ ✓✓✓ Nights: ✓ ✓✓✓
Total work shifts (8-hour periods) on intervention: **21**			
Average number of weight shifts/work shift: **5.76**			

Reprinted from CURN Project: *Preventing Decubitus Ulcers*. New York, Grune & Stratton, 1981, p. 32.

Intervention Recording Instrument: Example B

**INITIAL EACH TIME ACTIVITY IS PERFORMED
COMPLETE AND RETURN TO DESK**   **DATA PLATE**

	8 A.M.	10 A.M.	12 P.M.	2 P.M.	4 P.M.	6 P.M.	8 P.M.	10 P.M.	12 A.M.	2 A.M.	4 A.M.	6 A.M.
Day of O.R. *Date:*												
Deep breath & cough												
Turn												
Leg exercises												
1st P.O. Day *Date:*												
Deep breath & cough												
Turn												
Leg exercises												
2nd P.O. Day *Date:*												
Deep breath & cough												
Turn												
Leg exercises												
3rd P.O. Day *Date:*												
Deep breath & cough												
Turn												
Leg exercises												

Reprinted from CURN Project: *Preventing Decubitus Ulcers.* New York, Grune & Stratton, 1981, p. 32.

Data Summary Form: Decubitus Prevention

Trial Group _Postimplementation_

Risk Group _High Risk_

PATIENT		ASSESSMENT SCORE			DECUBITUS ULCER				INTERVENTION	
Name/I.D.	Data	1st	2nd	3rd	Present	Absent	None		No. Work Shifts on Intervention	Ave. No. Weight Shifts/8 Hrs.
John Doe 654321	Ca colon 68	15	13	12		✓			21	5.76
Totals: No. Patients ___		Average ___	Average ___	Average ___	No. Ulcers ___ Incidence ___ %				Average No. work shifts on intervention/pt. ___ Average No. weight shifts/8 hrs./pt. ___	

Reprinted from CURN Project: *Structured Preoperative Teaching.* New York, Grune & Stratton, 1981, p. 33.

APPENDIX I
TRAINING OF EVALUATORS

The preparation and training of the people who will serve as evaluators may vary depending on the nature of the tasks involved in the evaluation. Regardless of the complexity of the evaluation, the evaluators will require training and instructions regarding the sequence of the evaluation, orientation to the equipment and recording forms, and practice doing the evaluation in a consistent fashion. When special knowledge and skills are necessary to carry out the evaluation, the training will need to be more extensive. The people who will carry out this aspect of the research utilization effort should be familiar with the evaluation procedures before initiating the evaluation. If equipment is involved in the evaluation, the evaluators need an opportunity to learn how to operate it. Learning to record information accurately on the forms prepared for this purpose is also an important part of the preparation for evaluation. Identifying a person to whom evaluators can communicate their questions when collecting information is a useful strategy for keeping the evaluation running smoothly. It is also important for the evaluators to remain as objective as possible during the evaluation in order to record data in an unbiased fashion. Training evaluators to make and record observations systematically and objectively is essential to an accurate evaluation.

Practice sessions are an excellent way of preparing for an evaluation. Practice sessions help people feel comfortable with their assigned tasks. Questions can be answered and problems anticipated during these sessions. It is important to plan practice sessions that closely resemble the situation in which the evaluation will be done. The actual forms for recording the information to be

collected should be used by the evaluators during these sessions. Assembling the people who will do the evaluation for a training session makes it possible for everyone to hear the same explanations and instructions. During the training, inconsistencies among the evaluators can be identified and procedures standardized, thereby yielding more uniform data.

The practice session(s) should be held shortly before the evaluation to allow the training to be utilized before the details become less clear or forgotten. The practice sessions have been found to arouse a level of motivation in the evaluators that is needed for undertaking the tasks involved. Long delays tend to blunt enthusiasm as well as blur understanding.

To elicit staff cooperation during the process of evaluation someone will need to explain the purposes of the evaluation and in general terms decribe how the evaluation will affect staff and their daily routine. It is important to convey the message that this evaluation is designed to find out how to improve patient care. Staff should be encouraged to maintain as normal a care routine as possible so that the data reflect typical care. The emphasis on evaluation as a positive approach to improving care for patients can reduce concern of how the evaluation might reflect on the performance of any single individual. If the evaluation will require some adjustment in the way staff engage in their duties, some allowance for this and explanation will be needed.

APPENDIX J
CASE STUDY: CONDUCTING A TRIAL OF A PREOPERATIVE TEACHING PROGRAM

B ased on the results of a survey of patient care problems identified by the nursing staff in their hospital, the committee decided to conduct a trial of a research-based practice innovation designed to improve postoperative recovery.

DESIGNING THE PREOPERATIVE TEACHING PROGRAM

The committee developed the content and format of the teaching program using the research base, knowledge gained from contact with one of the original researchers, and materials used by the researchers. The committee designed a structured preoperative teaching program using the group instruction method and supervised practice. The basic content of the program followed the research-based guidelines described in the structured preoperative teaching protocol. The program was designed to teach groups of adult patients to perform deep breathing, coughing, turning and moving, and leg exercises. The content of the teaching program included the following:

Why the deep breathing, coughing, turning and moving, and leg exercises should be done

How to perform the exercises correctly

157

How to recognize if the exercises are being done correctly
When and *how often* to do the exercises pre- and postoperatively
Where to do the exercises

A script for the slide-and-tape presentation was prepared and a committee member was selected to make the voice recording. An outline of the material for each slide was developed using the rule of thumb that only one idea would be conveyed on each slide. A member of the committee with knowledge of photography and access to photographic equipment arranged for the slides to be taken. Volunteers, including patients and members of the nursing staff, were photographed so that the teaching program would appeal to both patients and staff.

The slides and tape recording were presented for critical review to the committee and were subsequently revised. When the revised version of the slide-and-tape program was available, it was shown to the appropriate nursing supervisors and administrators. Approval to use the material was obtained from the Nurse Administrators Group and the Patient Care Committee. The program was then presented to two influential surgeons and later at a surgical staff meeting, where it was endorsed for use with surgical patients.

The final version of the program was used to prepare the nurses who volunteered to teach the classes as well as the nurses on the pilot unit who would be holding the bedside practice sessions with the patients after the class.

PREPARING THE TEACHERS

Three staff development sessions for those nurses who volunteered to teach the structured preoperative teaching program to patients were held shortly before the trial by a member of the staff development department. The staff development instructor was also a member of the committee, was familiar with the research base, and had participated in planning for the preoperative teaching program.

During the first session, the teachers discussed their previous experience with patient teaching and patient groups, and were familiarized with the plan for the teaching program and how it was designed from the research base. At the second session, the teachers learned how to perform the deep breathing, coughing, turning and moving, and leg exercises and practiced them. They

were taught the principles underlying the teaching of skills. In addition, they learned how to operate the audiovisual equipment. The mechanism for getting patients to and from the classes was discussed. An outline describing how to conduct the classes was given to each nurse and teacher and was discussed. During the third session, the teachers "taught" each other how to perform the exercises. They practiced giving instructions and correcting errors, operating the equipment, and completing the recording forms. This practice session helped the teachers feel more comfortable about teaching their first classes of patients.

The committee member from the staff-development department who instructed the classroom teachers volunteered to be available during each teacher's first patient class as a consultant and for moral support. The teachers were encouraged to utilize this person for assistance. Communication with pilot unit staff was stressed in order to encourage patients to learn and to practice the exercises correctly and frequently.

PREPARING THE PILOT UNIT STAFF

When the baseline evaluation was completed, two staff development sessions were held by the head nurse for the nursing staff on the pilot unit. All of the unit's nursing staff (registered nurses, licensed practical nurses, and nurse's aides) were included in these sessions since all staff were expected to participate in implementation of the innovation, either as teacher or reinforcers of the teaching program. The head nurse was also a committee member, had helped to plan the teaching program, and was thoroughly familiar with the program and its research base. At the first session, the purpose of the teaching program and its relationship to the research base were discussed. The plan for pilot-testing the teaching program was presented and the need for a trial explained. At the second session, the nursing staff were shown the teaching program and taught how to perform the exercises. The need for participation of the staff in the bedside practice sessions was emphasized and the recording forms reviewed. The importance of communication between the teachers and the remainder of the nursing staff was emphasized to ensure that patients were learning the exercises. Staff were encouraged to contact the head nurse when questions or problems arose.

IMPLEMENTING THE TRIAL PROGRAM

After careful planning and preparation, the committee set a date for the trial to begin. All the adult patients on the pilot unit who were scheduled for elective surgery requiring a general anesthetic were included in the trial. Upon admission to the surgical unit, each patient received a brochure describing the preoperative teaching program and the deep breathing, coughing, turning and moving, and leg exercises. Patients were encouraged to read the brochure and were invited to attend a 30-minute class the evening before their surgery. The classes were held in a patient lounge at the end of the evening visiting hours. Each patient could invite one family member to attend the class if desired. Additonal family members could not be accommodated due to limited space in the classroom.

Before the classes began, the head nurse met with the teachers about scheduling of the classes and a rotation was established as a part of each nurse's assignment. Alternate teachers were scheduled for each class in case of an emergency or illness.

The classes were taught by a registered nurse using a series of 35-mm slides synchronized with a tape recording of the information to be learned. Following the slide presentation, the nurse reviewed the instructions, demonstrated the coughing, deep breathing, turning and moving, and leg exercises, and assisted each patient in performing them. Patients were encouraged to refer to the printed instructions in the brochure and were asked to repeat the exercises on two more occasions after returning to their rooms. Nursing staff from the pilot unit assisted the patients in doing the exercises twice before surgery and encouraged patients to do the exercises every 2 hours after surgery.

For each patient attending the class, the teacher completed the recording form describing how well the patient was able to do the exercises. The nurse returned the recording form to the nursing staff on the pilot unit, notifying them which patients had attended class and of specific consideration needed to assist each of the patients during the two practice sessions held at the bedside prior to surgery. A notation was made on each patient's hospital record regarding class attendance and the patient's ability to perform the exercises.

COLLECTING INFORMATION TO EVALUATE THE TRIAL

Before the baseline evaluation was conducted, the persons designated to collect information to evaluate the trial met for an orientation and training session with the coordinator of the trial. The evaluators learned to do the measurements and practiced recording the information. Interrater reliability was established among evaluators. After acquiring materials, informing others, and obtaining approval of the plans, the baseline evaluation was conducted while other members of the committee designed the teaching program. The baseline data collection period had to be lengthened when fewer operations than anticipated were scheduled following the Christmas holidays. However, the baseline data collection continued without interruption. Pilot unit nursing staff were cooperative and did not find that the evaluation interfered with their routine care. One evaluator was a member of both the pilot unit staff and the committee, a fact that facilitated the trial.

The evaluators for the baseline evaluation collected information about the effectiveness of the innovation. The same nurses from each shift were able to collect data about the patients' body temperatures, productivity of the cough, and chest expansion for 72 hours postoperatively for each patient who had received the preoperative teaching. The data were recorded using the same type of equipment.

The coordinator for the baseline evaluation also coordinated the evaluation conducted after the implementation of the preoperative teaching program. This continuity provided for great consistency during the monitoring of the trial. The committee met every 2 weeks to hear progress reports from those involved in the trial and to provide input when problems arose. One problem discussed by the committee was the mechanism for transporting patients to and from the classes. The plan to have the nurses' aides from the pilot unit escort patients to and from classes was not working effectively because of their other unit responsibilities. One committee member suggested that hospital auxiliary volunteers be asked to transport patients, and this was arranged.

The number and type of patients included in the baseline evaluation was similar to the number and type of patients included in the evaluation conducted after implementation of the teaching program. Thirty patients having abdominal surgery under general anesthesia were included in each evaluation period (total 60 patients).

OUTCOMES OF THE TRIAL

Both expected and unexpected events occurred once the teaching program was under way. The teachers were able to teach the classes as planned, and the patients learned to perform the exercises. Two patients refused to attend the classes. One patient had had surgery previously and knew how to do the exercises. The second patient decided she was not feeling well enough to attend the classes. Both the teachers and the patients who attended the classes were enthusiastic about the teaching program. Patients continued to do the exercises after returning to their rooms. Staff on the pilot unit reported that patients were performing the exercises correctly and noted that patients who had attended the classes were doing these exercises postoperatively.

The evaluation data collected during the trial was compared with baseline data and showed a decrease in the number of patients experiencing elevations in body temperature and a productive cough 72 hours postoperatively among the group of patients who received preoperative teaching. Average differences in chest expansion at 72 hours postoperatively did not differ appreciably for the two groups of patients.

The committee and the Director of Nursing discussed the results of the trial. The committee had discovered that the measurement of chest expansion was not performed accurately or consistently by the persons collecting this information during the trial. This may have influenced the lack of a difference in chest expansion between the two groups. This result, however, was not interpreted by the committee as a deterrent to adoption of the innovation, in light of other results that indicated the effectiveness of the practice innovation. The committee then considered the overall costs of personnel, materials, and monetary resources required to implement the program for all surgical patients admitted to this hospital. While the costs of the teaching program were considered moderately high, the committee recommended adoption of the program based on data describing the effectiveness of the innovation and the benefits received by patients.

The Director of Nursing requested that the committee submit a written report summarizing the major results of the trial and stating their recommendations. The final decision regarding permanent adoption of the innovation was made by the Director of Nursing after reviewing the report prepared by the chairperson of the committee.

The structured preoperative teaching program was adopted as originally designed.

Formal announcement of the results of the trial and decision to adopt the structured preoperative teaching program was made to the Nurse Administrators Group, the Patient Care Committee, and at staff meetings for nurses, physicians, and others. The cooperation and assistance of those involved in the trial was acknowledged personally by members of the committee and was given formal recognition in meetings where the results of the trial were announced. The committee then proceeded to plan for diffusion of the structured preoperative teaching program to other surgical units and for development of mechanisms to maintain the research-based innovation over time.

APPENDIX K
COMPILING AND ANALYZING
DATA

The results of the trial need to be compiled, analyzed, and interpreted if they are to be used to make a decision about the practice innovation. While the trial is being conducted, begin to compile the data on summary worksheets. Transferring data to summary worksheets permits large amounts of data to be scanned at a glance. Large quantities of numbers can create difficulties for those who wish to interpret them, as well as their intended audience, unless they are summarized and displayed in ways that make them more comprehensible.

First, total the scores for each item or category being evaluated. Begin with smallest sets of information you wish to have summarized. Record those totals and then continue totalling sets of information so you have totals available from the smallest to the largest set of information you desire. For example: In examining the data from summary worksheets noting when small shifts in body weights were done on patients, you may decide that you wish to have totals for each patient per shift, per day, and a grand total.

Second, decide which basic mathematical strategies will be useful in summarizing and describing your data. The mathematical strategies suggested here are called descriptive statistics. Descriptive statistics are useful because they provide a means of ordering large sets of individual (raw) data, and this ordering process helps us comprehend trends and relationships in the data that might otherwise go undetected. When the data from an evaluation procedure are examined, we are looking at the relationship between the nursing intervention and patient outcomes. The use of descriptive

statistics assists the examination by illuminating the relationships that are of interest among the data.

We believe that simple statistical strategies requiring only addition, subtraction, multiplication, and division are sufficient for the purposes of most clinical evaluation procedures. The descriptive statistical techiques listed below meet this requirement and will assist the evaluator in determining and demonstrating the meaning of the data obtained during a clinical evaluation.

- Frequency distributions
    Simple frequency distribution
    Cumulative frequency distribution
    Grouped frequency distribution
- Percent
- Graphs
    Histograms
    Frequency polygons
- Measures of central tendency
    Mean
    Mode
    Median

The following books discuss and describe the suggested statistical techniques in a straightforward manner. Most hospital and public libraries will have these or other statistics books in their collections.

1. Polit, D.F., & Hungler, B.P. *Nursing Research: Principles and Methods*. Philadelphia: J.B. Lippincott Co., 1978.
2. Welkowitz, J., Ewen, R.B., & Cohen, J. *Introductory Statistics for the Behavioral Sciences*. New York: Academic Press, 1976.
3. Spence, J.T., Underwood, B.J., Duncan, C.P., & Cotton, J.W. *Elementary Statistics*. Englewood Cliffs, New Jersey: Prentice-Hall, Inc., 1976.

BIBLIOGRAPHY

American Nurses' Association and American Hospital Association. *Quality Assurance Workbook.* Kansas City, Mo.: American Nurses' Association, 1976.

Babbie, E.R. *Survey research methods.* Belmont, CA: Wadsworth Publishing Co., 1973, pp. 131–158, 171–186.

Batey, M.V. Research: Its dissemination and utilization in nursing practice. *Washington State Journal of Nursing,* Winter, 1975, 6–9.

Bennis, W.G., Benne, K.D., Chin, R., & Corey, K.E. *The Planning of Change.* 3rd ed. New York: Holt, Rinehart and Winston, 1976.

Bloch, D. Evaluation of nursing care in terms of process and outcomes: Issues in research and quality assurance. *Nursing Research,* 1975, *24,* 256–263.

Cleland, V. Implementation of change in health care systems. *Journal of Nursing Administration,* 1972, *2,* 64–69.

CURN Project. *Using Research to Improve Nursing Practice.* New York: Grune & Stratton, Inc. Series of Clinical Protocols: *Clean Intermittent Catheterization* (1982), *Closed Urinary Drainage Systems* (1981), *Distress Reduction Through Sensory Preparation* (1981), *Intravenous Cannula Change* (1981), *Mutual Goal Setting in Patient Care* (1982), *Pain: Deliberative Nursing Interventions* (1982), *Preoperative Sensory Preparation to Promote Recovery* (1981), *Preventing Decubitus Ulcers* (1981), *Reducing Diarrhea in Tube-Fed Patients* (1981), *Structured Preoperative Teaching* (1981).

Haller, K.B., Reynolds, M.A., & Horsley, J.A. Developing research-based innovation protocols: Process, criteria, and issues. *Research in Nursing and Health,* 1979, *2,* 45–51.

Havelock, R.G. *A Charge Agent's Guide to Innovation in Education.* Englewood Cliffs, N.J.: Educational Technology·Publications, 1978.

Havelock, R.G. *Planning for Innovation through Dissemination and Utilization of Knowledge.* Ann Arbor, Mich.: Center for Research on Utilization

167

of Scientific Knowledge, Institute for Social Research, The University of Michigan, 1969.

Horsley, J.A., Crane, J., & Bingle, J.D. Research utilization as an organizational process. *Journal of Nursing Administration,* 1978, *8,* 4–6.

Ketefian, S. Problems in the dissemination and the utilization of scientific knowledge. In Ketefian, S. (ed.) *Translation of Theory into Nursing Practice and Education,* proceedings of the Seventh Annual Clinical Sessions, Division of Nursing, New York University, 1975, 10–31.

Krueger, J.C., Nelson, A.H., & Wolanin, M.O. *Nursing Research: Development, Collaboration and Utilization.* Germantown, Md.: Aspen Systems Corporation, 1978.

Lindeman, C. Nursing intervention with the presurgical patient: Effectiveness and efficiency of group and individual preoperative teaching— phase two. *Nursing Research,* 1972, *21,* 196–209.

Lindeman, C. Measuring quality of nursing care, Part 1. *Journal of Nursing Administration.* 1976, *6*(s), 7–9.

Lindeman, C., & Van Aernam, B. Nursing intervention with the presurgical patient—the effects of structured and unstructured preoperative teaching. *Nursing Research,* 1971, *20,* 319–322.

Lippitt, R., Watson, J., & Westley, B. *The Dynamics of Planned Change.* New York: Harcourt, Bruce & World, Inc., 1958.

National Institute of Mental Health. *Planning for Creative Change in Mental Health Services: A Distillation of Principles on Research Utilization.* Vol. 1. U.S. Department of Health, Education, and Welfare, 1971.

Polit, D.F., & Hungler, B.P. *Nursing Research: Principles and Methods.* Philadelphia: J.B. Lippincott Co., 1978.

Rogers, E.M., & Agarwala-Rogers, R. *Communications in Organizations.* New York: Free Press, 1976.

Rogers, E.M., & Shoemaker, F.F. *Communication of Innovations.* 2nd ed. New York: Free Press, 1971.

Rothman, J. *Using Research in Organizations: A Guide to Successful Application.* Beverly Hills, Calif.: Sage Publications, 1980.

Rothman, J., Erlich, J.L., & Teresa, J.G. *Promoting Innovation and Change in Organizations and Communities: A Planning Manual.* New York: John Wiley and Sons, Inc., 1976.

Rothman, J., Erlich, J.L., & Teresa, J.G. *Changing Organizations and Community Programs.* Beverly Hills, Calif.: Sage Publications, 1981.

Spence, J.T., Underwood, B.J., Duncan, C.P., & Cotton, J.W. *Elementary Statistics* (Ed. 2). Englewood Cliffs, N.J.: Prentice-Hall, 1976.

Welkowitz, J., Ewen, R. & Cohen, J. *Introductory Statistics for the Behavioral Sciences.* 2nd ed. New York: Academic Press, 1976, 15–37.

Zaltman, G., & Duncan, R. *Strategies for Planned Change.* New York: John Wiley & Sons, 1977.

INDEX

ISBN 0-8089-1510-X

90071
9 780808 915102